Danger and Defense

Danger and Defense
THE TECHNIQUE OF CLOSE PROCESS ATTENTION

A Festschrift in honor of Paul Gray

Edited by
Marianne Goldberger

JASON ARONSON INC.
Northvale, New Jersey
London

This book was set in 11 pt. New Baskerville by Alpha Graphics of Pittsfield, New Hampshire and printed and bound by Book-mart Press of North Bergen, New Jersey.

Copyright © 1996 by Jason Aronson Inc.

10 9 8 7 6 5 4 3 2 1

All rights reserved. Printed in the United States of America. No part of this book may be used or reproduced in any manner whatsoever without written permission from Jason Aronson Inc. except in the case of brief quotations in reviews for inclusion in a magazine, newspaper, or broadcast.

Library of Congress Cataloging-in-Publication Data

Danger and defense : the technique of close process attention / Marianne Goldberger, editor.
    p. cm.
  Honoring the 75th birthday of Paul Gray.
  Includes bibliographical references and index.
  ISBN 1-56821-583-5 (alk. paper)
  1. Psychoanalytic interpretation. 2. Defense mechanisms (Psychology) 3. Psychotherapist and patient. I. Goldberger, Marianne. II. Gray, Paul, 1918-
RC509.D36 1996
616.89'17—dc 20   95-17450

Manufactured in the United States of America. Jason Aronson Inc. offers books and cassettes. For information and catalog write to Jason Aronson Inc., 230 Livingston Street, Northvale, New Jersey 07647.

Contents

Acknowledgments	vii
Contributors	ix
Introduction by Marianne Goldberger	xiii

1. Defense Analysis and Mutative Interpretation
   Walter Todd Davison, Monroe Pray,
   Curtis Bristol, and Robert Welker
	1

2. Two Different Methods of Analyzing Defense *Monroe Pray*	53
3. Free Association and Technique *Fred Busch*	107

4. Use of the Close Process
   Attention Technique in Patients
   with Impulse Disorders
   James H. Hutchinson
	131

CONTENTS

5. The Importance of Facial Expressions in Dreams — 173
   Marianne Goldberger

6. The Clinical Use of Daydreams in Analysis — 179
   Marianne Goldberger

7. External Reality as Defense — 193
   Lawrence Inderbitzin and Steven T. Levy

8. The Envy Complex: Its Recognition and Analysis — 221
   Peggy B. Hutson

9. The Place of Empathy in Analytic Listening — 241
   Lucie S. Greenblum

10. Consciousness as a Beacon Light — 263
    Barry J. Landau

11. Common Ground, Uncommon Methods — 291
    Cecilio Paniagua

12. What's at Stake in the Truth Controversy? — 317
    Lawrence Friedman

13. An Interpretation of Transference — 337
    Jonathan Lear

Credits — 375

Index — 377

Acknowledgments

The most important acknowledgment goes to Gerda Gray, who conceived and lovingly nurtured the original Festschrift on which this volume is based. She thought it might be published and no one else believed her. Much appreciation also goes to all the contributors to this volume, not only for their excellent papers but also for their enthusiasm and cooperation in each stage of the planning.

Contributors

R. Curtis Bristol, M.D.
Clinical Professor of Psychiatry and Co-Director, Center for Post Graduate Studies of Psychiatry and Psychoanalysis, Georgetown University; and Faculty, Baltimore-Washington Institute for Psychoanalysis.

Fred Busch, Ph.D.
Training and Supervising Analyst, The Michigan Psycho-analytic Institute.

Walter T. Davison, M.D.
Clinical Professor of Psychiatry and Family Practice, Medical College of Wisconsin; and Training Analyst, Chicago Psychoanalytic Institute.

Lawrence Friedman, M.D.
Clinical Professor of Psychiatry, Cornell University Medical College, New York.

Marianne Goldberger, M.D.
Clinical Professor of Psychiatry, New York University Medical School; and Training and Supervising Analyst, The Psychoanalytic Institute at NYU Medical School.

Lucie Greenblum, M.D.
Clinical Assistant Professor of Psychiatry, Georgetown University; and Teaching Analyst, Baltimore-Washington Institute for Psychoanalysis.

James Hutchinson, M.D.
Teaching Analyst, Baltimore-Washington Institute for Psychoanalysis.

Peggy B. Hutson, M.D.
Clinical Professor of Psychiatry, University of Miami; and Training and Supervising Analyst, Florida Psychoanalytic Institute.

Lawrence B. Inderbitzin, M.D.
Professor of Psychiatry and Behavioral Sciences, Emory University School of Medicine; and Director, Emory University Psychoanalytic Institute.

Barry J. Landau, M.D.
Clinical Professor of Psychiatry, George Washington University; and Training and Supervising Analyst, Baltimore-Washington Institute for Psychoanalysis.

Jonathan Lear, Ph.D.
Professor of Philosophy, Yale University; and Clinical Affiliate, Western New England Institute for Psychoanalysis.

Steven T. Levy, M.D.
Professor of Psychiatry and Behavioral Sciences, Emory University School of Medicine; and Training and Supervising Analyst and Director-elect, Emory University Psychoanalytic Institute.

Cecilio Paniagua, M.D.
Lecturer, Universidad Complutense de Madrid; and Training and Supervising Analyst, Madrid Psychoanalytic Association.

Monroe Pray, M.D.
Clinical Faculty, Georgetown University Medical Center; and Clinical Faculty, Baltimore-Washington Institute for Psychoanalysis.

Robert Welker, Ph.D.
Clinical Assistant Professor of Psychiatry, Medical College of Wisconsin; and Candidate, Wisconsin New Training Facility.

Introduction

> It is a curious fact that the central, most necessary part of psychoanalytic technique is one of the least discussed, certainly one of the least well conceptualized aspects of psychoanalysis. I am referring to analytic listening or, more accurately, analytic perception. My main purpose in this essay is to examine and sharpen our idea of this aspect of technique in the analysis of adult neuroses.

With those words Paul Gray launched his first publication on psychoanalytic technique (1973), just a little over twenty years ago in the *Journal of the American Psychoanalytic Association*. Although some analysts were aware of the innovative nature of this paper, no one could have predicted the profound effect that his ideas would have on the psychoanalytic world, stirring up enormous interest and controversy about the important question of how the analyst listens. Until then it had been little discussed and ill-defined.

The most crucial ideas in this landmark paper include Gray's suggestion that the listening analyst adjust his perceptual focus to data limited essentially to *inside* the analytic situation. In elaborating this point of view, Gray illustrated the specific advantages it offers in the analysis of patient communications that refer to current or contemplated behavior *outside* the analytic situation (sometimes labeled *acting out*). He stressed that in view of the increasing understanding of the role of the ego, analysts need to diminish as much as possible the use of suggestion and persuasion and to increase their awareness of the importance of not pre-empting the patient's ego function during the course of the analysis. His goal was to improve analysands' capacities for eventual self-analysis. He asserted that if we are to increase the ego's autonomy through more effective analytic technique, we will have to learn more about the functions with which the normal ego can perceive itself.

All of these important ideas about technique have been developed in Gray's later publications (1982, 1986, 1987, 1990, 1991, 1992, 1994). They needed detailed elaboration because someone not fortunate enough to have discussed analytic material with him in person might find it difficult to grasp fully the effect of his perspective on analytic work. His 1986 paper, "On Helping Analysands Observe Intrapsychic Activity," was especially helpful in this regard. In 1987, he began publishing his views on the technique of analysis of the superego, a subject that had not previously been discussed in the literature in detail. In the 1980s, he began more and more frequently to refer to "the ego's superego activities." Using analytic evidence, he demonstrated the clinical usefulness of his conception of the superego as a defensive function of the ego.

Gray's effect as an educator preceded by far the publication of his important series of papers on analytic technique. The contributors to this Festschrift, as well as many others, have had the privilege of learning from Gray directly, and have had the chance to discover for themselves that his uniqueness as a teacher proceeds from his love of ideas and his capacity to imagine anything and everything. His unfettered imagination has been a major source of inspiration for his students, whom he has allowed to follow or question his thinking, and whom he has encouraged to pursue whatever explorations they wished. In addition, his genuine excitement about new ideas has been combined with an insistence on rigorous thinking.

Gray's contributions to the analysis of the superego are unique and would in themselves stand as a major technical advance. Not much has been written about specific technical approaches to the superego in clinical analysis. Most analysts are well aware of the regularity with which internal moral dicta of great variety are reexternalized in the analytic situation, and of the necessity of analyzing these externalizations of authority. Gray has recognized that the "optimal analysis of the superego . . . is achieved by perceiving and interpreting superego manifestations *mobilized during the analytic situation,* primarily as part of the *ego's* defensive activities" (1994, p. 120, original italics).

Thus, in describing *close process attention,* Gray made it possible for both patient and analyst to observe patients' use of reexternalized authorities from moment to moment in the analytic hour. Gray demonstrated the infinite variety of signs through which the analyst can notice a patient's sense of danger, especially as coming from the analyst, as well as the variety of defenses that may be used against the danger. His emphasis on *observing* instead of *using* the influence of that reexternalization completely changes the analytic atmosphere. The sense of danger applies to the analyst as well: Gray helps analysts become aware that their own sense of danger is most likely to rise when aggression is most fully expressed in the transference.

The effects Gray has had in bringing out the best in students and colleagues are apparent not only in the greater Washington area but all over the United States and Europe. The brief summaries (below) of the papers in this Festschrift bear witness to the many potentialities of his original contributions.

Walter Davison, Monroe Pray, Curtis Bristol, and Robert Welker joined forces to produce a detailed chapter on "Defense Analysis and Mutative Interpretation." It begins by reviewing definitions of terms frequently used in describing psychoanalytic process, including *resistance, repression,* and *working through.* Gray's technique of close process attention is defined and discussed, with an explanation of how and why one chooses the moment for making an intervention. The biases of the authors in making interventions are made explicit, together with suggestions for how to deal with patients in regard to these biases. This is followed by a description of a step-by-step analysis of defense interpretations. Finally, it offers a week of analytic process material to illustrate these techniques.

Monroe Pray's chapter presents a detailed study with a point-by-point comparison, "Two Different Methods of Analyzing Defense." He begins by explaining the two different methods, represented by Charles Brenner, who espouses analysis of "compromise formations," and by Anna Freud, who presented her new ideas in her 1936 monograph, *The Ego and the Mechanisms of Defense.* Pray's chapter further investigates Anna Freud's important departures from mainstream psychoanalysis, including a major change from the recommendation for "free-floating attention" to one favoring a specific focus of attention on the part of the analyst. The overall purpose of the chapter is to help analysts evaluate the analytic validity and research potential of these two technical points of view.

Fred Busch contributes a chapter that deals with the

orientation of analyst and patient toward the process of free association, called "Free Association and Technique." Busch contends that there are conceptual contradictions buried in the method of free association as currently practiced that lead to confusion in the method and goals of psychoanalysis. The author emphasizes the current differences in how free associations are viewed, not only among obviously divergent schools, but also among those who might be considered of similar orientation. As an example of the latter, he describes the subtle but important differences in the nature of what the analyst is looking for as revealed in the work of Arlow and Brenner on the one hand and that of Gray on the other. Arlow and Brenner (1990) are geared more to elucidating the meaning of the associations, while Gray is focused on the immediate conflict as seen in the *process* of associating.

James Hutchinson, in a foray into what he calls the "wider scope" of analytic treatment, writes about "The Application of Close Process Attention to Patients with Impulse Disorders." He first gives a picture of Gray's technique and then demonstrates its usefulness in the treatment of impulsive patients. The rationale for this technique is that it preserves the possibility of using insight as a curative force in the treatment of patients who are action-prone. Using detailed clinical vignettes, the chapter deals with the specific vulnerabilities of such patients. It then divides the technique derived from Gray into several principles in order to explain why it is useful with this group of patients.

Marianne Goldberger contributes two brief chapters, "The Importance of Facial Expressions in Dreams" and "The Clinical Use of Daydreams in Analysis." The first elaborates on the usefulness of facial expressions in dreams for the analysis of the superego. It expands on her 1989 paper on the analysis of defenses in dreams by emphasizing the fundamental importance of the visual sphere in the formation of the superego functions of the ego. She has found that dreams provide an especially useful opportunity to study the vivid reexternalization of various kinds of authority.

The second chapter deals with "transference daydreams," and emphasizes the defenses such daydreams evoke. This automatically involves superego functions, since the frequent desire to revise a daydream is importantly motivated by superego demands. Interpreting the defenses in a daydream often allows a patient to remember more details, or even an entire forgotten segment of the daydream.

Lawrence Inderbitzin and Steven Levy contribute "External Reality as Defense." They state that the meaning of the "grist for the mill" metaphor has shifted from "analyzing everything" to "everything is analyzable." This is used as a point of departure for exploring some of the multiple, complicated, and often unrecognized ways reality is used defensively by analyst and analysand. The point of view they present is in contrast to some current trends in psychoanalysis: emphasis on patient–analyst interactions, the analyst's contributions to transference, reality experiences as causation of psychopathology, and the role of the "real" relationship in the mechanism of therapeutic action.

Peggy Hutson writes a chapter that urges wider recognition, understanding, and analysis of "The Envy Complex." This complex commonly appears in the form of strong defenses against a drop in self-esteem, against shame, and against covetousness. She includes examples from the analysis of a patient with the envy complex, demonstrating her use of close process attention in the analysis of defenses against aggression. The details of specific fears of aggression are important in those patients who have unstable self-esteem and a propensity for experiencing shame.

Lucie Greenblum's chapter about "The Place of Empathy in Analytic Listening" illustrates two different ways for an analyst to utilize empathic understanding while listening to a patient's associations. The author presents brief vignettes from her own work, which is informed by the principles of the close process attention technique described by Gray. This is contrasted with the work of Evelyne Schwaber, which emphasizes the use of empathy for purposes of attunement.

Barry Landau studies the attribute of consciousness in a comparison of the topographic and structural theories in "Consciousness as a Beacon Light." He points out that with the development of the structural theory, the goal of analysis shifted from expanding consciousness to expanding the domain of the ego. Landau states that while the presence of a drive derivative in consciousness is evidence of *some* assimilation by the ego, it does not provide information about the *degree* to which the ego has integrated the drive. Therefore, it is crucial that the analyst distinguish those manifestations of the ego's functioning that are available to *consciousness* from those that are not. Patients defend against becoming and remaining conscious of their capacity to observe and "own" drive derivatives as they appear in consciousness. Working with patients' observations of their ego functioning also permits them to become more aware of the signs of inhibitions that the ego imposes on itself in an attempt to solve its conflicts and avoid anxiety.

Cecilio Paniagua brings his international experience to bear in the chapter called "Common Ground, Uncommon Methods," in which he asserts that analysts from different schools do *not* share the same clinical methods. He disagrees with Wallerstein's opinion that "our clinical interventions . . . reflect a shared clinical method," giving evidence to support his views. The importance of his assertions is brought into focus by comparison with the strong emphasis on the shared aspects of clinical theory and practice among analysts from different schools at the meeting of the International Psycho-Analytic Association in Rome in 1989.

Lawrence Friedman, in his chapter "What's at Stake in the Truth Controversy?," notes that many of today's analysts doubt that they deal in objective truths. He traces their doubt to the later Freudian theory of the mind, in which the meaning of "being realistic" became more complicated. He thinks that this subtlety makes the analyst's influence seem more substantive and therefore more manipulative than when the technique was first devised. He does not discuss the merits of the new relativism; instead, he tries to imagine what psychoanalytic treatment would evolve into if a different view became pervasive. He thinks it would be a very different treatment, since there would be an alteration in what he calls "the demand structure" of psychoanalysis, and perhaps would develop a new demand that the patient be creative, or that the patient cement a personal relationship with the analyst. He believes that new ideas should be evaluated in this practical way, as well as on their theoretical merits.

Jonathan Lear offers "An Interpretation of Transference." It begins with a reexamination of Socrates's therapeutic intent and Plato's revisions of psychological theory and technique in the light of Socrates's failure. In particular, Plato devised an account of a structured psyche, a theory of fantasy, and a complex "object relations" theory to account for dynamic interactions between psyche and social world. The chapter argues that these revisions embody a recognition of the phenomenon of transference—namely the psyche's characteristic of attempting to create a meaningful world in which to live. Freud's early conception of transference—as a transfer of psychological content across space and time—is criticized on the ground that it assumes that the world is already given, independent of any psychic activity. Freud's later conception of transference as a repetition is then explored in the light of the psyche's ability to create artifacts. It is argued that neurotic transference is the unconscious attempt to create an idiosyncratic polis, an *idiopolis*, in which to live. The resolution of the transference occurs because the analyst is made a citizen of the idiopolis, has learned the *idiolect,* and can speak in that idiolect about the fundamental conflicts within the idiopolis and their dynamic basis. A neurotic world cannot survive this internal recognition.

These chapters show that Gray not only has made important original contributions to our knowledge but also has inspired others to embark on doing the same. The papers brought together in this volume demonstrate the authors' feelings of gratitude and respect for Paul Gray. These papers were contributed to this volume (in slightly different form) to honor Paul Gray on his seventy-fifth birthday, and were presented to him at a dinner in Washington, DC on February 27, 1993. I would like to thank them for the considerable time and thought they devoted to modifying their manuscripts for this book. Thanks are also due to those colleagues and former students who offered manuscripts for this volume which, for reasons of time or space, could not be included.

Marianne Goldberger

References

Arlow, J., and Brenner, C. (1990). The psychoanalytic process. *Psychoanalytic Quarterly* 59:678–692.

Brenner, C. (1976). *Psychoanalytic Technique and Psychic Conflict*. New York: International Universities Press.

Freud, A. (1936). *The Ego and the Mechanisms of Defense*. New York: International Universities Press.

Freud. S. (1926). Inhibitions, symptoms and anxiety. *Standard Edition* 20:75–172.

Goldberger, M. (1989). The analysis of defenses in dreams. *Psychoanalytic Quarterly* 58:396–418.

Gray, P. (1973). Psychoanalytic technique and the ego's capacity for viewing intrapsychic activity. *Journal of the American Psychoanalytic Association* 21:474–494.

—— (1982). "Developmental lag" in the evolution of technique for psychoanalysis of neurotic conflict. *Journal of the American Psychoanalytic Association* 30:621–655.

—— (1986). On helping analysands observe intrapsychic activity. In *Psychoanalysis: The Science of Mental Conflict. Essays in Honor of Charles Brenner*, ed. A. S. Richards and M. S. Willick, pp. 245–262. Hillsdale, NJ: Analytic Press.

—— (1987). On the technique of analysis of the superego—an introduction. *Psychoanalytic Quarterly* 56:130–154.

—— (1990). The nature of therapeutic action in psychoanalysis. *Journal of the American Psychoanalytic Association* 38:1083–1097.

—— (1991). On transferred or approving superego fantasies: the analysis of the ego's superego activities. Part II. *Psychoanalytic Quarterly* 60:1–21.

—— (1992). Memory as resistance, and the telling of a dream. *Journal of the American Psychoanalytic Association* 40:307–326.

—— (1994). *The Ego and Analysis of Defense*. Northvale, NJ: Jason Aronson.

1
Defense Analysis and Mutative Interpretation

WALTER TODD DAVISON, M.D.,
MONROE PRAY, M.D.,
CURTIS BRISTOL, M.D.,
ROBERT WELKER, Ph.D.

When James Strachey wrote about the mutative interpretation, among the characteristics he identified were the following: it was a transference interpretation, it was done on a small scale, and it was mutative because it changed the analysand's superego (Strachey 1934). Strachey also said that he made more non-transference interpretations than transference ones. He described a therapeutic process that consisted of small scale transference and non-transference interpretations that examine unconscious superego prohibitions. The process he described seemed to follow along these lines: interpret small scale extra-transference conflicts until the conflicts are experienced in the transference; then interpret them there until their genetic determinants surface. Strachey was not thinking of defense interpretations, although the same guidelines may be applied to these.

In previous papers, we have examined some important aspects of small scale transference and non-transference interpretations that address superego attitudes and beliefs about thoughts, feelings, and fantasies (Davison 1981, Davison 1984, Davison et al. 1986, 1990).

Anna Freud (1936) suggested new ways to make transference and nontransference interpretations that affect the superego on a small scale not by internalization of a benign superego but by enhancement of reason. We will present an overview of a technique that uses her suggestions as viewed with the perspective of Paul Gray's (1973) ideas on close process attention.

In this chapter we present the following: (1) definitions concerning psychoanalytic process—namely, resistance, repression, and working through; (2) a description of close process attention; (3) ways of choosing the moment for intervention; (4) examination of four steps in defense analysis; (5) discussion of some implications for research; (6) enumeration of some biases inherent in making interventions from this perspective; and (7) an illustrative week of psychoanalytic process.

DEFINITIONS

In our study of the psychoanalytic process we use Gray's (1973, 1982, 1986, 1987, 1991) clinical hypotheses concerning analytic listening and intervention, which have come to be called *close process attention,* and Brenner's (1976, 1982) theoretical notions about defense being an inference in retrospect concerning a change occurring between two contents. The latter is an important part of our thinking because it suggests that defense is revealed not by a single content but by a transition from one content to another. We have adapted these ideas to Weinshel's (1984) definition of psychoanalytic process: "Those aspects of the unique relationship between the analyst and the analysand which permit and promote working through resistance to resolve repression." Psychoanalysis is an optimal condition for the analysis of resistance, which leads to understanding how repressions work as barriers, how they evolved in the patient's development, and why they remain in operation.

Resistance

Resistance is used here to mean a conflict about vocally expressing something in the analytic situation. We realize that limiting our definition in that way does not allow an exhaustive exploration of the subject, but there is precedent for this definition. Freud (1933) wrote "The objective sign of this resistance is that [a patient's] associations ignore or depart widely from the topic that is being dealt with. He may also recognize the resistance subjectively by the fact that he has distressing feelings when he approaches the topic. But this last sign may also be absent" (p. 68).

This definition of resistance is one which uses manifest data observable in close process attention. While resistance is frequently unconscious early in analysis, as analysis proceeds repression of the awareness of resistance is reduced, and analysands experience resistance. They become convinced that being acquainted with their resistances is useful in achieving insight. In termination, as in all phases of analysis, there is still resistance, but there is an increased ability to recognize it, to work through it, and to analyze it. We view resistance as a manifestation of defense in which shifts of feeling or subject are of sufficient magnitude to be experienced as reluctance to say something by the analysand.

Repression

Repression is fundamental to resistance and we believe it may be considered as a part of every defense. Repression is seen as a force that is stimulated by a quantum of aggressive energy. Repression is the unconscious equivalent to an injunction, "No, do not think of this mental content."

Early in his writing, Freud (1894) recognized that compulsive self-criticism had the effect of preventing criticism of others. Later (1914), he elaborated the concept of turning aggression from the object onto one's self. With the development of his structural theory, Freud (1923) identified the superego as the agency of intrapsychic self-criticism. Freud conceived the superego as retaining elements of its instinctual origin, more than other ego functions did. The superego is the agency that stimulates defensive activity in adult neurosis (A. Freud 1936).

In practice, we construe the ways in which the expression of one's thoughts and feelings in the analytic setting are inhibited, restricted, and delayed as resistance. We hypothesize that resistance is invoked by a quantum of aggressive energy emanating from the superego which activates the repressive part of each defense. This idea was stimulated by Freud's early (1910) idea that repression is like a negative judgment in the field of logic.

Working through

We have adopted Freud's (1914) idea that "One must allow the patient time to become more conversant with this resistance with which he has now become acquainted, to work through it, to overcome it, by continuing in defiance of it, the analytic work according to the fundamental rule" (p. 155). An important implication of this definition of working through is that it does not suggest a disappearance of resistance. Brenner (1976) made the point that working through is nothing special, it is just analyzing. We agree with his assessment, with the addendum that working through means analyzing what at an earlier time in the patient's analysis might have been fleeting or non-observable. As analysis proceeds, the patient can observe resistance and understand it. This contrasts with older ideas about overcoming resistance rather than respecting it as an indispensable part of analytic process.

CLOSE PROCESS ATTENTION ANALYSIS

Lawrence Friedman (1984) likened close process monitoring to an observer, on shore, watching a canoe move downstream. The canoe sometimes swerves away from an obstruction beneath the surface of the water. The observer, on shore, cannot see the obstruction and the paddler of the canoe also may pay no attention to what is happening beneath the surface. If the observer on shore were to call out to the person in the canoe, sometimes that person might recall that he had swerved and get a glimpse of what he had avoided. Later, the paddler may begin to register consciously the objects causing the swerves without much prompting from the observer. But that is only the beginning of the process.

Here is an example:

> *Patient:* I am so angry with Betty I could strangle her. ... (He elaborated for a while, then he became hesitant) ... on the other hand she has many fine qualities. ...
>
> *Analyst:* Now you are focused on her fine qualities. A moment before you were experiencing very different feelings. Then your feelings shifted. Can you see what happened there?

Patient: I was afraid you would think I was a brute for feeling so angry at her.

Often what begins as a clarification leads to a highlighting of transference.

Patient: I know it's not you. You have never asked me not to feel any way.

According to Strachey (1934), such a sequence is mutative at this point because the patient recognizes a difference between his automatic assumptions about the analyst and his knowledge of the analyst.

Patient: My mother always told me to think gentle thoughts about women.

To make the initial clarification one has to develop a sense of the swerves in the patient's verbal canoe. The defense is the equivalent of the patient's paddling. If the clarification of the swerves is clear, emergence of genetic material may occur easily.
Notice that defense analysis includes more than just pointing out a defense and asking the patient what comes to mind about it. Defense analysis includes an active attempt to find the superego imago transferred onto the analyst that makes it difficult to speak about one's thoughts and feelings, at the moment, to the analyst. In other words, an effort is made to uncover the transference fantasy (rock in the stream) that acted as a stimulus for the defense (paddling).

CHOOSING THE MOMENT

How one decides that this is the moment to intervene is a matter of the art of psychoanalysis, but we can specify a few guidelines that help us decide. In general, all the following are specific moments of resistance.

Turning aggression on the self

Turning aggression on the self when displayed in sufficient magnitude to be noticeable by the patient by a mere shift in attention may be a suitable time for intervention. However, there are exceptions. If the patient turns aggression on the self most of the time, pointing out each moment would make the analyst a nag. In such a case it is best to intervene when the analysand interrupts his usual process.

> *Patient:* I am so dumb, I should just stay in the corner all my life. . . . You know that is not true . . . I may be many things but dumb is not one of them.
> *Analyst:* There it is safe to stop berating yourself, at the thought of your intelligence. Can you sense what makes that seem more safe?

We used the recorded sessions of a patient for the research project that allowed us to delineate the six forms of turning aggression on the self outlined below. The recorded patient resembled the example above.

The point of working on this vicissitude of aggression is to permit the patient to experience aggression directed outwardly and then to move on from that. To get to love is a goal, but that may not feel safe until an individual learns to handle, mentally, his aggressive impulses.

Interruption of thinking about goals and ambitions

A patient often enters analysis with some life goals, or develops them while in analysis. The moment when thinking about such goals is interrupted can usually be conceptualized in close process attention analysis. What follows is from the analysis of a person who complained of losing interest in a pursuit just at the moment that success seemed imminent.

> *Patient:* I can make a difference at work with this project. I will complete it this weekend, but what a great time to lie in the sun and just relax.
>
> *Analyst:* Now you see yourself lying in the sun and just relaxing. A moment before you saw yourself making an impact, then just as success seemed within reach, you put your goal out of mind and relinquished the intention you held strongly just a moment before. Can you sense the risk in imagining yourself following through and making an impact at work?

Any silence of several minutes

Most silences of five minutes or longer are experienced as reluctance by patients. But what about the patient whose passivity has been a way of making those around him become active in one way or another? That can be addressed directly.

> *Patient:* (several minutes of silence)
> *Analyst:* Is this silence an invitation for me to become active?

Or the more usual kind of silence after a clearly conflicted content:

> *Patient:* It was one of the most rewarding meetings I have ever chaired. It would have been perfect if my boss hadn't stuck his two cents in just at the end. I could have tossed him out the window. [silence for several minutes]

Analyst: Do you feel reluctance as you are using your imagination to toss a man out of a window?
Patient: I was afraid you would think I'm a wild man, out of control.

Incongruent affect

If the patient had said, "Oh no, I wouldn't really want to toss him out the window. I was thinking of what a kind, generous man he is. He doesn't try to compete with me. It's a pleasure working with him. I can't wait to get to work in the morning," and then continued with a cheerfulness that belied his previous description of his boss as a man who seemed envious of his talents and who sought any excuse to destroy his chances at advancement, we might infer that the patient's cheerfulness was a reaction formation and was incongruent to his trend of thoughts about his boss. In this case, we might infer that the incongruent feelings marked a conflict about vocally expressing more critical observations and more aggressive feelings and fantasies about his boss in the analyst's presence at that moment, and we would intervene appropriately:

Analyst: Now you are speaking positively about him when just a few moments before you were examining him critically. Can you describe the feelings of danger in speaking about your critical observations?

Another patient was having difficulty speaking about her affectionate feelings for the analyst. When she hinted at them, she immediately switched to angry feelings toward other therapists she had encountered. The analyst saw this switch as uneasiness with her affectionate feelings toward the analyst. Exploration brought out the patient's fear of how the analyst might use her affection to influence her as she felt manipulated by her mother during her teenage years.

Posture of patient

During the expression of his cheerful view of his boss, the first patient mentioned crossed his legs, clenched his fists, and put them behind his head.

> *Analyst:* Now you are speaking cheerfully about a man who is generous and kind, but a moment before you clenched your fists, and crossed your legs, and put your hands behind your head, and you seemed freer to face feelings of frustration toward a man who was giving you a hard time.
>
> *Patient:* Goddamn it. Why don't you get off my back? I'd like to throw you out the window.

He continued for some time in an animated fashion. His last words were, "And don't think this has anything to do with anyone else either. You are the only person I have ever encountered who was such a pain in the ass." Then he became subdued.

Inhibition in time recall

(1) The patient gets stuck in the immediate experience with the analyst.

> The patient then said, "I don't ever remember feeling so irritated with anyone." Here the patient is clearly limiting his recall in time, because he had spoken in the session of very similar feelings toward his boss, and in the session before about similar feelings toward his father. One option is for the analyst to intervene in the following way:

> *Analyst:* (without irony) I seem unique in stimulating your angry feelings at this moment.

This intervention allows the patient to continue with his thoughts or feelings toward the analyst, or to insert the negative of this statement and to remember that he had said the same thing about his boss or his father. Which way he goes will depend upon the amount of split he has achieved between his experiencing and observing ego.

If the patient continues speaking about his feelings toward the analyst, a fuller transference picture will emerge. Eventually, the patient will find himself so far away from his actual experience of the analyst that his integrative functions will take over and he will attempt to find some time and place in his memory that will explain his experience better than does his experience with the analyst. This is a working relationship. It allows for dissonance and cooperation.

(2) The patient gets stuck in the remote past.

When the patient remembered an especially difficult time with his father, he continued for several sessions recalling a time in childhood when his father was home only sporadically. He remembered that when his father was present, he only criticized him. The analyst mostly listened. There were times that the patient paralleled his experience with his father and his experience with his boss. When he mentioned that his father gave him the silent treatment when he was really angry with him, the analyst said, "A silent man." The patient recalled how little the analyst had said recently, and turned his attention back to his more immediate experience.

(3) The patient gets stuck in the recent past.

At the beginning of the analysis, the patient complained at length about his boss and his spouse for their unavailability and their undercutting behavior. The above interventions did not lead to any recall of his experience in the analytic situation or in his remote past. After trying interventions such as those above, the analyst said, "Now you seem to be stuck in one time dimension, your recent experience outside of here. This is unlike what you showed when you were sitting up, when you were able to tell me about your experience with me and your memories from the past. Can you sense any reluctance to include more time dimensions in your thoughts?"

Avoidance of topics, lack of imaginative thoughts and dreams

There were long stretches of time in the analysis of the above patient when certain subjects were blocked. After two sessions when he had made repeated reference to "breaking in" a new woman at work and "poking" his ideas of management into her mind, the analyst pointed out that these references, which had been relatively frequent recently, would usually lead him to more imagery, but that just now he seemed to be limiting the picture part of his imagination. A similar approach was used with each avoided subject. The emphasis in the analyst's approach was to help the patient try to understand what risks he might be experiencing in the analytic situation that would make the restrictions seem necessary. Sometimes he said, "I had the image of screwing her several times, but didn't say it. . . . I didn't even think to say it." Then the analyst proceeded to investigate what may have interfered with his thinking to say thoughts closer to the imagery at these moments. Other times he would say, "Oh yes, it sounds sexual when you play it back to me. . . . I'm not sure why that didn't occur to me." The analyst proceeded to help him investigate why saying his thoughts closer to the imagery was inhibited. In doing so, the analyst does not necessarily take the patient's report of not having had the images before he intervened as truth, because if repression is working well, how would the patient remember whether he had the images or not? In addition, perhaps there was another layer of resistance that was not yet close to awareness that would contribute to the patient's distorting his report. All the analyst knows about the patient's experience is what the patient can say about it. What we can observe is when there appears to be a "change of direction in the patient's canoe" (Friedman 1984). Often we can detect a change when the patient cannot. There is no need to convince the patient other than by pointing out what we have observed in a sequence. When the resistance is experienced and the patient feels safe in examining it, he will. In this and in most analyses in the authors' experience, when the freedom to experience imagery is regained, dreams will be reported.

Rituals

The patient had the ritual of taking his shoes off to keep from soiling the analyst's couch, which was clearly protected against such occurrences. Nothing was said about this for many months, until he mentioned one day that it was curious that he was so careful with the analyst's couch and so indifferent to his furniture at home. Then the analyst began linking his taking off his shoes to starting the hour with a message, put into action rather than into words, that the patient was acting to reassure the analyst, "Don't worry, I will be very careful with you today." Taking off his shoes turned out to have many other meanings from all levels of psychosexual development. Later the ritual occurred only periodically and finally it was expressed only in words: "This is one of those days I feel like taking my shoes off. You must have irritated me yesterday."

Other ritual expressions were examined, such as routinely saying "and stuff like that," and were dealt with as they arose as markers of dangerous details in the context of the thoughts that came before and after.

Lateness, missing hours

Lateness or missing hours is not always indicative of resistance, of course, but when the patient is late several times in a row without thinking about the meaning of the behavior, the analyst might mention to him something like, "Usually after being late a few times in a row you might have thought about this as a sign of some self-depriving impulse, but for some reason recently you have not let the lateness enter the thoughts you express to me." Rationalized missed hours were dealt with similarly.

Not paying

This is dealt with as a message that is put into action because it is unsafe to put it into words.

Repetitive affect

For prolonged periods, it seemed that the patient experienced mostly rage. In our theoretical understanding, rage is an affect in which some aggressive impulse is mixed with anxiety about it and regression ensues. This theory influenced the analyst to avoid inferences about the patient's process while he was in a regressed state. During that period the analyst merely acknowledged the patient's thoughts and feelings without reference to shifts. When the patient felt comfortable again experiencing an evaluative stance toward the analyst, or toward others in the analyst's presence, attention to process was again experienced as helpful.

Acting out

Whenever possible the analyst hears all communication as expressions of the patient's moment-to-moment experience in the analytic hour. Sometimes the communication refers to what otherwise might be considered acting out or recall of important genetic material (Gray 1973). The analyst hears these associations much as he does any other in the analytic hour (Freud 1912). The equivocation here is deliberate. We think that analysts hear material with judgments that are immediately conveyed to the patient. True, the analyst probably does this in a more neutral way than anyone else in the patient's life. But when a patient plans to do something outside the hour that sounds as though it might be harmful to him or others, the analyst may question why the patient is presenting himself at that moment with more urgency than he might on other occasions. Additionally, there is a clear bias against acting in the analytic session. We justify this by thinking that in order to gain freedom of thought the patient must suspend action. Does such a bias make our work unscientific? Not necessarily. Modern science shows us that scientific observation always has a bias. The work of the scientist includes specifying rather than denying his bias.

RESEARCH IMPLICATIONS

If analysis of the archaic, punitive, superego functions is a priority, we assume that in the course of a successful psychoanalysis there will be a decrease in turning aggression on the self from the beginning of the analysis to the end. A complementary increase in instinctualized material may result from this. The decrease in turning aggression on the self and the increase in instinctualized material may even be a distinguishing characteristic between a successful psychoanalysis and a successful shorter-term psychotherapy. The authors studied a successful short-term psychotherapy by marking moments of turning aggression on the self and counted the words spent in that mode. We saw no appreciable change in the duration of turning aggression on the self, a measure of inhibitory superego function, from the beginning to the end of that case and predicted that despite significant life changes the patient would require further treatment. That prediction was subsequently confirmed. We are now testing this hypothesis on a psychoanalytic case.

Here is an example of how the case material is marked (from Dahl et al. 1988):

> Patient: Something that's been on my mind today is the relationship I have with the girl who is my assistant this year and was last year ... because of the other assistant having left, she's having to fulfill both of the functions to an extent and, and both of the teachers, myself and the other teacher, are to make adjustments too, so that she can help us both out. And today was the first day when she was really officially working for both of us. And I, I found all over again, I was beginning to react to her the way I had last year (**3a**) <u>which upset me very much because I know that some of it's</u>, is the way she is and, maybe I am annoyed by that kind of a person, (**1a**) <u>but some of it's got nothing to do with her. And I think it had something to do with just sharing her and. and the fear that she might prefer working with the other girl or being in the other room</u>. And, I think it also, when I'm faced with the aspect of sharing her, I, I also (**2a**) <u>have to face that perhaps sometimes I'm not treating her quite the way I should be. And. and this is another reason why I become almost jealous of who she works with</u>. [Sniff] <u>And then I think well. I will try to be fairer to her since it is something within me. It has nothing to do with her. but I still can't seem to maintain that. I still seem to treat her the same way I used to. And. I think I'm. well, I don't really know how she sees it. I don't know whether she thinks there's anything wrong with the way I treat her at all.</u>
>
> I think what I do to control her is to, um, through controlling what she does with the children in the classroom.

And I know I want to be the, the definite one in control in the classroom. And, and I know that I want to have a response from the boys that, as long as I have it, then it's all right for her to have it too. But I, I know I respond very much to any time that. . . .

The underlined words are those that we would consider to be in the turning aggression on the self mode, and the moments that initiated this mode are designated by the numbers and letters in bold (**3a**, **1a**, **2a**) and are summarized as follows:

1 (a)–Open aggression is directed at an object and then is shifted to the self.

"Jim is a jerk–but I am a jerk too."
"Jim is a jerk–he thinks I am a jerk too."
"Jim is a jerk–maybe I'm jealous."

(b)–Open aggression is directed at an object and then gives way to hesitancy, or silence, or a shift to a different mode or subject.

"John is a jerk . . . uh . . . er. . . . (silence)"
"John is a jerk. . . . What a lovely floral pattern on your carpet." (change of subject)

2 (a)–An open libidinal expression or a moment of pleasure gives way to self-criticism.

"I love the way she smiles . . . she probably thinks I'm a jerk."
"I really enjoyed the Knicks game on Saturday . . . I should go to more games."

(b)–An open libidinal expression or a moment of pleasure gives way to hesitancy or silence, or a shift to a different mode or subject.

"I love the way she smiles . . . I guess . . . uh . . . I don't know."

"I really enjoyed the Knicks game on Saturday . . . uh . . . what have you been doing?"

3 (a)—A positive or neutral perception of the self gives way to a diminished one or elevated view of another.

"I am talented at seeing the differences between what people do and what they say. . . . I wish I were good at something useful."

"I am talented at seeing the differences between what people do and what they say. . . . But you are ever so much better at that than I am."

(b)—A positive or neutral perception of the self gives way to hesitancy, silence, or a shift to a different mode or subject.

"I am talented at seeing the differences between what people do and what they say . . . er . . . uh. . . ." (silence)

4 (a)—Outwardly directed observations give way to self-criticism.

"I saw them walking and I noticed the leaves turning. . . . I wondered what's wrong with me that I pay attention to such stupid things."

(b)—Outwardly directed observations give way to hesitancy, silence, or a shift to a different mode or subject.

"I saw them walking and I noticed the leaves turning . . . er . . . uh . . . how's the family?"

5—A self-depreciation or self-derogation comes in response to the (a) therapist's comment or (b) some unknown stimulus.

(a) "How are you today?" "Crummy as usual."
(b) "Well, here I am again, as miserable as ever."

6—A strong feeling (often of sadness) quickly stimulates suppression of feeling experience and expression.

"Jill broke up with me and I miss her . . . but when the going gets tough the tough get going. . . . I have begun three new projects at work."

Four steps to a mutative interpretation

Step One: State what the patient is saying now.
Step Two: State what that seems to be a shift away from. If the analysand can hear these suggestions and follow them, then
Step Three: Inquire about the perceived risk or danger in holding the first thought or feeling. Listen for the transferred superego imago that was a stimulus for defense.
Step Four: Review the picture of the transferred superego imago.

The first two steps in a mutative interpretation done around a defense at the leading edge of a resistance are to identify moments when the patient turns aggression on the self, and then to play them back to him in a two-step process. A research project undertaken by the authors has identified six common forms of turning aggression on the self. Here are three of the most important ones:

Turning aggression on the self

Patient: I think John is a real jerk. . . .
Patient: I bet he hates my guts.

The patient began speaking of his outwardly directed aggressive impulses; then he experienced them as turned around on himself (by projecting the criticism and feeling on the receiving end of it).

> *Analyst:* Now you are thinking "he hates my guts" but just before you were freer to criticize John. Then something happened when you became uncomfortable looking at him critically. What do you think it was?

The other mechanism, other than projecting pique, is identifying with the onerous object:

> *Patient:* I dislike John intensely when he upstages me . . . of course, I probably do that myself. . . .

Here the patient first criticizes, then he steps into the picture on the receiving end of criticism.

The shower of "shoulds" (musts, oughts, have to's)

> *Patient:* I think John is a real jerk. . . . I really *should* have more patience with him.
> [The patient begins with an outwardly directed observation and then the shoulds move in.]
> *Analyst:* Now the "shoulds" seem to have moved in right after a moment of criticizing John. What do you think about that?

Catastrophizing

> *Patient:* I think John is a real jerk . . . but then . . . *I can never get along with anyone.* . . .
> [The patient begins with an outwardly directed observation and then catastrophe moves in.]

Analyst: Now you seem to be experiencing a sense of catastrophe just after you were criticizing someone else. *What is the danger in criticizing John?*

A unifying metaphor: a drop in self esteem

Patient: I went to the game . . . I felt good . . . *then I saw Carol. I know she hates me.*

All three types of patterns can fit into the general category of a fall in self-esteem, though the specific way it occurs is more descriptive for the patient's purposes than this more general description. Note that all the interventions begin with the ending statement (1) (Now you are talking about Carol hating you.) and end with the beginning statement (2) (But a few moments before you had achieved greater freedom in expressing feelings of pleasure). These are Steps One and Two.

Step Three attempts to elicit the patient's interest in finding out the risk or danger in speaking from the perspective of outwardly directed aggressive energy to the analyst at this moment. Notice that this is different from attempting to clarify an instinctualized transference. It is attempting to clarify an inhibiting transference. Step Three happens only if the patient can see steps one and two and can feel the shift in affect or the increased sense of risk in holding the former position.

Let us consider the question asked above: *What is the danger in criticizing John?* When the analyst asks this question, he knows there are a finite number of answers to it. Some include general dangers: he is concerned that he will leave the analytic situation and act on his aggressive feelings toward John; or he is afraid that if he gets in touch with his aggressive feelings they will linger as a distraction and he will not feel libidinal feelings toward John again; or he is afraid that thinking aggressive thoughts is as morally wrong as acting aggressively toward John; or he is afraid that if he thinks aggressive thoughts toward John something bad will happen to John or to himself; or he is afraid that he will be overcome by rage and will disintegrate emotionally.

Each can be analyzed in its adaptive and genetic origins. The addition of defense analysis is to analyze the externalized superego imago. That means the associations are considered to be a clue to how the analysand is experiencing the analyst. Often the patient will not be aware of how he is subliminally experiencing the analyst and how that experience is helping to shape his associations. He is not sure why he is tense about criticizing John, but some associations follow. How the analyst treats these associations is Step Four. *Whatever the patient says after the analyst asks the question about the danger or risk contains clues to the answer of that question. The analyst's job is to help the analysand learn to read these associations if an answer is out of awareness.*

> *Patient:* I am so angry at John I could spit. He is so irritating. How can he call himself a friend when he is so blatantly competitive? . . . Where is his sense of grace? . . . He is a graceless slug. . . . I don't know, I may be going too far. . . . He probably has some fine qualities that I am overlooking. . . .
>
> *Analyst:* Now you are looking for some fine qualities but a moment ago you looked critically at the man. Can you sense a risk in speaking to me about him critically?
>
> *Patient:* I feel uneasy. I had a dream last night. . . . I was in the garden when a dragon came after me. At first I thought of running, but then I had a sword and I stalked the dragon and it ran away.
>
> *Analyst:* Since these thoughts are in response to my question about risk, how might they be an answer?

Patient: I think I am afraid of being too cutting. . . . I might get caught up, be too competitive myself. It might ruin my friendship. I might want to have nothing to do with him. You might think I can't have friends.
Analyst: I would think of you as too competitive to have friends. I'd turn your criticism of him back on you. [here is Step Four: the analyst reviews his understanding of the risk]
Patient: Yes. Like my mother saying "Examine your own conscience before you blame others."

Here the analyst helps the patient translate his associations to answer the question about risk. By doing this *every time* the focus of inquiry is risk or danger, the analyst conveys a seriousness about answering the question. Even if the patient does not accept the assignment at first, if he can be encouraged to enter the quest for understanding risk he will learn an invaluable lesson for use in his self analysis: *The answer to what inhibits me is always on the tip of my tongue if I can learn to read my own associations.*

Later in the analysis, as the patient becomes progressively more attentive and able to translate the primary process for himself, the analyst may not be needed to remind the patient that these associations are an answer to the question of risk.

In attempting to do this work we have developed a set of biases that guide our use of defense analysis. This section is intended to begin a list of instructions that may be followed to make an effective, rational, mutative interpretation.

By "rational interpretation" we mean one which begins from data observable to both the patient and the analyst and offers an explanation as an hypothesis through one of the many possible windows of observation. We think that interpretations can be rational providing the analyst is attuned to his biases, understands the limits of what is observable, *assumes the fundamental hypotheses that thoughts following one another are causally connected,* and is aware that each interpretation is merely one of many possible ways to view the data.

To review, the four steps are as follows:

Step One: State what the patient is saying now.
Step Two: State what that seems to be a shift away from.
Step Three: Inquire about risk in speaking to the analyst, at this moment.
Step Four: Review the analyst's understanding of the risk.

Sometimes the patient will ignore the question about risk and just continue his associations. *In that case the analyst may return to the question after the patient has said what was on his mind*:

Patient: Bill is a jerk . . . uh . . . I don't know. (silence)
Analyst: Now you are more inhibited just after looking critically at Bill.
Patient: Yeah.
Analyst: Can you sense the risk in speaking critically of Bill?
Patient: When I was silent I was thinking of the time he stood me up for lunch and how unreliable he is.
Analyst: Now that you have been able to tell me those thoughts and feelings do you have any more sense of what made that difficult at first?
Patient: I was afraid you would see me as a whiny child, always bitching about something.
Analyst: Can you say more about that picture of me? [And the elaboration of the transference fantasy continues after that.]

Two variations on steps one and two

Variations of Steps One and Two are limited only by one's imagination. Two variations to Steps One and Two that we have found useful are the *camera* metaphor and the *two voices* metaphor.

The camera metaphor:

> *Patient:* I hate John. He probably is angry at me too; after all, I've done nothing but avoid him recently.
> *Analyst:* Now John has the camera and it is aimed at you. A few seconds before you had the camera and it was aimed at him and you were speaking of him critically.

The two voices metaphor:

> *Patient:* I am so angry at John I could spit. He is so irritating. How can he call himself a friend when he is so blatantly competitive? Where is his sense of grace? . . . He is a graceless slug. . . . I don't know . . . I may be going too far . . . he probably has some fine qualities that I am overlooking.
> *Analyst:* Now you speak to me in a voice of caution, reason, hesitation. Just before a voice of passion held the floor. Can you experience a risk in speaking to me in that voice?

It may be useful to restate what we view as our goal in psychoanalysis and why we think it is useful. We have several specific aims. (1) We are aiming to help the patient discover what makes it feel unsafe to say whatever comes to mind in the analytic setting. This is a slightly different aim than removing resistance. It is to understand reluctance to speak in the analytic hour. In doing this we aim to help the analysand develop a self-analytic capacity by analyzing inhibiting superego imagos. (2) This should increase the moments when a patient will focus attention on reluctance to speak in the analytic setting (and, with the use of a self-analytic capacity not confined to the analytic couch, to examine reluctance to behave optimally in other settings). (3) Saying what comes to mind is the behavior most likely to advance one's aims in the psychoanalytic setting, but probably not in most other settings. This is a distinction we help our patients make as soon as possible. We try to help our patients see how they are encumbering themselves by anachronistic restraints. In Gray's "Analysis of the Superego" (1987), he writes about two particularly important technical aims: "the first, a reclaiming of the uncompromised function of the observing ego from its altered role in superego formation; the second, a concurrent return of the defensively self-directed aggression to the ego's voluntary executive powers" (p. 152).

We hope that future research might prove scientifically that a person's thought processes can be freed significantly through a rigorously conducted analysis that focuses on restrictions of those processes imposed at earlier times (childhood) when feeling, thought, and fantasy were more ineluctably entwined with action than they are in adult life. What are we hoping will result from this improved self-observing skill?

1. Learning one's talents and how to use them to influence one's destiny. This is dependent upon freeing one's autonomous ego capacities of affect recognition, cognition, motility, perception, attention, and recall. Eventually, one's integrative capacity will synthesize these into something practical, such as talents. This process of freeing one's autonomous ego capacities may be directly attributed to the analyzing of inhibitions and restrictions of free association.

2. Freedom of feeling, thought, and fantasy in the analytic situation. With analytic intervention aimed at freeing one to say anything and everything that comes to mind, freedom of feeling, thought, and fantasy leads to a sense of imagination and creative capacities (Davison 1984). These first two goals are dependent upon helping the third goal.
3. Helping the analysand gain conscious understanding and control of the debilitating affects of anxiety, guilt, shame, and embarrassment. These affects are ones which may be conceptualized as containing relatively large amounts of aggressive energy turned against the self. These affects serve as signals for defense.
4. Learning and insightful understanding, the cornerstones of analysis. Debilitating affects are controlled through the analysand's increased capacity to reconstruct sequences of feeling, thought, and fantasy, leading to these affects and to being able to figure out how past experience is governing anachronistic present ones. The analysand knows, "I am never upset for the reasons I think." This knowledge permits reversing processes that lead to debilitating affects. Often after considerable conscious efforts the reversal becomes preconscious or automatic. However, the analysand is armed with the knowledge of a process that he may use either inside or outside the analytic setting, a self-analytic capacity that we consider crucial to analytic progress.

In making interventions that highlight anachronistic restraint to freedom of thought, as indicated by speech in the analytic setting, we have identified the following biases.

BIASES REGARDING A DEFENSE INTERPRETATION

Early in analysis intervene on the side of aggression first.

We have concluded that if you intervene in regard to aggression successfully, libido will be easier to deal with. If you think of aggression as arising from the frustration of libidinal impulses, then it is logical that understanding the aggressive side of a conflict will bring the libidinal impulses to the surface. Early in analysis a patient will feel more control after he becomes acquainted with his aggressive impulses. He will be less afraid of his affectionate and erotic feelings since he is more sure of his ability to tolerate frustration. Also, since we are trying to free self-observation and other observations it is crucial for aggression to be freed, because aggression when sublimated leads to discriminating observations. A typical example of an early analytic intervention is as follows:

> *Patient:* I'm sorry to be late. My supervisor, the clod, just had to tell me about his weekend in excruciating detail. I really wanted to be here, but I hate to be rude to him. I am such a wimp [and he continued a litany of self-deprecatory comments in a childlike voice].
>
> *Analyst:* Now you are portraying yourself as weak; a moment before you had begun with strong feelings about your supervisor.
>
> *Patient:* Yes, I guess I did say he was a clod. I might sound too harsh. . . .
>
> *Analyst:* To me?
>
> *Patient:* You might think I was too harsh if I told you how irritated I get with my boss. After all, he has been really good to me and I appreciate the way he has helped me get ahead. He has been a real booster of mine and here I am criticizing him.

Analyst: Are you experiencing me as a person who wouldn't want you to look critically at someone you like and someone you feel has been a help to you?
Patient: You'd think "How ungrateful can you be?" My father had a great sense of humor. When I gave him a hard time sometimes he would laugh and say, "How sharper than a serpent's tooth is a thankless child." He was kidding, but I sometimes worried that I hurt his feelings.

In this example, addressing the inhibition of aggressive impulses reveals the fear that the analyst would think him ungrateful if he looked too closely at a reasonably pleasant person, but it also uncovers affectionate feelings for the supervisor and his father. Analyzing the conflict over aggressive impulses often reveals libidinal motivations and, after all, that is the whole point: to let patients feel the force of their aggressive impulses, not so they will be more aggressive but to help them sublimate these impulses, making subtle distinctions so they can see others clearly and feel safe experiencing their libidinal impulses.

Intervene first with a focus on process, not on content.

In the above example, the analyst focuses on process and not one specific content. This approach has the advantage of sending the patient the message that the analyst's interest is in how the patient's mind works without suggesting a preference for elaboration of any particular content. In so doing he tries not to give the patient the idea that he expects the patient to favor any particular set of thoughts or feelings toward his boss, just that he is attempting to help the patient not to limit any expression in the analytic setting that come from irrational or anachronistic fear. Also, by maintaining this perspective the analyst gives the patient the message that the analyst is more interested in the patient's mental processes in the analytic situation than he is in how the patient behaves or feels toward his supervisor outside the analytic situation. If the patient were to model his self-analytic stance after the analyst's he might learn to *look upstream* in his train of thoughts and perceptions when attempting to answer the question: Why do I feel tense right now?

Emphasize the shortest possible time interval.

As in the above example, the analyst's intervention should be experienced as rational because all the data are available for the patient's scrutiny, assuming the patient does not repress immediately after saying something. Many patients do repress immediately, at times, and when they do, they will not find process interventions any more rational than any other kind.

Emphasize a polarity and a transition.

When the analyst says, "Now you are criticizing yourself. A few moments ago you were criticizing your supervisor. Can you see that shift?" And later: "Is there something less safe about speaking the outwardly directed critical observations?" the analyst is showing the patient a polarity in perception—outwardly directed observations as opposed to inwardly directed observations. The analyst points out the polarity and a transition. After the patient can observe the shift, the analyst tries out a causal hypothesis (is there something less safe?) about what makes the transition seem necessary. This puts the data in sharp relief for the patient. This is recommended rather than: "I think you are having some difficulty criticizing your supervisor." If repression has been working just a little bit, the patient may not remember that he had been previously criticizing his supervisor and the analyst's rational observation may seem quite irrational to the patient.

Before looking for the risk that makes a resistance seem necessary, make sure the patient can experience, or find reasonable, the shift that the analyst is seeing as a manifestation of defense.

This is illustrated in the sequence on page 28. The process as it is spelled out there is one that we frequently find. It is also in keeping with what Strachey predicted: if one deals with the first part of the mutative interpretation well, then the genetic material may follow almost automatically. When the adaptive experience with the analyst is focused upon after the dynamic process is recognized and can be experienced by the patient, the patient will often switch to the genetic perspective to understand his adaptation. It is often necessary for the analyst to thoroughly explore only the adaptation that the patient is making to the analyst's presence and the genetic investigation seems to proceed automatically. In previous writings, we have emphasized that it is important for the analyst to refrain from initiating the genetic inquiry lest the patient think the analyst is discouraging continued perceptions of his behavior (Davison 1984). By continued elaboration of his fantasy about the analyst, the patient will get farther away from the perceptions that stimulated his fantasy. Eventually the dissonance will stimulate him to look elsewhere for the roots of his fantasy. This will often cause a transition to genetic inquiry.

Admit your bias.

Sometimes a patient will be more interested in his perspective than in the analyst's inferences about how his mind works. The patient above may have responded as follows to the analyst's initial intervention:

> *Patient:* Why do you focus on that transition? I was trying to talk about how I get wimpy toward superiors whom I sense like and support me. I should keep some back-

bone with them. George [his supervisor] uses me to affirm his existence without caring what I have on my mind. I wish I knew a way to be more assertive with him without hurting his feelings.

Sometimes the analyst may say explicitly that he recognizes he is speaking from "only one of many ways your thoughts and feelings may be understood." Other times the elaboration of the patient's feeling about the analyst's bias is all that is necessary. In this example the analyst does neither, but merely stops interfering in the patient's initiative, which includes the patient's achieving with the analyst what he thought he could not achieve with his supervisor. For the analyst's part, it is very important for him to feel comfortable with his bias.

Analyst: More assertive in that you don't let yourself become distracted from your goal, like you were able to keep me from doing to you just there.
Patient: Hmm... I guess I was. I don't see you as touchy as he is. He can't really seem to tolerate a different point of view.

Here the analyst does not push his perspective if the patient does not find it useful. Highlighting intrapsychic conflict is a bias that the analyst superimposes on what is being said to him.

The patient is always correct about an intervention's usefulness.

In the above sequence the analyst does not attempt to make his bias more precious than the patient's. If the patient does not find the perspective useful, it is important to learn more about what the patient does experience in order to be most useful.

If the patient is stuck in a regressed transference experience, he will not find process interventions very useful because the urgency of his feelings will be a more prominent priority.

At those times it is most helpful if one tries to understand the details of that regressed experience better. Stick with his metaphor. Do not try to introduce another one until he is feeling stronger. At these moments showing him what has been regressed *from* is of no use to him.

Focus on the vicissitudes of perception.

Perception is one of the autonomous ego functions. References to perception are ubiquitous in analytic material. Framing one's interventions in the idiom of perception often is optimally neutral: "Now you are criticizing yourself, a moment ago you were able to *look* in your supervisor's direction, then your focus of observation turned on yourself . . . (later) Can you observe what stimulated this shift in the focus of your observations as you were speaking to me?"

This intervention and the series of interventions on page 28 use the perception metaphor. One advantage of the perception metaphor is that it suggests a sublimation of one's aggressive impulses into seeing, looking closely, and observing carefully.

Emphasize identification, projection, and repression.

These defenses are the building blocks of more complex defenses, such as identification with the aggressor or projective identification. We have found it useful to use the most elemental shifts. They are easiest to grasp in the throes of dissonant affective forces.

> *Patient:* I am angry at him for not taking me into consideration. . . . He always keeps me waiting . . . (she

became quiet for several minutes) but then I am not always so Johnny-on-the-spot myself. I guess I am as inconsiderate as he is [pause].

Analyst: Now, it is you who are inconsiderate, but just before that you seemed to evaluate him as inconsiderate.

Patient: Hmm. Yes, I can see that.

Analyst: Can you experience what got in the way of holding that outwardly directed, evaluative stance in my presence, just now?

Patient: You were three minutes late today. I was annoyed. I wondered if you were angry at me. When I came in here I forgot all about it, but when I started talking about my boyfriend's lateness I began to feel that you would remember the time I stood him up and even though he did it to me this time you would think that I was easily as inconsiderate as he was.

When the evaluation of a man as inconsiderate came dangerously close to an evaluation the patient might have had of the analyst—that is the repression necessary for her displacement began to break down—she invoked a second line of defenses: projection and identification. She projected her anger at the analyst onto the boyfriend and identified with the inconsiderate one, the former object of her derision. After uncovering this sequence, which includes inferences of both projection of pique and identification with the object of former criticism, the analyst investigates each: "What makes it seem safer to let me (the analyst) have the blaming feelings just there?" and "What makes it seem necessary for you (the patient) to step into the picture on the receiving end of scrutiny just as you were allowing yourself to look more critically?" If the patient forgets about the more active thoughts and feelings then the analyst will focus on motives for repression:

Analyst: Now it is you who are inconsiderate, but just a moment before you were evaluating him.
Patient: What do you mean? I wasn't evaluating anyone.
Analyst: Have you blocked from your mind that you were angry at him for not taking you into consideration?
Patient: Yes, I forgot.
Analyst: Perhaps we can understand why forgetting the more outwardly directed thoughts and feelings seemed safer in my presence, just now?

One additional point: analyzing repression of a perception is a good way to *avoid* focusing on displacement as moving away from a subject which is often experienced by patients as an irrational, paradoxical injunction against free association.

Respect displacement.

One of the most important defenses to manage properly is displacement. *Free association depends upon ease of displacement.* Sometimes a patient will begin to speak about some feeling toward the analyst and then speak of a much stronger similar feeling toward someone else. It often is best to deal with the vicissitudes of the feeling or impulse toward the object in the displacement as preliminary to the eventual experience of that feeling in the transference. Trying to pull the focus back into the transference when the patient is expanding his freedom to experience a feeling toward someone in displacement may be experienced as undermining autonomy. Sometimes the feeling worked out in displacement is not worked out in the transference.

Intervene on the down slope of the assertive-retractive curve.

In our experience, patients tend to become assertive and then unassertive in their communication when they are freer to express their feelings and when they are free to be attentive to the presence of a listener. (See Figure 1-1.)

If the analyst intervenes on the up slope (A) he is likely to be experienced as undercutting the patient's initiative, dismissing the patient's strong feeling, and discouraging the experience of the full force of a drive derivative. If he intervenes on the down slope (B), he will be more likely to be experienced as someone who does not discourage the patient from experiencing the full strength of his impulses. Another reason that we think it is better to intervene on the down slope of the curve is that it does little to discourage expansiveness, outwardly directed perception (including scrutiny of the analyst), and positive feeling about oneself. *This bias is diagnosis-dependent. We assume we are talking about technique with a neurotically inhibited adult as opposed to someone prone to action or hypomanic overstimulation.*

Use the most neutral language you can think of. An analyst's timing must be sharp, but his language is dull. An individual intervention is best when it is not memorable.

To gain access to rational discourse, speak the language of reason. Every one of the previous interventions has illustrated optimal dullness. Another way that analyst's interventions are best not memorable follows: Imagine a young woman complaining that her analyst had not smiled that day in greeting

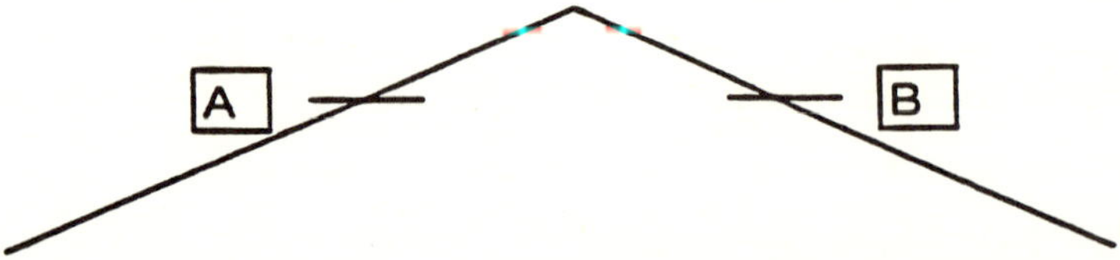

I could strangle the .... Maybe I am too harsh

Figure 1-1.

her. She paused, then turned her focus to complain of her sourpuss mother. When she paused again, the analyst considered intervening. One way to do so was, "Maybe it's easier to complain about your mother than it is to complain about me, because of some danger you experience here." While there is nothing inaccurate about that intervention, it runs the risk of providing an opportunity for the patient to turn on herself because of the phrasing. She might lament her always trying to find "the easy way," and remember childhood experiences of parental injunctions against that. Such an experience involves an ego regression, stimulated by the analyst's intervention. Even if that was not the analyst's intent, which may be clarified and analyzed, it may be more difficult for the patient to believe in the analyst's neutrality than if the analyst used another approach. An alternative intervention, choosing words less likely to be considered as an invitation to self-derogation, is: "Now you are complaining about someone at some distance, but a moment before you were examining those feelings about me. Can you experience what got in the way of your speaking about me?" This intervention makes it more difficult for the patient to believe that the analyst was calling her lazy and emphasizes the analyst's foremost interest in learning more about how to free her mental capacities in the analytic hour. Later in the analysis it may only be necessary to say, "Now you are experiencing those feelings toward someone at a distance." The patient will have developed the skill to search backwards in his or her thoughts and fill in the memory loop. The preferred of these two interventions invites a view of restricted freedom in the use of the mind as opposed to what may be construed as an invitation to view a deficit. The wording suggested here avoids the pitfall of attracting superego injunctions.

Gray (1985) stated that "when we choose our words most wisely, we manage to lessen the burden on patients' rational listening, comprehension, and observation in three ways. First, we respect their egos by choosing language that does not strain their fund of knowledge; second, we choose words that do not stimulate their conflicted instinctual drives; and third, we try not to attract their superegos into substituting a judgmental attitude for an objective one." An awareness of all three factors helps us choose wording less likely to invite turning aggression on the self.

We like to think of the analyst serving a function of an assist man rather than the star on a basketball team. His function is to get the ball near the hoop, not to make the "slam dunk."

Aim to free the patient's mind so any thought, fantasy, or feeling is acceptable to be spoken in the analytic setting.

In all the previous interventions, we have tried to make it implicit (if not explicit) that the type of behavior we are attempting to influence is freedom of the autonomous ego functions, including articulating one's thoughts, feelings, and fantasies in the analytic setting.

Aim each intervention at turning aggressive energy away from the patient's self.

This principle was abundantly illustrated above. We use the question, "Is this intervention likely to encourage or discourage the instinctual vicissitude of turning aggression on the self?" for the final tuning of our interventions. This point was central in a previous paper (Davison et al. 1986).

Once you have asked the question "what is the risk?" a collaboration to find an answer, even one constructed from the patient's associations, ensues.

>   *Patient:* I feel like laughing . . . but such jocularity probably isn't appropriate. . . .
>   *Analyst:* Does it feel like that prohibition comes from me?

Patient: Yes, I know it's not, but you looked pensive when I came in today. . . .
Analyst: And the risk in laughing with someone pensive?
Patient: I had just come in from a baseball game. I was the winning pitcher. I was laughing and bragging to my mother. She was trying to be congratulatory, but something was wrong. Later that night my father told me that her father died earlier that day. I felt so bad for laughing while she was so sad.
Analyst: So the risk with me might involve a fantasy?
Patient: Maybe you lost someone close to you. . . .

Most patients who appear to be unable to use process interventions will develop the capacity to use them in time if the analyst keeps making process interventions.

Some patients who use repression as their main line of defense will show adeptness at process recognition less quickly than patients who isolate affect as a primary line of defense. Other factors also affect how well a patient can use a process orientation. Most adult neurotics can use process interventions very well.

Some conflicts are not experienced in the transference.

When asked, "Is that shift influenced by my presence?" sometimes the patient will say, "No, it's my wife who wouldn't want to hear that." In this case we accept that the patient does not experience the analyst as inhibiting in that way at this moment, and remember that *the patient is always correct about the usefulness of an intervention.*

Some patients rarely can use close process monitoring.

There are some patients who can rarely use close process monitoring. We do not know why this is so. It is not entirely intelligence-dependent. We need more experience to answer that question. With such people we use it sparingly.

A CASE EXAMPLE

Here is a week of analytic work that shows the process described above in action. The Thursday before the first of these analytic sessions the analyst announced that he would be away on Monday eleven days hence. No direct reference to that announcement was heard on Friday of the previous week.

Monday

> *Mrs. M.:* It was not a good weekend. I was stuck inside with C [her daughter]. David [her husband] is covering some goings on in California. I had a dream. There were two vials of medicine that I was supposed to give C. I had to give her a shot. Then a doctor appeared and took them from me. He said, "Here, let me help you." I was so relieved. I really wanted some adult companionship this weekend but I didn't want to have to look for it. I wanted someone to come to me. [Her voice dropped in pitch and volume] I was awful with C. I screamed at her for the first time in a long time. [Long pause then more quietly] Then I felt guilty and invited her into bed with me. I know that isn't right. [With vehemence] It reminds me of my own goddamn mother always blowing cold until I cried and then she became mamma cuddles. The stupid bitch. [pause] I probably shouldn't complain about her [longer pause].
> *Analyst:* Can you sense the risk in telling me?
> *Mrs. M.:* Sure. I've left myself wide open. I'm the one who screwed up over the weekend and you could nail

me for it at any time. That reminds me of those vials of medicine. My father took us to the dentist. He demanded that we hold perfectly still while we were injected with anesthetic. Brit [her sister] and I did but not Tony [her brother]. He kicked and screamed like a tiger. I wanted to be so good for my father so I did just as he said. I was a fool. If I had it to do again I'd make Tony look like a pussycat. They'd think they had the Incredible Hulk on their hands [pause] [Less animated]: I could go on like this, but you could bring me down with any remark that points out something I haven't thought of.

Analyst: You would feel put down if I had a thought in addition to yours?

Mrs. M.: Is there an echo in here? That's what I just said. Anyway, don't sound so innocent. That's how you keep this racket going, isn't it? By convincing people that you have some great wisdom that they don't have?

Analyst: Something I said?

Mrs. M.: What about [mocking] "Something I said?" What are you, a clone from the Hal factory? Have you made any exciting correct-time recordings lately? [pause, reflectively]: It sounds like I want to pick a fight with you. No, that's not right. I know you won't fight back and I can needle you all I want. I guess I just feel like needling you.

Analyst: If you experienced yourself on the receiving end of that, at an earlier time, then doing it to me may seem natural to you.

Mrs. M.: I remember how still I was. What a fool. I want to please you but I won't hold still for that—not the needle—not ever again, not even for you.

Analyst: You experience me as needling you following a moment when you were freer to think of doing that to me.

Mrs. M.: Yes, your calmness seems insulting, even condescending, like you are saying to me, "I have calmness and you don't." Damn it. It makes me mad. . . . I felt like I needed you this weekend. You were probably home with your wife [pause] If that fat-mouthed law student gives me a hard time today he's going to get a fat lip. [She delivered a short punch to the air.]

Analyst: Now you are punching someone outside the room, just before you were thinking of doing something to me; can you sense the danger there?

Mrs. M.: Are you a glutton for punishment? Would you feel better if I thought of giving you a chubby jowl? I feel really wound up today and I guess I don't want to take it all out on you. I don't know when David will be home. I need him. C needs him too. I guess I am afraid that if I am too hard on you, you won't be there for me.

[*Ideally, the analyst might restate that idea*]

Tuesday

Mrs. M.: I am jittery today. David is coming home this weekend. I'm looking forward to seeing him but I am nervous. He has been such a help when he is home. He was working on the roof last . . . I don't like to see him on a ladder. I hope he doesn't extend himself too much for me. I had a dream last night. I slammed a laundry hamper closed, then noticed that the belt of David's bathrobe was sticking out. I felt frightened when I awakened. I'm reminded of a baby's umbilical cord. [Her voice trailed off; a minute or so passed.]

Analyst: Does your hesitation include a feeling regarding the dream imagery?

Mrs. M.: Yes. It's sexual. It makes me nervous. David stopped using condoms. I have to use a diaphragm. I hate it. I feel exposed, like I'm the one making the first move toward sex. [A few moments silence] That belt may have to do with a [mumble mumble] hanging out.

Analyst: Some tension about that word.

Mrs. M.: Uh huh. [She clenched her fists and put her hands behind her head. She sighed] It sounds like I want to cut someone's penis off.

Analyst: And maybe you feel concern about speaking of that wish in my presence.

Mrs. M.: You might think I was after you. Maybe I am. I have been cutting to you lately.

Analyst: And the risk involved in speaking of cutting me?

Mrs. M.: Just that if I am cutting to you, you may be sharp with me. [pause] Sometimes when David gets on top of me his penis slips out and bends back. He shrivels up. Men seem so brittle to me. So delicate. [Mockery replaced concern.] It probably wouldn't take much to break one off. [pause] That reminds me I had a fantasy last weekend that David was home and he tied my hands and had intercourse with me. I was surprised that it didn't hurt which is weird because I don't remember a time when intercourse hurt though suddenly it seems possible. Like I might not be able to stretch enough. [She shuddered.]

Analyst: One way to view this train of thoughts is that uncertainty about your elasticity and being tied up follows a moment when you spoke of advantage over a man.

Mrs. M.: Well, I can't do much damage with my hands tied, can I? When I was eleven, coming home from school, a man in a telephone booth stepped out all exposed. He said, "Come get a look at this, little girl. Bigger than daddy's, eh?" He had an enormous erection. He grinned, zipped up, and got in his car. It had a ladder strapped to the top. What that penis might have done to my little body! Now, of course, one good karate chop could ruin his whole day. [She slashed her hand through the air and giggled.] The ladder . . . I just remembered my worry about David and the ladder . . . afraid he'd hurt himself. You know, I was afraid to tell mother what happened because she was down on all men anyway. So I waited 'til father came home and told him. He just puffed out his jowls like he always did. He said, "It couldn't be old Sam," or whatever the man's name was who did odd jobs in the community, and then left the room like he thought it was just a figment of my dirty mind.

Analyst: Is that a moment when reference to a man's jowl seems unfamiliar to you?

Mrs. M.: I called you chubby jowl, didn't I? Yesterday, wasn't it? You know what? When I told my mother she was sympathetic . . . chubby jowl . . . I thought I saw that man's car following me home from school every day for weeks. . . . You are behind me every day. You could shove some big earth-shattering idea on me that would make me think that I am just a dirty minded . . . but words are my meat. I can twist a person's words until they scream for mercy.

Analyst: And you may worry about what you could do to something I showed you.

Mrs. M.: Yeah, you do talk funny sometimes. You seem to measure what you say so much that I just want to say, "Spit it out. Stop beating around the bush. Get to the point!"

Wednesday

Mrs. M.: I had the best time ever in bed with David last night. He came home early. It was beautiful. You really have helped me a lot. I feel very grateful to you. But the phone rang. He had to leave right then. I was sick to my stomach. I got drunk. Today all I wanted was a woman to nurse me . . . to cuddle me in bed like a baby.

Analyst: Now you speak of yourself as an infant with a woman following a moment of pleasure as an adult with a man.

Mrs. M.: I just saw myself slamming that clothes hamper on the belt. . . . I'm afraid I'll ruin it with a man. Some night David is going to come home and hear me screaming like I do at you sometimes or like I used to at C. When he hears what comes out of my mouth he will just turn his back and keep walking. I wish I could have screamed as a kid, then maybe I could spare you some of this.

Analyst: As if you might have to concern yourself with sparing me?

Mrs. M.: I know, but it's hard to believe that anything's different. Only boys were allowed to raise hell. I'm afraid that I might spew all this resentment out all over David for leaving me last night. . . . I just pictured myself as a big penis spewing all over him. He has trouble with my raising my voice. Someday you may just leave me too. How much of this can you put up with?

Analyst: You imagine yourself a special burden to me?

Mrs. M.: My father thought so. Why am I saying that? I don't know why I am concerned.

Thursday

Mrs. M.: When I said goodbye yesterday you looked so tired and sallow. I thought you must really be sick. Could you have cancer? Maybe that was why you were wearing all that awful smelling cologne, to cover up the smell of your shrinking and dying.

Analyst: I am growing smaller in this fantasy, linked to a smell of something described as cologne.

Mrs. M.: Yes, but it was probably air freshener like they use in a hospital. I am angry at you for your comments about my diminishing myself yesterday when I wanted to talk about suckling at a woman's breast. You weren't in touch with what I was talking about.

Analyst: I missed your point and you were reluctant to tell me that at the time but now you can talk about it.

Mrs. M.: Yes. I was talking about how women are ever so much more reliable than men. Men just come and go as they please. I felt challenged by you, like you were saying, "Stop feeling sorry for yourself. Stand up on your own two feet." I felt vulnerable, too. I am revealing all my fantasies and I am afraid that you will die and leave me. Why would you come to work when you are obviously so sick?

Analyst: Is that a moment when in addition to having a fantasy about me you are additionally burdened with the belief that the fantasy might be true?

Mrs. M.: Not really, but it wouldn't help if you push yourself, you know. That's all I need—for you to die and leave me when I need you so much.

Analyst: Now you are imagining yourself as needy, but a few moments ago you were speaking of yourself as the strong observer of me as a weakened man. This moving into the position of the weakened one occurs around the subject of leaving.

Mrs. M.: You said that you would be away Monday, didn't you? Maybe you need the rest. Maybe you are getting treatment for cancer. If you had cancer then I wouldn't have to be angry at you. Yesterday I had a thought that I couldn't tell you. After I got drunk I threw up and smelled up the whole bedroom. I guess I feel stinking and rotten . . . unless I might have done that to myself rather than complain to you how unfair it is of you to just announce you are leaving with absolutely no hint of why or where. It has always bothered me that I tell you everything and you share almost nothing of yourself with me.

Analyst: Something that seemed dangerous to complain about before that now seems safer.

Mrs. M.: I have complained about it before but yesterday the way you looked startled me. I think I was worried that you might really be sick. Then it would be unfair to burden you with my complaints. I really did a job on myself. It affected my work. I had to give a lecture that I have given many times before but it seemed that I had forgotten something and couldn't get emotionally in touch with what I was doing.

Analyst: Something difficult to get in touch with. Something forgotten.

Mrs. M.: Well, I never saw anyone look the way you did yesterday when I left. Certainly my father never looked that way. He was big, brown, robust, NOT shriveled. . . .

Analyst: If he was *not* shriveled then you would not have to worry about speaking of feelings associated with something shriveled.

Mrs. M.: Absolutely! He was NOT shriveled! He was healthy looking even when he was sick. He kept pushing himself, going to work every day up until the last week. . . . Then he just withered before my very eyes. Everything but his jowls, they remained fleshy and baggy. When I was left in the room with him there were times when his genitals were exposed. I was nervous about looking. What a time for mother to leave us alone. For years she couldn't stand for us to be together without her, then she leaves me with him as he is just about gone. He looked to me for comfort. I felt awkward being near him. I didn't know how to help him. I felt so alone. It's a similar feeling that I have with you sometimes when you miss the point. . . . I try to go along with your direction but I resent it so much and feel so alone. I saw his genitals . . . his penis and testicles were all shriveled . . . not big like I expected. It was awful.

Friday

Mrs. M.: I had a dream last night. I had a skinned, bloody beagle under my arm. It came to life. It was like a penis becoming erect. I hate to see dead bodies, any kind of dead animal. Yesterday you looked dead [silence].

Analyst: Some difficulty with speaking of thoughts of me dead.

Mrs. M.: I can't stand the image in my mind of you like that.

Analyst: Are you concerned that I can't stand it?

Mrs. M.: I don't see how you could . . . it's that fleshy, flabby . . . I just remembered being in the bathtub with my brother . . . he turned toward me. His flabby penis became erect. Mother was out of the bathroom. I see that dead beagle. It looks like a piece of meat. That's a way of saying you just want to use someone sexually. He's just a piece of meat to me. I can see myself in the bathtub with Tony yanking his penis off. Then I can raise hell and get away with it. Where was my mother when I really needed her! I just feel all boxed in.

Analyst: Immediately following a moment in which you spoke of more active thoughts.

Mrs. M.: You must think I am a castrating bitch.

Analyst: Because there was a time in your life that you thought of a penis as a key to freedom.

Mrs. M.: I remember a fantasy I had last night. David will be home this weekend. He will probably do some work on the roof so he will be up on the ladder. In the fantasy he falls and I take him to the basement and bind him to a beag ... I mean bed and use his body for my own pleasure [silence for several minutes].

Analyst: In that pause is there tension about speaking of your slip of the tongue?

Mrs. M.: Mmm hmm. I thought about my beagle, Earl. Mother had him castrated. He died from the operation. Sarah, my roommate in law school, had an alley cat with a big bushy tail. I think she called him Tom. He used to go on three-day binges with the girl cats in the neighborhood. We were trying to get away to the beach one weekend but Tom disappeared. Sarah swore that she would have him "fixed" when he came home to discourage his three-day binges. Tom may have been an alley cat but he wasn't stupid. He didn't come back. I saw him a few times after that. . . .

Analyst: A cat on a three-day binge?

Mrs. M.: [chuckle] You're going away for three days. Guess what I have in store for you when you return ... if you dare? [She made a slashing motion in the air.]

Analyst: There you express something in action that may seem dangerous to put into words.

Mrs. M.: I'll cut your nuts ... your penis too [she said with considerably less anxiety than on Monday].

Analyst: Now that you have told me that fantasy, could we look at your anxiety over it?

Mrs. M.: I really care for you ... and it's hard to believe that you won't withdraw from my cutting thoughts.

SUMMARY

In this chapter, we reviewed definitions of some of the important terms in the psychoanalytic process, including *resistance, repression,* and *working through.* We described close process attention analysis. We listed some ways of choosing the moment for intervention. We described some research implications. We specified four steps in making a mutative interpretation with defense analysis. We presented some of the biases we hold in making interventions. Finally, these techniques were illustrated with a week of psychoanalytic process.

References

Brenner, C. (1976). *Psychoanalytic Technique and Psychic Conflict.* New York: International Universities Press.

—— (1982). *The Mind in Conflict.* New York: International Universities Press.

Dahl, H., Kachele, H., and Thoma, H., eds. (1988). The specimen hour. In *Psychoanalytic Process Research Strategies,* pp. 15–28. Berlin, Heidelberg, New York: Springer Verlag.

Davison, W. T. (1981). The mutative interpretation reexamined. *Journal of the Philadelphia Association for Psychoanalysis* 8:111–122.

—— (1984). Reflections on the mutative interpretation, defense analysis, self analysis. *International Review of Psycho-Analysis* 11:143–149.

Davison, W. T., Bristol, R. C., and Pray, M. (1986). Turning aggression on the self: a study of psychoanalytic process. *Psychoanalytic Quarterly* 55:273–295.

—— (1990). Mutative interpretation and close process monitoring in a study of psychoanalytic process. *Psychoanalytic Quarterly* 59:599–628.

Freud, A. (1936). *The Ego and the Mechanisms of Defense: The Writings of Anna Freud*, vol. 2. New York: International Universities Press, 1966.

Freud, S. (1894). The neuro-psychoses of defence. *Standard Edition* 3:45-61.
—— (1910). The psycho-analytic view of psychogenic disturbance of vision. *Standard Edition* 11:211-218.
—— (1912). Recommendations to physicians practicing psychoanalysis. *Standard Edition* 12:111-120.
—— (1914). Remembering, repeating and working-through. *Standard Edition* 12:147-156.
—— (1923). The ego and the id. *Standard Edition* 19:12-66.
—— (1933). New introductory lectures on psychoanalysis. *Standard Edition* 22:5-182.
Friedman, L. (1984). Pictures of treatment by Gill and Schafer. *Psychoanalytic Quarterly* 53:167-207.
Gray, P. (1972-1992). Personal communication.
—— (1973). Psychoanalytic technique and the ego's capacity for viewing intrapsychic activity. *Journal of the American Psychoanalytic Association* 21:474-494.
—— (1982). "Developmental lag" in the evolution of technique for psychoanalysis of neurotic conflict. *Journal of the American Psychoanalytic Association* 30:621-656.
—— (1986). On helping analysands observe intrapsychic activity. In *Psychoanalysis: The Science of Mental Conflict. Essays in Honor of Charles Brenner*, ed. A. D. Richards and M. S. Willick, pp. 245-262. Hillsdale, NJ: Analytic Press.
—— (1987). On the technique of analysis of the superego—an introduction. *Psychoanalytic Quarterly* 56:130-154.
(1991). On transferred permissive or approving superego functions: the analysis of the ego's superego activities. Part II. *Psychoanalytic Quarterly* 60:1-21.
Strachey, J. (1934). The nature of the therapeutic action of psychoanalysis. Reprinted: 1969. *International Journal of Psycho-Analysis* 50:275-292.
Weinshel, E. M. (1984). Some observations on the psychoanalytic process. *Psychoanalytic Quarterly* 53:63-92.

2

Two Different Methods of Analyzing Defense

MONROE PRAY, M.D.

INTRODUCTION

Until Paul Gray's recent, detailed, still evolving examination of ego analysis in a series of papers (1973, 1982, 1986, 1987, 1988, 1990, 1992), there were no clearer descriptions of the ways in which defenses work than in the writings of Anna Freud and Charles Brenner. If we add Fenichel's systematic contributions on analyzing defense, we have the guiding influences in the fifty-year development of ego-analytic technique.

Looking back, we see that the technique for analyzing defense branched in the middle 1930s, one branch becoming trunklike, while the other, Anna Freud's, did not begin to grow into importance until much later when Gray (1973, 1982) described the ego's capacity for viewing moments of intrapsychic conflict. Not widely recognized today, but standing out as truly original, is the method she described in *The Ego and the Mechanisms of Defense* (1936) of doing defense analysis by focusing "microscopically" on moments of conflict and defense occurring at the *conscious* surface.

Mainstream analytic thinking at that time did not incorporate Anna Freud's method, although her close attention to details at the surface was adopted briefly by a few theorists such as Rapaport (1944–1948) and Hartmann and Kris (1945). Open interest in the method essentially disappeared from the literature, including Anna Freud's own writing. Then, starting in the early 1970s, Gray described using what he has come to call "close process defense analysis." While Anna Freud did not write more about the technique, she did not change her mind about the existence of this "window" on the unconscious. We shall see that she became even clearer and firmer in her assertions concerning conflict at the surface in her Hampstead Clinic conversations with Joseph Sandler (1980–1984, 1985) when they "revisited" *The Ego and the Mechanisms of Defense*. She did not expand on her methodology. The purpose of this paper is to do that.

We all know that Freud's (1923, 1926) structural propositions had offered new possibilities for seeing and representing conflict more clearly than before. His structural model made it possible to demonstrate analytic premises about patients' conflicts in more understandable form. Theorists saw new hope for technical progress. In the 1930s the ego's strength grew relative to the id, and the importance of defenses to the understanding of neurotic symptoms and character traits grew apace. Fenichel said everyone was talking now about analyzing defenses but no one was saying how to do it—a job he himself proceeded to tackle with enormous skill and tenacity. His systematic approach held the center ground in classic technical thinking and is the base on which traditional defense analysis stands today, as exemplified by Brenner's writings on technique.

Fenichel was vitally concerned with trying to reduce the magnitude of suggestive influence in psychoanalytic work, where a weak and passive ego is vulnerable to an authority imbued with magical powers (1944a). He said that the patient's critical, evaluative capacities have to be safeguarded to combat his natural longing for "magical protection" and "participation in omnipotence." This means that what the analyst presents to the patient's perception and judgment should be demonstrably close to awareness and not require submission to the authority of the analyst for him to "believe in" the analyst's interpretations (1941, 1944b).

At approximately the same time that Anna Freud proposed her "conscious conflict" perspective, Fenichel, with his interest in reducing "hypnotic" influence in technique, advocated moving the aim of interpretation closer to the surface—as close as one could get: "it makes no sense to give 'deep interpretations' (however correct they might be as to content) as long as superficial matters are in the way" (1934, p. 334). He went on to say that the analyst "directs the patient's attention to something preconscious which he had not noticed (and to a 'something more')" (p. 342).

While this may sound as if Fenichel is very near Anna Freud's conscious surface, he is not. He says that *manifestly what the patient says disguises unconscious conflict.* "Psychoanalysis is a psychology that strips disguises" (p. 320). We "deduce what the patient actually means" and tell it to him in the form of what we call "interpretation" (1935, p. 322). What the words of the patient actually allude to requires "an intense empathy with the personality of the patient—the tool of the analyst is his own unconscious" (p. 324). "The forces which at one time opposed each other are now wasted in the useless and hardened defensive attitudes of his ego; the conflict has become latent" (1940, p. 190). "Dynamic interpretation" means finding things not mentioned by the patient spontaneously—though they are "shown involuntarily"—finding where the "decisive conflicts are located." Fenichel focused the analyst's interest on the ways *unconscious conflict* is pervasively influential on manifest behavior and on "hardened defensive attitudes of his ego." Fenichel did not find Anna Freud's formulation helpful. He felt that the analyst had to "break through to the rejected instinct" (p. 189), stripping the disguise concocted by the defending ego. Anna Freud's manifest surface point of view was either not seen clearly or, if understood, was not deemed useful.

THE GOALS OF THIS CHAPTER: WHY IS A COMPARISON PERTINENT?

This chapter compares Anna Freud's 1936 ideas on analyzing defense with mainstream traditional psychoanalytic thinking, represented here by Charles Brenner's views in *The Mind in Conflict* (1982) and other writings, as well as the views of other analysts consistent with his point of view. Anna Freud and Charles Brenner agree with Ernst Kris (1938) that "psychoanalysis is human behavior viewed as conflict," but they differ fundamentally about how to recognize intrapsychic conflict and how to show their conflicts to patients.

First, we will compare their observational stances and compare the ways each would choose to intervene. Second, we will use a detailed clinical example by Martin Silverman (1987) for comparison, which was first published in *Psychoanalytic Inquiry*. Third, we will discuss more about the differences between the two approaches and why Anna Freud's approach caught the eye of so few analysts. Ultimately, the purpose is to begin a discussion that will lead to an evaluation of the analytic validity and research potential of the two points of view.

We will see especially clearly in her conversations with Joseph Sandler that Anna Freud's views about conflict at the conscious surface seem (to him) to deny the advantages that modern structural theory has provided for understanding the ubiquity of unconscious influences and compromise formations. She responds that modern theory may say what he says it does, but that it thereby contributes to the loss of a sense of immediacy in analyzing, to overlooking the *experience* of powerful clashes within one's personality, and to a dwindling interest in the ways thought processes actually work. She felt hers was the "classical" viewpoint and that modern theory erred in neglecting topographic considerations.

In her 1972–1973 Hampstead Clinic Conference discussions with Sandler (1980–1984,1985) about *The Ego and the Mechanisms of Defense*, Freud tried to make it clear that she used topographic concepts to detect conflict. Growing up with the topographical theory as she did, she said that she had incorporated structural concepts only gradually: "I definitely belong to the people who feel free to fall back on topographical aspects whenever convenient. . . . By the way, this bad habit of mine of living between the two frames of reference—the topographical and structural—is much to be recommended because it simplifies thinking enormously and simplifies description when necessary" (pp. 31–33). Once she had learned to be comfortable with structural theory she used both concepts as tools: "To think of unconscious, preconscious, and conscious as qualities now instead of as topical areas did not seem to give them second place; on the contrary, these qualitative factors seem to offer the only real explanation for the struggle between the parts of the mind being such a muddle" (A. Freud's letter to Lawrence Kubie, 1955, quoted by Young-Bruehl, 1988, p. 162). She indicates that the ego only cares about a threatening impulse *when it becomes conscious.*

THE TWO BRANCHES: CONSCIOUS CONFLICT AND UNCONSCIOUS CONFLICT

The following short clinical excerpt from Silverman's (1987) long example to come (see pp. 105–109) will be useful in beginning to illustrate the differences between the two points of view:

> *Friday*
> The rain woke me up early this morning. It was beating down on my air conditioner so loudly it woke me up. I looked at the clock. It was 5:30. I thought in an hour I have to come here. I didn't want to come today. I've been mad at you all week. It's not that I'm mad at you. I wanted to stay away from all this stuff I think I feel here. I also got angry at R. [her roommate] yesterday. In the bathroom, she takes two towel bars and a hook. And I just have one towel bar. I didn't say anything for a long time. I finally got up the courage and told her we have to change the arrangements in the bathroom. It sounds so silly. I get so worked up over such things. I get so angry. [p. 151]

"Only for a few moments at a time," Anna Freud said (1936; see also Sandler with Anna Freud, 1985), "can the analyst observe 'fresh conflict.'" The analyst observes an instinctual impulse, a drive derivative expressed and then opposed. The analyst can observe the clash, the dynamic opposition, in the ego's inhibiting, defensive effort to reduce uneasiness aroused by that instinctual expression.

> "I've been mad at you all week. → It's not that I'm mad at you."
> "I finally got up the courage and told her we have to change the arrangements in the bathroom. → It sounds so silly. I get so worked up over such little things."

If the defensive effort is successful, she said, a compromise formation is achieved: "Peace reigns once more in the psyche—a situation most unfruitful for our observation" (1936, p. 10). This statement draws the line clearly between the two positions on defense analysis.

Charles Brenner (1982) says that the analyst can look at conflict from Anna Freud's moment-to-moment viewpoint but that it "gives too limited a picture of the psychic phenomena one is trying to describe and to understand" (p. 111). For example, rather than attending closely to what he hears at the patient's conscious surface, he might perceive the patient's anger and indignation as serving defensively to prevent awareness of sexual interest in the analyst, and to push away the idea of missing him when he is on his upcoming vacation. He says that the id, ego, and superego are involved in extremely complex unconscious, conflictual interactions. There are varying proportions of expression, satisfaction, and restriction, and different degrees of unpleasure produced. The "guiding principle is: as much satisfaction and as little unpleasure as it is possible to attain" (p. 111). Brenner centers analytic interest on the compromise formations that are outcomes of unconscious psychic conflict of infantile origin.

ANNA FREUD'S VIEW OF CONFLICT AT THE SURFACE IN MORE DETAIL

In 1936, Anna Freud introduced four new ideas. The first, as we have indicated, was that the analyst can observe moments of intrapsychic conflict at the conscious surface, when repressed elements surface and the ego then opposes them. In discussion with Sandler (1985), she said:

> Of course the whole of psychoanalytic therapy is based on the fact that the reconciliation between opposing ten-

> dencies can happen only when they are lifted into consciousness. Why should we try so hard to make them conscious if they could be brought into harmony while they are unconscious? One of our basic presuppositions in analytic therapy is that conflict exists only in the conscious ego. [p. 301]

The second idea was that these small pieces of clinical material can be used to great effect in the technical process of gradually and systematically uncovering the vast realm of unconscious contents. When these moments of conflict are analyzed, she said, it is discovered not only that a repressed impulse has surfaced but that the patient falls back on old modes of defensive functioning. These moments provide opportunities for studying the transference of defense. The motives for the defenses, the defensive rationale, and the defensive repertoire light up the past. Her third idea was that analyzing conflict solutions (compromise formations) was not helpful for seeing the ego's defensive functioning.

The fourth departure from prevalent thinking was that the analyst's observational stance required very sharp attention to moment-to-moment variations in what the patient actually says, not a matter of free-floating attention or listening with the third ear.

She apparently believed at the time that there was nothing new in her interest in the superficial layers of the mind, but later she said to Sandler (1985):

> I was interested to hear how very strong the reaction of older analysts was at the time, when the value of an analyst was thought by many people to be measured by the distance from the surface of the area he was exploring. So the idea that I advocated at the time, that the analyst's position should be equidistant from the id and the ego, from the depth and the surface, was not a popular attitude at all, at a time when the whole tendency was to go

deeper and deeper into the unconscious. From the beginning I felt that this was maligning analysis, because analysis was always the exploration of conflict, the examination of the defense neurosis. . . . The depths alone could never produce a neurosis. This can only happen in interaction with the surface. [p. 523]

On the other hand, she was aware that her idea that these very small pieces of clinical material could transferentially light up the past *was* new. She said that the concept of transference of defense "was for some reason not generally recognized at the time" (Sandler with A. Freud, 1985, p. 41).

To go back for a moment to the clinical vignette, Anna Freud "listened" for intrapsychic conflict first by catching a drive derivative being expressed and then by watching for the collision of forces as the ego "objects" to the drive.

"I finally got up the courage and told her we have to change the arrangements in the bathroom. → It sounds so silly. I get so worked up over such little things."

In this example, the patient speaks up actively and aggressively for a moment, and then a second "voice" (after arrow →) stops (controls) the impulse with self-ridicule. These two voices represent parts of the mind relatively closer on the one hand to the id and on the other to the ego/superego.

Anna Freud sees this internal dialogue as the way "normal" associative thinking and expression work. For the purpose of identifying conflict, she tries to make the distinctions between the parts of mind, the "id" and "ego" voices, easily recognizable and familiar. The id-like part is bent on wish-fulfillment at any price without regard for consequences. It is self-centered, impassioned, wants what it wants "now." The ego she describes has "an innate disposition against the drives." She says, "This is what the ego was meant to do from the beginning. That is why it was set up at all, to control, to impede the id" (Sandler with A. Freud, 1985, p. 61). It is able to rein in, frustrate, and guide the instinctual impulses in directions that avoid "danger" at that moment, with relative gratification later as its goal.

Interpersonal considerations are vitally important to the ego and not the job of the id. Evolving personal "rules," a map or chart of what it is safe or dangerous to say or do or to "think" (when thought leads immediately to action) is a critical task for the developing ego as it deals with both environmental "dangers" and "dangers" from within [drives]. Using trial-and-error methods, the child, like an experimental scientist, creates charts that he or she will come to depend on more and more, gradually making these charts the basis of automatic interpersonal adaptive adjustments and defensive efforts. The outcome, inevitably, is that there are repeated, uniquely personal tendencies in "conflict [and conflict-solving] within each person, as the aims, ideas and ideals battle with the drives to keep the individual within a civilized community" (A. Freud, 1974, letter to J. C. Hill as quoted by Young-Bruehl, 1988, p. 457).

A map, however, is only dependable within its borders. Anna Freud recalled one of Freud's comments about how we bring up children—supplying them with maps of the Italian lakes and sending them off as adults to the North Pole (Sandler with A. Freud, 1985, p. 343). In analysis, our study of the ego's "map" is all-important. Rapaport (1960) wrote:

> Human beings in dealing with each other repeat the patterns they have developed in their relations to "significant others," and these patterns of relationships *ultimately* go back to those which the individual has developed toward the earliest "significant others": father, mother, siblings, nurses, etc. Such repetitions of relationship patterns are the empirical referents of the transference concept. Transferences are ubiquitous in everyday life, but

so far the psychoanalytic methods are the only ones for observing them systematically and for tracing their genetic roots. [p. 125]

She admitted that simplifying the picture of the "parts" of mind was too much for some people's comfort, but she herself embraced personification. Her simplifying was consistent with a major purpose of Freud's when he proposed the new structural model as a replacement for the topographic model;[1] it puts life into the description of mental conflict that fits the ways people experience opposing parts of their minds—"struggling." Her viewpoint suits "everyday" observation if we recall what Grossman and Simon (1969) write about the interior dialogue we all engage in. They write of the "natural language of introspection" and the usefulness of "anthropomorphism." People naturally experience inner conflict in terms of oppositional "voices."[2]

---

[1]Freud (1933 [1932]) wrote: "We are warned by a proverb against serving two masters at the same time. The poor ego has things even worse: it serves three severe masters and does what it can to bring their claims and demands into harmony with one another. These claims are always divergent and often seem incompatible. No wonder that the ego so often fails in its task. Its three tyrannical masters are the external world, the super-ego, and the id. When we follow the ego's efforts to satisfy them simultaneously—or rather, to obey them simultaneously—we cannot feel any regret at having personified this ego and having set it up as a separate organism. It feels hemmed in on three sides, threatened by three kinds of danger, to which, if it is hard pressed, it reacts by generating anxiety . . . " (p. 77).

[2]Grossman's and Simon's basic idea about the "natural" language of introspection is that "the experience of conflicting [parts of mind] is rendered in anthropomorphic language and is intimately connected with certain commonly accepted and popularly held views about the division of mind, such as the division into a moral part, a reality-oriented part, and an animal-impulsive or a childish part [p. 97]. So long as the only processes of which we speak are wishing, intending, and needing, and their defensive counterparts, there is no other language available" (p. 108).

The metaphors introduced by the structural model come "closer to our immediate understanding . . . the anthropomorphism corresponds to human experience" (Hartmann et al. 1946).

In the following two clinical examples (Silverman 1987, Dahl et al. 1988) we hear an "id-like" voice and then a more reasoned, balanced, "ego-like" comment that controls the first voice and changes the perspective:

> 1. "*—I thought of saying 'thanks for asking' to him because I was so grateful he'd asked,* → but I decided not to say it. Because I'd have been calling attention to her never asking." [Silverman, p. 152, emphasis added]
> 2. "—And, and he just didn't say anything, except sort of mutter under his breath. And so I got *furious at him and* → [*sniff*] *I imagine I'm doing–in a way–the same kind of thing that my father always is doing*" [her father whom she had described as weak and childish]. [Dahl et al., p. 21, emphasis added]

Anna Freud takes the structural model and aims at making things so clear and logical that anyone can understand—including patients when their psychodynamics are identified for them. She personified and concretized the parts of mind. The id and ego, she said, "are not only at cross-purposes with each other but also speak different languages and act out their intentions in a totally different medium" (from her letter to Lawrence Kubie, January 1, 1955, quoted by Young-Bruehl, 1988, pp. 161–162).

She makes manifest *consciousness* an operational "stage," visualizing the parts of mind as actors who speak and clash. In her conflict model, the ego is innately predisposed to oppose, supervise, and regulate the id. An impulse being expressed may be thought of as "consciousness-syntonic" (but not ego-syntonic) for varying amounts of time. Watching for conflict, she prefers not to think of an impulse as "ego-syntonic" because she wants to keep in mind that the two agencies, the ego and id, pursue entirely different aims (Sandler with A. Freud, 1985, p. 48). Of course, the other way around, during times when compromise has been achieved, when conflict is not evident, she sees that the ego shapes and guides the id's impulses toward "safe" satisfaction. She writes:

> On the one hand, the ego is of enormous help to the instincts. By knowing the outside world, it can guide the instincts towards fulfillment and particularly towards safe fulfillment. The ego takes regard of reality. It is not any more owned by the pleasure principle. But, on the other hand, by interposing these thought processes and by insisting on safety, reality, and good sense, it holds up and inhibits wish fulfillment. So while on the one hand the ego is the friend of the id, on the other it seems to be the enemy of the id. [1952, p. 34]

In advocating her observational stance, she would not agree with Fenichel (1940, 1941) who says that to ferret out the unconscious id and defensive ego we "need first of all an ally accessible to us, the reasonable ego, which must be separated from the defending element" (1940, p. 189). Watching manifest expression of previously unconscious bits as she does, Anna Freud does not need to ally one way or the other. (Here is the basis of her famous dictum that the analyst should analyze from a position "equidistant" from the id and ego: he waits until both are evident at the surface.) Watching intently, she sees the ego's efforts to get the id under control. She sides neither with the rational ego against "unreasonable" defenses, nor with the superego to gain leverage in confronting infantile impulses (as Freud suggested at one point). We will see the use of such "leverage" in the long clinical example to come.

Technically, Anna Freud is *reconstructing* conscious—or recently conscious—sequences of thought, not really *interpreting* unconscious contents at all. Rather than interpreting she *points out* conflict (1936, p. 15).

CHARLES BRENNER: CONFLICT SOLUTIONS/ COMPROMISE FORMATIONS

As opposed to an interest in moments of "fresh conflict," primary attention is paid to unconscious infantile conflict; the analyst observes compromises, multifaceted conflictual *outcomes*. He infers and interprets the unconscious forces and tendencies of id, ego, and superego. The task involves interpretively dissecting these compromises.

> It is compromise formation one observes when one studies psychic functioning. Compromise formations are the data of observation when one applies the psychoanalytic method and observes and/or infers a patient's wishes, fantasies, moods, plans, dreams, and symptoms. Each of these is a compromise formation, as are, indeed, the entire range of psychic phenomena subsumed under the heading of material for analysis. [Brenner 1982, p. 109]
>
> All psychic activity, including neurotic symptoms and character traits, is a compromise among drive derivatives, anxiety and depressive affect, defense and superego. One cannot ask, therefore, "Is this defense? Has this to do with castration or loss of love? Is this gratifying? Is this self-punitive?" The answer will always be "Yes" to each question. What one wants to know is the answer to the question, "Which determinant of the compromise formation is it most useful to interpret to this patient at this time?". [Brenner 1987, p. 167]

ANNA FREUD AND BRENNER'S ANALYTIC "LISTENING" IN PRACTICE

Hypothesis: Brenner tries to recognize (relatively enduring, persisting) *defensive postures* that bar threatening contents from access to the patient's awareness, while Anna Freud tries to observe conflict in process at the manifest surface.

Analyzing "postures"

About analyzing "postures," Brenner (1976) writes:

> To put the matter succinctly, a defense is not a thing, it is a posture, specifically a mental posture. To ask, "What happens to defenses in analysis? Do they disappear? Do they go away?" is like asking, "What happens to your lap when you stand up?" "A lap" is not a thing any more than a defense is. Both are useful concepts that refer to a posture, the one to a physical posture, the other to a mental one. Thighs are thighs, whether they are vertical or horizontal. Their function, however, is (or can be) different, depending on their posture, and "a lap" refers to one of their possible functions when they are horizontal. The same is true for ego functions. When they serve one purpose, they are executants of drive derivatives. When they serve another, they are defenses against them. [pp. 77–78]

An analyst can analyze the mind in its "sitting posture" to identify and explain a part or parts of the compromise formation: instinctual elements, superego influences, defensive efforts, and considerations of reality as it is perceived.

Analyzing changes in posture—that is, analyzing "process"

In the technical model Anna Freud describes, the analyst might ask the patient to look back, to recall "standing" just moments before, to try to look into what was going on right there when she sat down. Recalling that, the patient might be able to recognize clearly and feel again a sense of annoyance that had become uncomfortable.

> *Patient:* "I've been mad at you all week. → It's not that I'm mad at you."

(A. F. might comment: You are saying you don't feel that way now, but the feeling was there a moment ago—did some discomfort stop your saying more about it?) Clinical material in this "process" model might find the patient "standing" and "sitting," again and again, as drive derivatives surface, become conflicted, and get resolved. These operations occur rapidly and repeatedly.

THE DEFENSES THEMSELVES

Brenner (1982) indicates: "Defense is an aspect of mental functioning which is definable only in terms of its consequence: the reduction of anxiety and/or depressive affect associated with a drive derivative or with superego functioning" (p. 73).

"There are no special ego functions used for defense and for defense alone. There are no specialized defense mechanisms" (pp. 74–75). The twists and turns, the augmenting, diminishing, or silencing of attention, perception, thinking, memory, and affect, that is, plainly and simply the usual ego functions, perform defense. The ego can use "anything that comes under the heading of normal functioning or development" (p. 75).

All defenses have in common that they "oppose." In defense, by definition, there is "an element of denial or negation, in the colloquial meaning of those words. Every defense against a drive derivative arousing anxiety and/or depressive affect is a way of saying, 'No,' to some aspect of it" (pp. 75–76). "Every defense denies something" (p. 78).

Anna Freud (1980b) writes that because "dangerous impulses . . . are more difficult for the child to combat when they are perceived, acknowledged, and remembered, . . . defense turns not only directly against the id derivatives themselves but simultaneously . . . *puts the relevant ego functions at least partially out of action*" (p. 143, emphasis added). She implies that we will see a patient's sharp, direct, incisive observations become softened, or blurred, or contradicted when the ego objects to the "sharpness" or "aggressiveness" of the observation (the drive derivative). But, in addition, when such an impulse is opposed, defense includes "impairment" of the ego function that might recognize the impulse—self-perception is blocked. Such ego functions as perception, attention, memory, reason, and reality testing get impaired as part of the control effort.

While Brenner does not appear to use his operational definition of defense for studying regularly recurring fluctuations in the associative process, his descriptions of defensive operations are compatible with analysis of moment-to-moment conflict and defense—the technique Anna Freud proposed. A patient's shift from present to past tense, or vice versa, can restore a sense of balance that had seemed precarious moments before (i.e., "I've wondered if you understand me. I think that less than I used to"). Changes in the scope or direction of the patient's attention avert "danger." All the subtle changes of tone, emphasis, attribution, and so on, that move uncomfortable thoughts out of awareness help in regaining a "sense" of safety. By means of simple variations in what the patient is attending to from moment to moment, the ego reduces conflictual anxiety.

Brenner indicates that id derivatives can break through to the surface under certain conditions that encourage the return of the repressed. But in Anna Freud's listening, breakthroughs "naturally" occur over and over again and while they are conscious they run into opposition by the ego.

AN ILLUSTRATION OF MOMENT-TO-MOMENT LISTENING FOR CONFLICT

The following are excerpts from the fully transcribed fifth hour of an audiorecorded analysis (Dahl et al. 1988). Defensive "shifts" are indicated by arrows: →.

1—At the beginning of the hour:
[3-minute silence, occasional stomach rumbles] Something that's been on my mind today is the relationship I have with the girl who is my assistant this year and was last year. And [sigh] well, it took me quite a while to get used to her last year and I imagine it was a **variety of reasons.** → **But** at the beginning of this year things were going quite nicely and I was quite pleased with the kind of things she can do and not feeling at all annoyed by her, which was part of the trouble I had last year, although at times she's a, a type of person that I **don't feel completely sympathetic with.** → **I guess. And uhm,** because of the other assistant having left, she's having to fulfill both of the functions to an extent and, and both of the teachers, myself and the other teacher, are to make adjustments too, so that she can help us both out. [p. 16, emphasis added to indicate moments when the ego opposes an impulse being expressed.]

2—Because I, I [chuckle] was just thinking I probably do the same thing with David. Last night in particular, I was talking **with him about** →—**I don't know.** I just seemed to be in a funny mood by the time he got home. He got home sort of late, and it wasn't that he was late, because I knew he would be. But I guess he didn't immediately respond to me in the way I **wanted him to or** →—**I don't**

know what it was, because I imagine that somehow I was already in some kind of a mood.—I was upset about something I'd done and I didn't want him just to listen to me say it. I wanted him to actually react to it, and either suggest another course of action or, or approval that well, I guess that in the circumstances that wasn't that bad a thing to do. And, and he just didn't say anything, except sort of mutter under his breath. And so I got **furious at him and** → [**sniff**] **I** imagine in a way it's the same kind of thing that my father always is doing [i.e., that she, like her father, is weak—"always asking for reassurance"] [Pause, stomach rumble]. [pp. 20–21, emphasis added]

3–[Analyst comments] Is there any connection? Does it follow perhaps that uh you [stomach rumble] have some criticisms of me that have occurred to you?

[Pause] I think if I had, I would have [nervous chuckle] suppressed them too much to admit them. [Clears throat, sniff, pause] Uh, perhaps one. I'm starting with one that's less [nervous chuckle] personal, one that I'm sure still is occurring to me **at times.** → **although** I don't think it functions as much in my thinking now as it might have—is uhm, sometimes wondering if all this really does get anywhere, and [sniff] you know, if it isn't some sort of a **hoax.** → **But** that's partly because I was brought up to think of it as being something that really didn't do any good for anybody and just costs a lot of **money.** → **I don't think** that occurs to me as much now. [p. 25, emphasis added]

BRENNER'S LISTENING

Brenner writes, "The balance between defense and drive gratification is a mobile one, not a static one. For example, in a revery, a dream, or a slip of the tongue, a drive derivative often emerges into conscious awareness or is given verbal expression only to be forgotten, repudiated, or ignored moments later" (1982, p. 110).

While he indicates that one may analyze moments of impulse expression and defense, he sees a bigger picture that is far more important for analysis. His perception of the relationship of repressed drives to manifest mental operations is that the repressed *"regularly gains access to consciousness and influences conscious mental life and behavior while it is repressed."* As Brenner listens to clinical material, *ubiquitously* there are profound influences on that material from unconscious, deep, long-standing infantile conflicts. These are the targets of his analytic work.

> The phenomena of our daily mental life, our fantasies, our thoughts, our plans, and our actions, are compromises among the forces and tendencies of id and ego and, later, of the superego as well. The parts of the id Freud called the repressed are among the determinants of the phenomena of daily psychic life—not true only for those relatively atypical phenomena called neurotic symptoms. ... They constantly influence every patient's thoughts enough *so that they can be inferred with some certainty* by the listening analyst. [p. 114, emphasis added]

The analyst holds the compromise formation model in mind as he infers wishes, fears, fantasies, moods, and plans. Brenner (1976) writes, "It [may be] obvious, for example, that a patient is bending every effort to remain unaware that he is so angry that he wants to kill everyone in the world" (p. 60). At another point, he draws on a clinical example of defense analysis in which the "patient regularly blamed himself and was angry with himself in order to avoid knowing he was angry at someone who offended him" (pp. 54–57). He indicated that while "the main emphasis in each interpretation was on the fact that the patient was blaming and criticizing himself in order to divert his attention from his critical and angry thoughts about someone other than himself, the fact is that each interpretation contained some reference to the drive derivative being warded off as well as to the defense employed for that purpose" (pp. 60–61).

Thus, Brenner describes one patient who is "bending every effort to *remain unaware*" and another who is "angry with himself *to avoid knowing*." In the second instance, Brenner essentially interprets to the patient what is "unthinkable," beyond his awareness, disguised within his defensive posture: "Which determinant of the compromise formation is it most useful to interpret to this patient at this time?" (Brenner 1987, p. 167). Brenner emphasizes the importance of considering what the patient has been talking about in that hour and previous ones, particularly the importance of an overall understanding of the patient's dynamics and most important conflicts. He says:

> Having understood what these conflicts are as best we can on the basis of the patient's history, current symptomatology, and analytic material, including various transference reactions, we interpret whichever components of the conflicts are both important and accessible as determinants of a patient's current associations and behavior in analysis. Our framework, so to speak, is our knowledge of the patient's conflicts. Our focus within that framework is what the patient says and does in a particular analytic session. [p. 169]

In 1990, Arlow and Brenner wrote:

> The analyst determines the specific contribution made by each of the components of the patient's conflicts. Wish, unpleasure, defense, moral imperatives, and realistic considerations are represented in varying degrees. The analyst's interventions serve to clarify for the patient

the interplay of these various components, to indicate the purpose each serves, and to trace their origins to their sources.

What the analyst communicates to the analysand serves to destabilize the equilibrium of forces in conflict within the patient's mind [which]—leads to growing awareness of the nature of their conflicts and facilitates the emergence of additional material—and so forth. [pp. 679–680]

In summary, Brenner (with Arlow) describes interventions that name components of the compromise formations that make up thoughts, plans, attitudes, fantasies, and emotions. He judiciously selects elements of the "postures" he sees before him. The element he names is not conscious at that moment to the patient, nor was it conscious moments before, as is true of the data addressed by Anna Freud's reconstructions. Naming contents that are at a greater depth, Brenner "sees through" the defense into the compromise, rather than catching the defense in the act as Anna Freud does.

ANNA FREUD'S "TECHNICAL TASKS"

Anna Freud's (1936) first technical task is to recognize the drive derivative and then, the moment that it meets resistance. The next task is to undo what has been done by the defense—revive the impulse in its most recent context by reconstructing the sequence. The third task is to investigate the resistance encountered by the impulse (p. 14). The fourth is to focus on the linkage between that id derivative and that specific defense, to study the repetitive defensive methods of the ego (p. 20). She says, "Not only do we fill in a gap in the patient's memory of his instinctual life as we . . . do when interpreting the first, simple [id] type of transference, but we acquire information which completes and fills in the gaps in the history of his ego development or, to put it another way, the history of the transformations through which his instincts have passed" (p. 21). Hartmann and Kris (1945) wrote a paper particularly relevant to Anna Freud's model ("The Genetic Approach in Psychoanalysis"). They describe a two-step technical sequence of first recognizing a conflict and then moving to analyze the epigenetic-adaptive history of that specific conflict and defensive outcome.[3]

Brenner uses his total experience with the patient to study what initially appears to be a far more complex, largely unconscious picture. In a sense, Anna Freud is trying, with William Blake, "to see a world in a grain of sand." Brenner, deductively, comes to know on the basis of his broad experience what the patient's world contains, and by naming its components in a timely way helps the patient see what is there. His patient can associatively confirm and expand his understanding.

---

[3] In "The Genetic Approach in Psychoanalysis," Hartmann and Kris (1945) elaborated their clinical understanding of the dynamic investigation followed by analysis of the causal (genetic) factors. In an example, they write of "the man who tends to drop his effort whenever an immediate competitor appears." (We can imagine how that can become manifestly apparent as the patient associates.) The analyst, they say, will take the opportunity "to establish a causal relationship between the individual's retreat pattern in conflict situations and [in] earlier experiences, in which the pattern was gradually formed" (p. 19). Learning theory applies. The analyst "will inquire when retreat from competition was learned or adopted as a solution; why, when the competitors were father or sibling, that conflict was solved by retreat; and what experiences . . . in which different behavior was attempted . . . failed in response to parental disapproval or feelings of guilt. The pattern was learned through failure (and via alternative defensive/adaptive *success*." Dynamic propositions "are concerned with the interaction and the conflicts of forces within the individual and with their reaction to the external world, at any given time or during brief time spans." The genetic propositions are "concerned with the explanation of these behaviors by an investigation of their origins, how any condition under observation has grown out of an individual's past, and extended throughout his total life span" (pp. 11–12).

CLINICAL EXAMPLE

Neither Anna Freud nor Brenner offers us specific, detailed clinical material. There is help in trying to understand Brenner's clinical thinking, however, in his paper, "A Structural Theory Perspective" (1987), written as a critique of Martin A. Silverman's (1987) meticulously recorded clinical paper.

We will assess Silverman's (and Brenner's) method from two standpoints: (1) How might an analyst listen to develop inferences about impulses, defenses, and superego influences from compromise formations? (2) When the analyst forms a conjecture about something that a patient is *not* permitting himself to think, how is it possible to demonstrate that picture to the patient in a way which is both understandable and tolerable to him? With each question, I will speculate about the ways that applying Anna Freud's technical point of view to the study of conflict and defense would change the picture.

FROM "CLINICAL MATERIAL" (SILVERMAN, 1987)

> Miss K., 25 years old, was referred for analysis by a psychiatrist with whom she had been in psychotherapy in college in another location. She showed sexual and social inhibitions, masochistic tendencies, as well as chronic, neurotic depression. Throughout her childhood and adolescence, she indicated, she had been unhappy, restricted in her self-expression, and a homebody who clung to her family. She had always felt unappreciated and mistreated, both at home and outside of it. The details which she presented amounted to a litany of complaints and grudges over injuries and slights she could neither forget nor forgive. Her parents had gone away together on frequent business trips each year during her childhood, including her birthday, which still infuriated her. Her

father and older brother always had had a special, intellectual relationship with one another, centering largely on word games and word play, from which she had been excluded, since she was too young to keep up with them. She had always considered herself "dumb," even though she had been an excellent student in elementary school.

Her father was an emotionally restrained man with a quiet but quick temper. He had a way of explaining things unclearly but was impatient with her and intolerant when she failed to understand him. She had developed a kind of pseudostupidity with him so that she found herself incapable of answering even his simplest questions and ended up in tears. She had looked up to and loved her father, with whom she had subjected herself to repeated disappointments and pain. She described her parents as angry people who compensated for resentments, insecurities, and low self-esteem, stemming from unhappy childhoods, by derogating and disparaging other people, whom they perceived as their inferiors. Miss K. described her older brother as a pampered, favored child who in her parents' eyes could do no wrong. He was condescending and disparaging with her, when he paid her any attention at all. Miss K. had always loved, revered, and hated her older brother.

She always had clung to her mother while complaining bitterly about her favoritism toward her older brother. She repeatedly expressed hurt and disappointment at her mother's dependence upon her father and her failure to appreciate herself as a woman. [pp. 147–148]

Silverman describes the analytic work as it progressed from the beginning of analysis, and then expands on the year of analysis that leads up to the "Sample Sessions" presented in full detail. He begins with the Friday session. Thoughts which occur to him and his verbalizations to the patient are in parentheses and observations about the patient's affect or about background data are in brackets.

Friday
The rain woke me up early this morning. It was beating down on my air conditioner so loudly it woke me up. I looked at the clock. It was 5:30. I thought in an hour I have to come here. I didn't want to come today. I've been mad at you all week. It's not that I'm mad at you. I wanted to stay away from all this stuff I think I feel here. I also got angry at R. [her roommate] yesterday. In the bathroom, she takes two towel bars and a hook. And I just have one towel bar. I didn't say anything for a long time. I finally got up the courage and told her we have to change the arrangements in the bathroom. It sounds so silly. I get so worked up over such little things. I get so angry. *She* was talking about being all worked up because someone called her for a date. She hardly listened to what I was saying. She's so self-centered. Her boyfriend came, and he was there two minutes and he asked about my cousin. She never asks about my cousin. She only thinks of herself. I thought of saying "thanks for asking" to him because I was so grateful he'd asked, but I decided not to say it. Because I'd have been calling attention to her never asking. I get so mad at her. I thought about something else in the car on the way here. I went to have my hair cut and it was to be cut at seven o'clock. But I had to wait and wait till nine o'clock. I got angrier and angrier. I told the girl when I paid (she'll get a bill from me in a few days, and it's the end of the week and she has to wait two days to see me again on Monday—like the two hrs. for the hairdresser—and in two weeks I leave for vacation, and she'll have to wait a month for me) that I was angry. I told her that I can go to someone else to get my hair cut—or I can wait for him. I don't like either alternative. I don't even know why I go there. I don't fit in. They're mostly older women. But I didn't say anything to *him*. I'm intimidated by him the way I'm intimidated by M. [the tennis pro]. I don't know why. He's not big and tall like M. He's good-looking, but he's not my type. He's married and has children (so does her father). He has their

pictures up. With M., I think it has something to do with my knowing nothing about tennis and his knowing so much about it. And I couldn't understand when he was telling me what to do. "Hold it this way" and "turn that way," and I couldn't understand anything he said. It was just like with my father all my life. He thinks he gives such good directions and clear explanations, as I said yesterday, but he doesn't. I get intimidated with men. I always feel that they know they have the knowledge. They have the brains, and I'm dumb. And I always feel like I don't know anything and I can't understand and I get intimidated. It's the same thing here, I keep feeling like asking you, "What does it mean?" I always feel like you know. I feel like asking you now. I know you've told me you don't know anything until I've told it to you, but I don't feel that way. I feel you're always a step ahead of me. You *know*, because you're smarter than I am and all the training and experience you have. (I speak: I don't think that's what it is. I think you feel I know because I'm a man, that as a woman you don't have the brains.) I get intimidated by men. [anxiously] Do you think I signal it to them and that drives them away? So they think, "Who wants her!" I think it started in a way when my father said to me, "Every man is going to want the same thing from you." I got so angry. Why? Why would he expect that of me? What right does he have? I heard R. and her boyfriend kissing just outside the door. She *likes* it! When my father said what he did, first I was mad at them for wanting sex eventually, and then I got mad if I thought they wanted to kiss on the first date. Then I started getting mad that they'd *ever* want to kiss. I got so *angry*. I'm such an angry person. (I speak: As you've said, you get mad to push away other feelings.) With A. [the young man she had met on a singles weekend trip, at which she had relaxed her usual guarded stiffness and had danced and smiled and joked, and who had become interested in her and arranged to come in from out of town to spend two days with her, only to stand her up when she went to meet him] I told him when he said he would come down here that he could stay at my apartment. And he got all excited about it and eager to come. And then I got frightened about what I'd said to him, and I said, "Wait a minute," and I made it clear to him I meant he could sleep over at my apartment—on the couch—not with me. [with emotion] Do you think that's why he didn't show up? Did *I* chase him away? Men intimidate me. It's like with my father. It's a mixture of excitement and pain and hurt and fear. But wait a minute. It's not only men who intimidate me, I get intimidated about money. Paying and tipping intimidates me. I avoid it if I can. Until lately, when I've been thinking about it here and trying not to avoid the things I tend to avoid. When I left the hairdresser's I looked for the girl who'd shampooed my hair to give her a dollar. But I'd have avoided it if I could. If they had a can with tips in it I would've put it in there. I was too intimidated by the hairdresser who cut my hair and I was intimidated about tipping the girl who shampooed my hair. Why? [slight pause] I can't figure it out. There's no rhyme or reason. I don't understand it. (I speak: So long as you take that attitude, so long as you don't think it out and find out the rhyme and reason . . .) Well, *he* cut my hair. He *cut* me. But she just put her fingers into my hair. I don't understand. (I speak: He stuck scissors into your hair and she stuck fingers into your hair. You were talking before that about avoiding sexual excitement. Scissors and fingers into your hair *sounds* sexual. You turn away and avoid the excitement, pain, and hurt with men, and when you turn away from men altogether and turn toward a woman you get scared all over again.) Yes. But there's something that doesn't fit. I had no problem about tipping the woman who gave me the manicure. And she massaged my fingers. And didn't get me anxious. I like it. It's relaxing. I thought of something. I told you about it a long time ago and then dropped it and avoided it. It's a masturbation fantasy. [Now her voice changes, becomes more hollow, tending toward a chilled monotone, drained of all emotion. She speaks this way for much of the remainder of the session, constantly pausing between words. I found her slow, start-and-stop delivery agonizing, and have tried to convey it on the page by the use of dashes to indicate her briefer pauses, reserving the word *pause,* in brackets, for the longer ones.] There's—a doctor—a mad scientist—and his nurse and—he ties me down to—do things to me. I don't know what this has to do with being intimidated by the hairdresser and feeling inhibited tipping the girl who washes my hair but not the manicurist. It makes no sense [pause] (I speak: You've blocked yourself from hearing the answer you gave: the hairdresser sticking scissors in your hair and cutting you; the young woman preparing you for the haircut; they're the mad scientist doctor and his nurse.) The fantasy had to do with—something—it had to do with getting bigger breasts. It's foolish—I feel sheepish [pause] It's so silly [pause] (I speak: There's nothing silly about it; you mobilize those feelings to push away and avoid looking into the fantasy and the feelings.) I'd try not to think the fantasy. I didn't want to dig into it. You're right. I feel sheepish to push it away. (I ask: And what happens to sheep?) They get sheared, their hair is cut off. (I say: And so do "fallen women.") In old times, they did. I know about that. The hairdresser was cutting *my* hair off. Maybe it was my "crowning glory." And sheep certainly get their hair cut off. When I was in New Zealand, I saw the sheep getting sheared. There was one brown one I remember. They held it and sheared it, and piled the wool, and all that. (The emotion's gone from her voice; she's shearing the sheep to pull the wool over our eyes.) (I speak: You're getting away to avoid uncomfortable feelings.) You're right. That fantasy makes me very uncomfortable. The mad scientist would do something to give me bigger breasts. I wanted bigger breasts very much [pause]. (I speak: Notice you're interrupting yourself, stopping yourself?) I don't want to talk about it, think about it: I'm afraid you'll think I'm foolish. I had to submit to the mad scientist, like I was his slave and he was my master. When I'm intimidated by men, it's like I have to put up with anything. [pp. 151–155]

WHAT CAN THE ANALYST LISTEN FOR TO DEVELOP INFERENCES ABOUT UNCONSCIOUS CONFLICTS UNDERLYING COMPROMISE FORMATIONS?

Sometimes material that is manifestly concerned with others in the patient's life contains recognizable, logically connectable, apparently "unconscious" *allusions and references* to important objects (the analyst, her father, etc.). Analytic theory sees this in terms of *unconscious displacements* that operate to keep her from knowing about her impulses, feelings, or fantasies (at root), or knowing that they are intended for her analyst or important others.

> *Example 1:* But I had to wait and wait till nine o'clock. I got angrier and angrier. I told the girl when I paid (*she'll get a bill from me in a few days, and it's the end of the week and she has to wait two days to see me again on Monday–like the two hrs. for the hairdresser–and in two weeks I leave for vacation, and she'll have to wait a month for me*).
> *Example 2:* He's married and has children (*so does her father*).
> *Example 3:* I don't know what this has to do with being intimidated by the hairdresser and feeling inhibited tipping the girl who washes my hair but not the manicurist. It makes no sense. [pause]
>
> *Analyst:* You've blocked yourself from hearing the answer you gave: the hairdresser sticking scissors in your hair and cut-

ting you; the young woman preparing you for the haircut; they're the mad scientist doctor and his nurse.
Patient: The fantasy had to do with—something—it had to do with getting bigger breasts. It's foolish—I feel sheepish. [pause]
Analyst: *There's nothing silly about it; you mobilize those feelings to push away and avoid looking into the fantasy and the feelings.*
Patient: I'd try not to think the fantasy. I didn't want to dig into it. You're right. I feel sheepish to push it away.
Analyst: *And what happens to sheep?*
Patient: They get sheared, their hair is cut off.
Analyst: And *so do "fallen women."* [Silverman 1987, pp. 151–155, emphasis added]

In other instances there is manifest clinical material in which she denies knowledge of something Silverman understands—her underlying impulses, wishes, and fantasies. Her negation is manifestly evident in the form of reaction formation, denial, blocking, ignoring, naiveté, and getting mad.

Example 1: I keep feeling like asking you, "What does it mean?" I always feel like you know. I feel like asking you now. I know you've told me you don't know anything until I've told it to you, but I don't feel that way. I feel you're always a step ahead of me. You *know,* because you're smarter than I am and all the training and experience you have.

Analyst: *I don't think that's what it is. I think you feel I know because I'm a man, that as a woman you don't have the brains.*

Example 2: I got so *angry.* I'm such an angry person.

Analyst: As you've said, *you get mad to push away other feelings.*

Example 3: Patient: With A. [the young man she had met on a singles weekend trip, *with whom she had relaxed her usual guarded stiffness and had danced and smiled and joked, and who had become interested in her and arranged to come in from out of town to spend two days with her only to stand her up when she went to meet him*] I told him when he said he would come down here that he could stay at my apartment. And he got all excited about it and eager to come. And then I got frightened about what I'd said to him, and I said, "Wait a minute," and I made it clear to him I meant he could sleep over at my apartment—on the couch—not with me. [with emotion]

Example 4: Why? [slight pause] I can't figure it out. There's no rhyme or reason. I don't understand it.

Analyst: So long as you take that attitude, so long as you don't think it out and find out the rhyme and reason....
Patient: Well, *he* cut my hair. He *cut* me. But she just put her fingers into my hair. I don't understand.
Analyst: He stuck scissors into your hair and she stuck fingers into your hair. You were talking before that about avoiding sexual excitement. Scissors and fingers into your hair sounds sexual. You turn away and avoid the excitement, pain, and hurt with men, and when you turn away from men altogether and turn toward a woman you get scared all over again. [Silverman 1987, pp. 151–155, emphasis added]

TECHNICAL SCHEME—ANALYZING COMPROMISE FORMATIONS

Brenner (1987) writes:

> Silverman and I function as analysts in essentially the same way. We try to understand a patient's symptoms and characterological problems as compromise formations ... [that], we believe, originated in childhood and have persisted throughout the patient's life in various forms right up to the present time. [p. 169]
>
> As I read the protocol, [the] patient is a sexually inhibited, masochistic woman who, at the time of the report, wished to stay in the same sort of relationship to Silverman that she'd had for years with her father: one which was unconsciously gratifying in a masochistic, submissive way ("You teach me; you tell me what to do.") and at the same time was not consciously sexually exciting. To that end, Silverman tells us, she avoided any contact with suitable and available men or, when she made contact with one, arranged to push him away in a fashion that enabled her to feel rejected by the man, righteously indignant at him, hopelessly unattractive, and ready to give up on men forevermore and to hate them all. In particular her anger, we are told, served an important defensive function. In addition, Silverman believes that his impending departure on vacation played an important role as a determinant of his patient's emotions and associations at the time reported: she would miss him and was angry with him for leaving her, both feelings she energetically warded off. [p. 168]

Silverman and Brenner see two principal currently obvious themes underlying this clinical material: (1) the patient was unconsciously angry about the analyst's impending vacation but prohibited herself from being aware of that fact, and (2) she had active unconscious sexual impulses and interests in men, including the analyst, that she energetically defended against knowing about. These conflicted underpinnings, including "unconscious gratification" of some aspect of the wishes involved in the conflicts, are beyond surface recognition.[4]

FORMING CONJECTURES ABOUT THE COMPONENTS OF COMPROMISES

Silverman's knowledge of his patient's typical conflicts and defenses allows inferences into the patient's compromise formations in which displacement and negation effectively defend her (1) against experience (and awareness) of her unacceptable impulses; (2) against knowledge of the defensive maneuvers she employs; (3) against the nature of her "moral" prohibitions (superego) that operate against knowledge of, or expression of, those impulses; and (4) against the ways in which she experiences "reality" as a consideration in her behavior. One assumption is that her impulses are being "unconsciously gratified." The patient "wished to stay in the same sort of relationship to Silverman that she'd had for years with her father: one which was unconsciously gratifying in a masochistic, submissive way ('You teach me; you tell me what to do.') and at the same time was not consciously sexually exciting."

---

[4]By tradition, to infer or "tease out" psychic conflict and defensive activity, an analyst asks himself *three questions*: (1) What is the patient's hidden wish? (2) Of what is she afraid when she wishes that? and (3) When she is afraid, *what does she do to* reduce the 'danger'? "What the patient *does* when she is afraid" is a compromise formation that has a defensive purpose and effect. For instance, Brenner (1976) describes a patient who "regularly blamed himself and was angry with himself in order to avoid knowing he was angry at someone who offended him" (p. 60).

Silverman looks at her struggling in terms of hidden, "unthinkable" sexual conflict. Her displays of ineptitude, refusals to "think," momentary aggressive disagreements, and eventual submission, are all assumed to be part of a sadomasochistically gratifying enactment.

Why? [slight pause] I can't figure it out. There's no rhyme or reason. I don't understand it.

> *Analyst: So long as you take that attitude, so long as you don't think it out and find out the rhyme and reason....*
> *Patient:* Well, *he* cut my hair. He *cut* me. But she just put her fingers into my hair. I don't understand.
> *Analyst: He stuck scissors into your hair and she stuck fingers into your hair. You were talking before that about avoiding sexual excitement. Scissors and fingers into your hair sounds sexual.* You turn away and avoid the excitement, pain, and hurt with men, and when you turn away from men altogether and turn toward a woman you get scared all over again.

I don't know what this has to do with being intimidated by the hairdresser and feeling inhibited tipping the girl who washes my hair but not the manicurist. It makes no sense. [pause]

> *Analyst: You've blocked yourself from hearing the answer you gave: the hairdresser sticking scissors in your hair and cutting you; the young woman preparing you for the haircut; they're the mad scientist doctor and his nurse.*
> *Patient:* The fantasy had to do with—something—it had to do with getting bigger breasts. It's foolish—I feel sheepish [pause]. . . .

—They held it and sheared it, and piled the wool, and all that. (*The emotion's gone from her voice; she's shearing the sheep to pull the wool over our eyes.*) [Silverman 1987, pp. 151–155, emphasis added]

ANNA FREUD'S TECHNICAL SCHEME

Here is the beginning of the clinical material again, looked at from Anna Freud's point of view. We see drive derivatives expressed for a few moments and then "counterattacked"— via defensive efforts that reduce conflictual danger (bold-face; arrows indicate defensive "shifts"):

> Friday
> *Patient:* The rain woke me up early this morning. It was beating down on my air conditioner so loudly it woke me up. I looked at the clock. It was 5:30. I thought in an hour I have to come here. I didn't want to come today. I've been **mad at you all week.** → **It's not that I'm mad** at you. **I wanted to stay away from all this stuff I think I feel here.** → **I also got angry at R.** [her roommate] yesterday. In the bathroom, she takes two towel bars and a hook. And **I just have one towel bar.** → **I didn't say** anything for a long time. I finally got up the courage and **told her we have to change the arrangements in the bathroom.** → **It sounds so silly. I get so worked up over such little things.**

—I've been mad at you all week. It's not that I'm mad at you.

—we have to change arrangements.
                                    It sounds so silly.
                                    I get worked up over such
  Aggressive drive derivative is   little things.
                conscious   ↓
    _____
                          ego defends

Figure 2–1.

Simple defenses in the forms of negation and displacement in person and time are evident in these examples of conscious drive/defense contiguity. She says, "I've been mad at you all week," and, immediately, "I'm not mad—." One "voice" and then another, a drive-controlling, anxiety-reducing, "quieter" one. She complains more openly about R. (a displacement away from the analyst as her target), but then says, "I *didn't say anything—*" (she uses her *memory* defensively—by recalling holding back her criticism in the recent past, reassuring herself and the analyst about her "control" of her anger, she reduces anxiety) Then she becomes freer, for a moment, to renew her complaint, but quickly labels her feelings "silly" and overdone.

The material further along in the hour, gives us the opportunity to watch moment-to-moment editions of a kind of "aggressive expression → masochistic submission." She brakes her active aggressive[5] comments by turning to self-observation and criticism.

> —and I said, "Wait a minute," and I made it clear to him I meant he could sleep over at my apartment—on the couch—**not with me. [with emotion]** → **Do you think** that's why he didn't show up? Did *I* chase him away? Men intimidate me—

---

[5] In this clinical material we are looking primarily at aggressive drive derivatives encountering conflict. There are also libidinal conflicts, though not at the same frequency. For instance, she describes a man's interest in her and, moments later, she stops that presentation of herself [as if stifling any display of her "sexual, competitive" urges.].

—Her boyfriend came, and he was there two minutes and **he asked about my cousin.** → **She never asks** about my cousin. She only thinks of herself. I thought of saying "thanks for asking" to him because **I was so grateful he'd asked,** → **but I decided not to say it.** Because I'd have been calling attention to her never asking. [Competitive impulses become conflicted—a triangle in which she gives way to her friend.]

—I always feel like you know. **I feel like asking you now.**
→ **I know you've told me** you don't know anything until I've told it to you,—

—then I got mad if I thought they wanted to kiss on the first date. Then I started getting mad that they'd *ever* want to kiss. **I got so *angry*.** → **I'm such an angry person.**—[In this example, she shifts from active anger at "them," to deprecating herself.]

Anna Freud might intervene after the patient has regained her equilibrium via the defensive effort. She observes where the patient stands at the current moment, "just as the conflictual anxiety has been reduced."

—I always feel like you know. **I feel like asking you now.**
→ **I know you've told me** you don't know anything until I've told it to you,—

What if Anna Freud said, "You're thinking of how I might comment—Are you getting control of your urge to ask me by answering for me? What if you were to let your question stand? continue with it?—whatever! Can you sense a risk right there?"

Speculatively, if that kind of conflict had been worked on before, the patient might say that she notices again ["now"] that she is feeling uncomfortable. As she recalls saying, "*I feel like asking you now!*" she says that she feels again very uneasy! She feels frustrated with him but imagines the analyst ridiculing her for not thinking things through. There is a range of fantasies we might imagine the patient sensing or noticing that involve the analyst's "reacting" to her being more aggressively demanding—his reproach, even disdain, or "teasing" her, or his judgments about her lack of self-reliance, and so on. One advantage in looking at this as fresh conflict is that both the analyst and patient can see directly how she gained control over her impulse to demand an answer—an impulse that was conscious, became dangerous, and can be recalled immediately. By mobilizing the fantasy of her analyst disapproving of her question, she controlled the impulse and reduced her "anxiety." Submitting, she is on safe ground.

Anna Freud points out "in-situ" moments of conflict and conflict resolution. She invites the patient to look back at the moment when the impulse became dangerous and asks the patient, by implication, to hold herself there in that precarious position again—to see what she, the patient, notices looking her impulse right "in the eye" to experience the sense of danger—to sense whatever she can in her imagination, feelings, and memory that are linked to that danger.

Repeated conflict occurring on a small scale with a short time span is the focus. Conflictual anxiety is related to the "danger" of the drive derivative remaining conscious for a moment more. Her approach deals with very small quanta of resistance which can be sharply experienced, and confronted in ways that drive derivatives can "grow" to whatever size the patient can tolerate.

If we examine closely the ways in which conflicts arise and are "solved," we can demonstrate to her this tendency to be submissive in order to stop an aggressive impulse—her "masochistic" solution. We can still assume that there are unconscious gratifications within observed compromises, but in this model the "evidence" might not support the observation that she "*wished to stay* in the same sort of relationship to Silverman that she'd had for years with her father: one which was unconsciously gratifying in a masochistic, submissive way." Instead, we seem to observe over and over again, for moments at a time, that she is *attempting* different behaviors.

This segmented, incremental, or "fractal"[6] picture of

---

[6]"Fractals," in this context, are self-similar repetitions that occur on the same as well as larger and smaller scales of magnitude. The theory is that changes produced in manageable "bits" result in large effects. A symp-

tendencies, attitudes, character traits, and symptoms is consistent with what Hartmann and Kris (1945) and Rapaport (1944-1948,1951) describe.[7] A character trait seen up close seems to be made up of repeated conflicts and their solutions. For moments at a time, the patient demonstrates *active* aggressive behaviors and then controls them in her characteristic fashion. If we were to help the patient study these moments of conflict, we would invite her to look into the "dangers" experienced at those moments (before restraint), to look into why her aggression needs restraining, how she tames it, the rationale for handling it the way she does, when she learned to do that, with whom in childhood some attempted behaviors failed while others worked. In what ways did her solutions represent the most adaptive outcome? (Hartmann and Kris, 1945).

As the Friday hour continues, the patient's "denial" is interpreted by Silverman in a variety of contexts. She finds her disagreements with him more and more dangerous. Her "defensive" efforts grow—this is marked by relatively small capitulations initially, but she gradually moves toward a larger-scale regressive masochistic submission. This is manifestly

---

tom or trait will be altered by systematically "interfering," with the "normal" sequence of events (with conflict solving that is currently automatic).

[7]Two contrasting hypotheses (of many): (1) Conflict and conflict-solving (regulation) are going on simultaneously at every moment. "Effective regulation" is the rule and moments at which we glimpse imbalance are rare. (2) Thought is advanced in tiny increments. Conflict and conflict-solving is an "event" that occurs incrementally over and over again. (One could use as a metaphor the description of the way the brain works neurochemically, the recurring activation and inhibition that occur at the neural cleft.) As listeners, we are only aware of impulses that are relatively less "controlled" or "balanced," and that will vary clinically with diagnostic type and developmental level, as well as all sorts of factors like fatigue, illness, "permission," "seduction." etc.—described by Arlow and Brenner (1964).

evident in her recalling her slave-master fantasies. The clinical material quoted in this paper stops with the beginning of this regressive slide, before its full degree is demonstrated.

DISCUSSION

In Ernst Kris's review of *The Ego and Mechanisms of Defense* for *The International Journal of Psycho-Analysis* (Vol. 19, 1938), Anna Freud's "method of observation" caught his attention. He wrote that innovations, in analytic circles, "are generally received with proper skepticism.... Great misunderstandings dictated by resistance often proceed from efforts to modify its technique." In this instance, however, he said, "I am much more inclined to think that the opposite danger exists: *the change in the mode of observation might pass unnoticed.*" He went on, "There is no need to insist what an advance it represents if we follow Anna Freud's lead in the technique of interpretation, first revealing the whole extent of a type of behavior, the activity of the ego, and only then penetrating into the deeper layers.[8] This method promises to bring us decisively nearer our therapeutic goal ... but—and I say this simply to prevent misunderstanding—it is only *one* step in interpretation." He adds, "It is desirable to emphasize what insight acquired in this way must mean for the *theory* of psychoanalysis, for *psychoanalysis as psychology*: the superficial layers of the mind, those functions of the psychic apparatus that are bound up with ego, have for long remained beyond the reach of psychoanalytic psychology" (pp. 347–348).

---

[8]Kris's comment here showed that he did see the extent to which Anna Freud's technique avoided the need to "penetrate" to the deeper layers (by restricting attention to what keeps coming from the depths to the surface).

Both Otto Fenichel and Ernest Jones also contributed reviews of her 1936 book to the 1938 *International Journal.* Neither indicated that he saw how different the *"change in the mode of observation"* really was.

Based on watching very closely what the patient actually says, Anna Freud's method of observation did not follow the suggestions of Freud, and others, including Fenichel, that one's attention should be "evenly suspended" or "hovering" or that one's unconscious is his tool. She indicated that when derivatives surface they come right up to the observer. (She says that we have less trouble observing *others'* ids—"dangers" external to ourselves—because it is adaptively useful for survival. Observing inner "dangers," our own impulses, is a different matter; for example, the child's perceiving and remembering her own aggressive impulses makes control more difficult and "peace of mind" unlikely [A. Freud, 1980a,b]). Anna Freud then watches the ego's reaction to the expressed impulse very closely. How much will be expressed? How long will it go on before the ego takes action?

Her concentrated attention on what the patient actually says was something even her close colleagues found difficult to grasp. We can look again at what she said in her 1972 to 1973 Hampstead discussions with Sandler (1980–1984, 1985). She tries to make it clear. In the following quoted transcription, the controversial portion, in italics for emphasis here, was omitted when the discussions were published in book form in 1985, in *The Analysis of Defense: The Ego and the Mechanisms of Defense Revisited.*

> *Anna Freud:* Of course the whole of psychoanalytic therapy is based on the fact that the reconciliation between opposing tendencies can happen only when they are lifted into consciousness. Why should we try so hard to make them conscious if they could be

> brought into harmony while they are unconscious? One of our basic presuppositions in analytic therapy is that conflict exists only in the conscious ego.
>
> *Sandler:* Not in the unconscious ego? [1985, p. 301].
>
> *Anna Freud:* No, the conflict only arises there. *The opposing elements are in the id, but they don't conflict with each other—they simply exist as opposites.*
>
> *Sandler: I think we are running into some difficulties, Miss Freud. . . . Don't you think it a great mistake to equate all that is unconscious with the id?* [Sandler with Anna Freud 1980–1984, 1982, p. 311].
>
> *Anna Freud:* Yes, you are right. The better way would be to say that in primary process functioning there is no conflict, but with secondary process functioning there is. Then it becomes a secondary question of whether the conflict is in full consciousness, or is preconscious. . . . [1985, pp. 301–302]

By contrast, if the analyst focuses on unconscious conflict, he is freer to listen with his unconscious, to listen for allusions, to interpret deductively, to be guided by empathy or intuition or to use countertransference as a guide.

The two methods also define *resistance* differently. Anna Freud (1936) says that we see "resistance" when "defense mechanisms intervene in the flow of associations." Resistance is defined as an event occurring for only moments at a time. In the compromise formation model, resistance is large scale and virtually ubiquitous. It refers to a panoply of forces that keep infantile conflicts and their solutions out of awareness.

In the clinical example that follows, Anna Freud would consider the patient's disagreements with the analyst as "*not-*resistance." In contrast to a view that the patient's objections represent "resistance," Anna Freud might say that resistance appears only after the patient becomes "anxious" about contradicting the analyst, speaking of pleasure at the hands of a woman. Identifiable *resistance* occurs when she stops disagreeing, becoming painfully self-critical, and regresses.

There are indications that Silverman may need to employ more "authority" or "influence" to overcome resistance because his technique requires interpreting unconscious conflicts and their resultant compromises. A degree of "insistence" appears to be necessary. The "resistance" to awareness of unconscious contents is considerably greater than to the conscious or barely preconscious contents Anna Freud addresses. On the basis of our limited material, it is not possible to assess how much the "authority" of the analyst is necessary to get the patient to consider his interpretations. Brenner and Silverman would want to analyze thoroughly any behavior in which a patient deferred masochistically. But it is possible, ironically, that when Silverman analyzes something the patient cannot see or evaluate directly, he introduces a dilemma for the patient in which submitting to his "authoritative suggestion" may be unavoidable.

> When I left the hairdresser's I looked for the girl who'd shampooed my hair to give her a dollar. . . . I was too intimidated by the hairdresser who cut my hair and I was intimidated about tipping the girl who shampooed my hair. Why? [slight pause] I can't figure it out. There's no rhyme or reason. I don't understand it.
>
> *Analyst:* So long as you take that attitude, so long as you don't think it out and find out the rhyme and reason. . . .
> *Patient:* **Well, he *cut* my hair. He *cut* me. But she just put her fingers into my hair. *I don't understand.***
> *Analyst:* He stuck scissors into your hair and she stuck fingers into your hair. You were talking before that about avoiding sexual excitement. Scissors and fingers

into your hair *sounds* sexual. You turn away and avoid the excitement, pain, and hurt with men, and when you turn away from men altogether and turn toward a woman you get scared all over again.

Patient: **Yes. But there's something *that doesn't fit.* I had no problem about tipping the woman who gave me the manicure.** And she massaged my fingers. And didn't get me anxious. I like it. It's relaxing. → **I thought of something. I told you about it a long time ago and then dropped it and avoided it. It's a masturbation fantasy. [Now her voice changes, becomes more hollow,** tending toward a chilled monotone, drained of all emotion.]

The two techniques have different goals. Brenner's interventions (and, even more clearly stated, Arlow's [1985]) aim at "destabilizing the equilibrium of forces in conflict within the patient's mind" for the purpose of healthier restabilization (Brenner, 1976, chap. "Defense Analysis"; Arlow and Brenner, 1990, pp. 679–680). A desirable result might include reports of various new conflict solutions evident in the form of compromises. In the hour itself, new attitudes and access to new memories and fantasies would be good signs. "It is the compromise formation that changes, not this or that defense" (Brenner, 1976, p. 74). Insight into and familiarity with the mechanics of thought processes, of conflicts and defenses, of the "voices" representing the ego, id, and superego as entities would not be likely—nor important. It might develop as a side-product but is not required for good results.

Anna Freud (1980a) was convinced about the curative importance of *insight*: "It is the knowledge of the unknown inner life that cures" (p. 161). All the rest—the relationship to the analyst, transference, etc.—are adjuncts to that aim. "Insight" is defined as "the extent of the individual's knowledge of his own psychic processes, especially the communication between the ego and the id" (p. 139). Her technique objectifies whatever is being called impulse and defense. The patient can see, and is invited to look into whatever the analyst is considering "evidence." Whenever the analyst hypothesizes conflict and defense, it is immediately subject to the patient's critique. She aims at the patient's being able to hold her ego and id apart in order to get a clearer look at their interaction—and in an attempt, as well, to postpone and inspect those id-regulating strategies of the ego that involve pain and personality restriction. This perspective helps the ego "face" more and more intense drive derivatives. It is clear that the ego, including the "rational" ego, is never expected to give up its fundamental guidance of impulse expression— its basic interest in regulating impulses.

These are dramatically different techniques. Yet we know, as Kris warned, that the major differences were not really noticed. Anna Freud analyzed manifestly expressed dynamic interactions of id and ego. In his conversation with her, Sandler (1985) reacts to her comment that it is possible for an analyst to directly "hear" the id speak![9] (Not possible if we only "hear" compromises). In the transcript (1980–1984), Sandler appears at first to have "misheard" what she said (in the following, the portion italicized is, again, not included in their 1985 book):

> *Sandler:* I was intrigued by the fact that one can think of the ego in terms of depth, in terms of distance from con-

---

[9]"In favorable cases the ego does not object to the intruder but puts its own energies at the other's disposal and confines itself to perceiving; it notes the onset of the instinctual impulse, the heightening of tension and the feelings of unpleasure by which this is accompanied and, finally, the relief from tension when gratification is experienced.... The ego, if it assents to the impulse, does not enter into the picture at all" (A. Freud, 1936, pp. 6–7).

sciousness, and that the deeper strata of the ego can be seen as being the location of earlier modes of functioning. It does seem to be worth noting, Miss Freud, that the "deeper" functions of the ego were regarded by you as those which relate to an earlier time in the life of the child. [1985, p. 29]

In considering this chapter we come up against a question which we have discussed before, namely the role of the ego in relation to instinctual impulses. We agreed last time that to say that the ego stands aside or is silent is simply a way of speaking, and in fact no derivatives of the id can come through without the collaboration of the ego. In this regard, perhaps it could be that the id and its derivatives come to the surface with the collaboration of a deeper or more infantile part of the ego, in the form, for example, of a slip. Would that be correct?

Anna Freud: I want to emphasize that I meant in our discussion last time, that even though the ego may lend itself to the instinctual wish and its fulfillment, and by lending itself lend its particular way of functioning, **this does not help the observation of psychic structures.** *When what goes on is unified and harmonious, then we do not know in our observations what belongs to the id and what belongs to the ego. It is only when the two clash that their different modes of functioning become obvious. I wanted to clarify this and it is also related to your question.*

Sandler: I think you have made it very clear that it is conflict that shows us the psychic institutions, or rather enables us to conceptualize things in terms of the psychic institutions. Nevertheless statements of the sort we discussed last time, such as "the ego standing aside and allowing the id to act" would, I think, be phrased differently now. [1980–1984, p. 8, emphasis added]

I should like to go straight to a point on which I would very much like to hear your comments, a point relating to the role of the unconscious ego. If I am correct, with the introduction of the structural theory, the replacement of the unconscious dynamic system by the id represented an attempt to deal with problems that had been confronting Freud in regard to the topographic model. . . . [p. 8; 1985, p. 29]

While Anna Freud might agree that her description of the id acting without the ego's participation "*would* be phrased differently now (by many analysts)," would she agree with him that they *should* "be phrased differently"? I believe that is very doubtful.

Sandler seems to insist on a compromise-formation model. Anna Freud views the ego as initially permitting expression of a drive derivative, and then objecting and acting to stop this expression. She puts a spotlight on the ego first and then goes back to the id. She is "simplifying," studying them individually, trying to describe their activities in ways that are highly focused.

Gray (1982) generalizes the problem analysts have had with understanding her point of view. He attributes it to a "developmental lag" inherent in the prodigious difficulty we all have in trying to observe and understand the ego's functioning—including our own.

There is another possibility. These two different ways of viewing intrapsychic conflict are scientifically and philosophically different worlds, with very different theoretical and technical languages. They are not easily reconciled.

Why didn't her point of view attract more attention—other than that of Kris, Hartmann, and Rapaport? Was one of the problems (!) with her approach that it was radically better for appreciating dynamics in an analytic situation and cast into virtual irrelevance the investigation of dynamics using the other method? The appearance of being able to understand conflict that is out of sight, at some distance in time, was being taken for a reality. Analysts don't (and apparently can't) recognize that they are using such an awkward instrument for analyzing dynamics. As soon as she made her position clear, did it render the prevailing view obsolete?

In trying to stimulate discussion of ways to measure the usefulness of these two clinical approaches to conflict, I suggest that it might hang on which way of organizing the clinical data "works better" scientifically. Does Anna Freud's approach seem to be more consistent with current scientific theory and research methodology?

Hers is a style of thinking we can associate with modern science. First, she sees that the fundamental problems in psychoanalysis cannot be understood unless they are epistemically sound; particularly so with respect to the meanings of "dynamics" and "intrapsychic conflict." Second, the way she views conflict puts it on the level of perceived "reality"—it fits with natural introspection (Grossman and Simon, 1969)—she does not put it beyond or behind sense experience. And third, her method of observing conflict is described in terms of its usefulness as an "instrument": she says to Sandler, *"I want to emphasize that I meant, in our discussion last time, that even though the ego may lend itself to the instinctual wish and its fulfillment, and by lending itself lend its particular way of functioning, <u>this does not help the observation of psychic structures</u>."* In other words, she says, "you can hold, if you wish, to the model of unconscious conflict and compromise formation, but then you won't be able to 'see' the id and ego as separate! You won't see the struggle between the parts of the mind, between voices 'speaking different languages and acting out their intentions in a totally different medium.'"[10]

The essential differences described between the two approaches to analyzing defense involve: (1) the analysis of "fresh" moments of conflict (characterologically determined)

---

[10] Scientific models have limited domains of validity and their value is measured by their utility. It is fundamental to understanding the use of such models that "scientific truth" is not possible to establish.

versus analysis of compromise formations ("infantile" conflict-solutions); (2) the use of very short time-span reconstructions versus interpretation of components of compromise; (3) the supposition that analysis-created *insight* into the relations between the id and ego will be "curative" versus a belief in the fundamental importance of stimulating new compromise formations—often, without "insight" as a factor; and (4) the comparative ease or difficulty each method presents as to demonstrability, analytic utility, and research potential.

One of the astonishing aspects of Anna Freud's thinking about conflict is the consistency of her outlook over the years after her 1936 revelation. She drew a line as clearly as one can be drawn and remained convinced about her side of it, wondering still in 1980 what had become of the idea that insight was the vehicle of cure. Her side offers possibilities for treatment and research that were not really noticed until Gray marked it out in 1973. We have the chance now to evaluate the two techniques.

Table 2-1. Comparison of the Two Methods

	Charles Brenner	**Anna Freud**
A. *Observation* ["*Listening*"] *Intervention*	Free floating Interpretation	Focused Demonstration by immediate reconstruction
Transference Addressed	Id > defense	Id = defense
"*Method of Free Association*"	Not as essential	Requisite part of method
B. *Drive Addressed*	Unconscious, "Infantile" intensity reduced by interpretation	Conscious → preconscious, "Infantile-adult" intensity may grow or diminish depending on "safety"
C. *Defensive Ego*	Unconscious	Unconscious/conscious, named, studied, identified as id-regulator/guide
	Worked on analytically but diminishing in importance as it offers less resistance	Significance not diminished
D. "*Rational*" *Ego*	Allied with	Named; identified as id-regulator
E. *Superego*	Allied with [partly]	Components named [i.e., in reexternalized defensive/ transference forms] Identified as id-regulator employed by ego
F. *Outcome/Goals*	New equilibria/new compromise formations	Equilibria postponed [to → Insight]
G. *Insight into Structure and Mechanics of Thought Processes*	Not essential	Crucial to "cure"

References

Arlow, J. (1985). Interpretation and psychoanalytic psychotherapy: a clinical illustration. In *The Transference in Psychotherapy*, ed. E. A. Schwaber, pp. 103–120. New York: International Universities Press.

Arlow, J., and Brenner, C. (1964). *Psychoanalytic Concepts and the Structural Theory*. New York: International Universities Press.

—— (1990). The psychoanalytic process. *Psychoanalytic Quarterly*, 59:678–692.

Brenner, C. (1976). *Psychoanalytic Technique and Psychic Conflict*. New York: International Universities Press.

—— (1987). A structural theory perspective. *Psychoanalytic Inquiry*, 7:167–171.

—— (1982). *The Mind in Conflict*. New York: International Universities Press.

Dahl, H., Kachele, H., and Thoma, H., eds. (1988). The specimen hour. In *Psychoanalytic Process Research Strategies*, pp. 15–28. New York: Springer Verlag.

Fenichel, O. (1934). Concerning the theory of psychoanalytic technique. In *The Collected Papers of Otto Fenichel*. First series, pp. 332–348. New York: W. W. Norton.

—— (1935). Psychoanalytic method. In *The Collected Papers of Otto Fenichel*. First Series, pp. 318–330. New York: W. W. Norton.

—— (1938). Review of *The Ego and the Mechanisms of Defense*. *International Journal of Psycho-Analysis* 19:116–136.

—— (1940). The study of defense mechanisms and its importance for psychoanalytic technique. In *The Collected Papers of Otto Fenichel*. Second series, pp. 183–197. New York: W. W. Norton.

—— (1941). *Problems of Psychoanalytic Technique*, tr. D. Brunswick. New York: Psychoanalytic Quarterly.

—— (1944a). Brief psychotherapy. In *The Collected Papers of Otto Fenichel*. Second series, pp. 243–259. New York: W. W. Norton.

—— (1944b). Psychoanalytic remarks on Fromm's book *Escape, from Freedom*. In *The Collected Papers of Otto Fenichel*. Second series, pp. 260–277. New York: W. W. Norton.

Freud, A. (1936). *The Ego and the Mechanisms of Defense*. In *Writings*, 2. New York: International Universities Press, 1966.

—— (1952). *The Harvard Lectures*, ed. and annotated J. Sandler. Madison, CT: International Universities Press, 1992.
—— (1980a). "Insight" symposium, chaired by Lampl-de Groot. *Bulletin of the Hampstead Clinic* 3:139–193.
—— (1980b). Insight: Its presence and absence as a factor in normal development. In *Writings*, 8, pp. 137–148. New York: International Universities Press.
Freud, S. (1923). The ego and the id. *Standard Edition* 19:1–66.
—— (1926). Inhibitions, symptoms and anxiety. *Standard Edition* 20:75–176.
—— (1933 [1932]). New introductory lectures on psychoanalysis. *Standard Edition* 22:3–182.
Gray, P. (1973). Psychoanalytic technique and the ego's capacity for viewing intrapsychic conflict. *Journal of the American Psychoanalytic Association* 21:474–494.
—— (1982). "Developmental lag" in the evolution of technique for psychoanalysis of neurotic conflict. *Journal of the American Psychoanalytic Association* 30:621–655.
—— (1986). On helping analysands observe intra-psychic activity. In *Psychoanalysis: The Science of Mental Conflict. Essays in Honor of Charles Brenner*, ed. A. Richards and M. Willick. Hillsdale, NJ: Analytic Press.
—— (1987). On the technique of analysis of the superego—an introduction. *Psychoanalytic Quarterly* 56:130–154.
—— (1988). On the significance of influence and insight in the spectrum of psychoanalytic psychotherapies. In *How Does Treatment Help?*, ed. A. Rothstein. Madison, CT: International Universities Press.
—— (1990). The nature of therapeutic action in psychoanalysis. *Journal of the American Psychoanalytic Association* 38:1083–1097.
—— (1992). Memory as resistance, and the telling of a dream. *Journal of the American Psychoanalytic Association* 40:307–326.
Grossman, W. I., and Simon, B. (1969). Anthropomorphism: motive, meaning, and causality in psychoanalytic theory. *Psychoanalytic Study of the Child* 24:78–114. New York: International Universities Press.
Hartmann, H., and Kris, E. (1945). The genetic approach in psy-

choanalysis. *Psychoanalytic Study of the Child* 1:11–30. New York: International Universities Press.

Hartmann, H., Kris, E., and Loewenstein, R. (1946). Comments on the formation of psychic structure. *Psychoanalytic Study of the Child* 2:11–38. New York: International Universities Press.

Jones, E. (1938). Review of *The Ego and the Mechanisms of Defense* by Anna Freud. *International Journal of Psycho-Analysis* 19:115–116.

Kris, E. (1938). Review of *The Ego and the Mechanisms of Defense* by Anna Freud. In *The Selected Papers of Ernst Kris.* New Haven, CT: Yale University Press, 1975.

Rapaport, D. (1944–1948). The scientific methodology of psychoanalysis. In *The Collected Papers of David Rapaport*, ed. M. Gill, pp. 357–367. New York: Basic Books, 1967.

—— (1960). The Structure of Psychoanalytic Theory: A Systematizing Attempt. *Psychological Issues*, Monograph 6, vol. 2, no. 2. New York: International Universities Press.

Sandler, J., with Freud, A. (1980–1984). Transcripts of their discussions about *The Ego and the Mechanisms of Defense* in 1972–1973. *Bulletin of the Hampstead Clinic* 3/4 through 7/4.

—— (1985). *The Analysis of Defense: The Ego and Mechanisms of Defense Revisited.* New York: International Universities Press.

Silverman, M. (1987). Clinical material. *Psychoanalytic Inquiry* 7/2: 147–165.

Young-Bruehl, E. (1988). *Anna Freud: A Biography.* New York: Summit Books.

3

Free Association and Technique

FRED BUSCH, PH.D.

Freud's method of free association, labeled the "fundamental rule" of psychoanalysis in 1912, and part of his psychoanalytic technique by 1892, remained unchanged as a technical precept from its elaboration in *The Interpretation of Dreams:*

> We therefore tell [the patient] that the success of the psycho-analysis depends on his noticing and reporting whatever comes into his head and not being misled, for instance, into suppressing an idea because it strikes him as unimportant or irrelevant or because it seems to him meaningless. He must adopt a completely impartial attitude to what occurs to him, since it is precisely his critical attitude which is responsible for his being unable, in the ordinary course of things, to achieve the desired unraveling of his dream or obsessional idea or whatever it may be. [Freud 1900, p. 101]

There is little doubt that, at present, most analysts would agree with Kanzer's assessment that, "Free association remains the essential instrument of psychoanalytic investigative techniques" (Panel 1971, p. 104), or Kris's (1990b) observation that "free association is the hallmark of psychoanalytic treatment conducted by analysts of every stripe" (p. 26). When one is listening to colleagues present clinical data, it does not appear as if there have been significant changes in the *intent* or *tone* of the instructions given to analysands since Freud's original description. While the words may be different, Moore and Fine's (1990) description of "free association" some 85 years later defines the expectations for the analysand as essentially the same:

> The patient in psychoanalytic treatment is asked to express in words all thoughts, feelings, wishes, sensations, images, and memories, without reservation, as they spontaneously occur. This requirement is called the fundamental rule of psychoanalysis. In following the rule, the patient must often overcome conscious feelings of embarrassment, fear, shame, and guilt. His or her cooperation is motivated in part by knowledge of the purpose for which he or she is in analysis—to deal with conflicts and overcome problems. [p. 78]

It is difficult to know what to make of Lichtenberg and Galler's (1987) survey of analysts' presentations of the fundamental rule. A skewed sample, giving variable responses (in terms of detail), can only give one an impressionistic view of some analysts' current perception of how they practice. While the authors are impressed with the diversity of responses they received, I am impressed with their similarities to the guidelines suggested by Freud. With some exceptions, the numbers of which are difficult to determine, the *intent* of the instructions often remains the same. "I hope you will express yourself as freely as possible because the more you can do so, the more likely it is that we will be able to work usefully . . . I'd like you to tell me as fully as you can everything as it enters your mind, and I will try to help you as best as I can" (pp. 64–65). Lichtenberg and Galler's characterization of the tone of the guidelines given to patients as "gentle exhortation" (p. 63) captures a current dilemma for many analysts. The strident nature of Freud's view of the method of free association seems alien, thus the "gentle" component. Yet we still believe it necessary to "exhort" our patients to hold back as little as possible. One gets the impression from this study, and from informal discussions with colleagues, that subtle changes in the method of free association are being made. However, the reasons for such changes, and their implications for technique, have not been made explicit.

This chapter, then, is in the spirit of the conclusion of a panel on this topic which ended with the thoughts, "Free association, so basic to the science of psychoanalysis, is far from being a closed book, . . . despite the further delineation of the conceptualization of it; thus far we are still on the threshold of the exploration of its many mysteries" (Panel 1971, p. 109). It is my contention that there are conceptual contradictions buried in the method of free association as currently practiced, which lead to confusion in the method and goals of psychoanalysis. Recent advances in understanding the ego have given us the potential for a view of the method of free association that is subtly different from Freud's. But these different views, and why they are necessary, have not been fully explicated. For some, my argument will have a familiar ring in that older and newer models of the method have been blended together and differences between them have become blurred. However, I shall explore the distinction between Freud's view of the method, and the problematic view of the psychoanalytic process it fosters, and some current views of psychoanalytic technique rooted in the structural model which have important implications for the method of free association.

FREE ASSOCIATION AND RESISTANCE ANALYSIS

Freud's discovery and elucidation of free association stems from a time when he viewed anxiety as the result of dammed-up libido, and his model of the mind was the topographical one. These views cast a long shadow over the method of free association. The purpose of free association was to get out in the open something that was unconsciously being held back. While Freud understood and appreciated resistances, and wrote about them, at times with a clinical sensitivity enviable even today (see Breuer and Freud 1895, p. 269), his technical handling of resistances relied primarily on suggestion, education, and the influence accrued to the analyst via the positive transference. The method of free association as first developed was geared to *overcoming* and not *understanding* the resistances. In his instructions to patients, Freud (1913) included the following *injunctions against holding anything back:*

> You will be tempted to say to yourself that this or that is irrelevant here, or is quite unimportant, or nonsensical, so that there is no need to say it. You must never give in to these criticisms, but must say it in spite of them—indeed, you must say it precisely *because you* feel an aversion to doing so. Later on you will find out and learn to understand the reason for this injunction, which is really the only one you have to follow.... Finally, never forget that you have promised to be absolutely honest, and never leave anything out because, for some reason or other, it is unpleasant to say it. [p. 135]

This recommendation was repeated in 1923: "They were to communicate these ideas to the physician even if they felt objections to doing so, if, for instance, the thoughts seemed too disagreeable, too senseless, too unimportant or irrelevant" (p. 195). Freud's view of the technical significance of this prohibition against holding thoughts back is captured in the following: "It is very remarkable how the whole task becomes *impossible* if a reservation is allowed at any single place" (Freud 1913, p. 135, emphasis added). On another occasion, referring to the prohibition against holding thoughts back, Freud referred to it as his "sacred rule" (Freud 1917, p. 288).

It becomes clear that the very essence of the method of free association was geared toward overcoming rather than analyzing resistances. When a resistance developed, the patient was instructed to push on in spite of it. Freud saw the work of analysis as "impossible" as long as resistances were in evidence—this, in spite of the fact that he saw resistances as an inevitable part of the analysis. I believe this is another crucial component in the "developmental lag" of integrating resistance analysis into clinical technique that Gray (1982) and I (Busch 1992) have pointed to, while also contributing to a critical attitude toward resistances on the part of many analysts. While analysts generally agree that resistances are the ego's response to distressing affect as first described by Freud (1923, 1926), and that resistance analysis is a cornerstone of the psychoanalytic method, *our technique of analyzing as expressed in our instructions to patients is geared toward bypassing the importance of these affects and the ego's responses to it.* This seems to be a factor in why so many analysts persist in seeing their purpose as "getting out" the strangulated affect or unconscious fantasy in spite of seemingly sophisticated views of the resistances (e.g., Greenson 1967, pp. 299–300). The basic mission of analysis, as defined by the original intent of the method of free association, is to have the patient hold back as little as possible. While this contradiction exists (i.e., we believe the analysand should not hold back anything while considering it crucial to work with those reasons why he inevitably holds back), confusion over goals and methods of analysis must exist. We cannot continue to ask the patient "to say what comes to mind no matter how painful" without acknowledging the impossibility of the task, and the importance of understanding the reasons for its impossibility. Our understanding of resistances dictates that instruction in the method of free association needs to be updated.

Until recently there have been few critiques of the method of free association. As Mahony (1979) notes, many of Freud's original ideas on this subject get "reiterated in the psychoanalytic literature with very little advance beyond them" (p. 163). A. Kris (1992) observes that even through the height of the ego-psychological approach to psychoanalytic technique, insight remained intertwined with the lifting of repression and the topographic notion of making the unconscious conscious. Thus the method of free association, when emphasizing the pushing away of resistances so that the unconscious could be observed, was quite compatible with this approach. An exception was the work of Loewenstein (1963), who noted, as Freud did, the "possibility of complying with such a request is severely limited" (p. 455), and quietly changed the focus of the associative process, suggesting, "the patient is expected to observe and express emerging thoughts as well as *his reluctance to perceive or verbalize them*" (p. 454, italics added). With this additional focus, the resistance is brought to center stage in the associative process. The analysand's focus is equally on the emerging thoughts and those barriers to thought. Loewenstein, however, did not note the slight but significant alteration in perspective, seemingly because of his belief in Freud's "insistence on the importance of analyzing resistances" (p. 254). While this is correct from one perspective, as noted above, Freud's view of analyzing resistances relied heavily on suggestion and persuasion.

Some analysts have argued that directing the analysand to hold nothing back exerts a type of superego burden which the patient cannot meet (Blum 1981, Epstein 1976, Kanzer 1972). That the analysand's attempt to meet the demands of free association was doomed to failure was well known to Freud. In discussing free association, Freud (1913) states, "Later, under the dominance of the resistances, obedience to it weakens, and there comes a time in every analysis when the patient disregards it" (p. 135). In presenting free association as a demand upon the analysand to "say everything that comes to mind," without any stated modifications regarding this difficult task, we shall likely contribute to an effect opposite to the one intended. We are consigning the patient's efforts to inevitable failure, with each individual's response based on his or her particular psychology (i.e., some patients will become secretive, some will be rebellious, or passive). This is not to say that giving the correct instructions will do away with reactions to the associative process. However, as we well know, there are important differences between the reality of being asked to comply with an impossible task and a fantasy that this is what is being asked.

A fresh approach to the method of free association is found in the work of A. Kris (1982, 1983, 1990a, 1992) and Gray (1973, 1986, 1990, 1992). Instead of seeing resistances as a barrier to free association, they see free association as a method by which resistances can become the centerpiece of the analytic process. For A. Kris (1990a), "the first aim of the method is to help diminish through understanding the *unconscious* restrictions that limit the associations" (p. 27). The key component of this approach is that "through understanding" the inevitable resistances are worked on, with the goal to increase the analysand's conscious acceptance of his thought. No longer are the resistances an impediment that makes treatment "impossible." "A major goal of the analytic process is to help the analysand gain full access to those habitual, unconscious, and outmoded ego activities that serve resistances" (Gray 1986, p. 245). In an attempt to correct what Gray (1986) characterizes as a "paucity of methodology for achieving this goal" (p. 245), both authors focus on the *process* of free association rather than its "hidden content." The heart of their technique involves listening for the moment in the associations when a resistance is in operation. Gray has likened it to an apple picker watching a conveyer belt for bad apples. One's attention is on the flow of material, looking for a change that indicates the flow of thoughts has been blocked. This is the moment of the resistance, and the point at which the analysis of the resistances begins. The advantages of this method over searching for the "hidden content" (i.e., either by directing patients to tell us what they were holding back, or via the analyst interpreting what was not said) have been known for some time (see Searl 1936), and recently have been brought to our attention by Gray. In essence, investigating the resistances to free association rather than circumventing them has been shown to be an ego-strengthening rather than weakening technique. While there are significant differences between Kris and Gray in their techniques for investigating the resistances, and in the specifics of how they see this process as helping the patient, both have given psychoanalysts a way of thinking about working with free associations in a manner that corrects one of our oldest methodological inconsistencies, and fits with our understanding of the workings of the mind as modified by our knowledge of the unconscious resistances. Before, analysts had to resolve how we could implore patients to follow the "basic rule," while also believing that working through resistances was a cornerstone of analytic technique. This has had a profound effect on the methods and goals of psychoanalysis.

Gray's (1986) instructions, which include the expectation that resistances to the method of free association will occur, could serve as a useful model.

> I make clear that I am talking about an effort toward free association, since interferences regularly take place while we are working to carry out this task. I point out that it is precisely the study of these interferences and the obstacles to putting the observations into words that provides us with greater access to what is now out of reach and which contributes to the patient's problems; and that the nature of the obstacles to free association will be intimately connected with the nature of the problems or conflicts that brought the patient to treatment. [p. 248]

With this addition to the "basic rule," conveyed in whatever language and with whatever timing the analyst deems best, we tilt the method of free association toward the study of resistances. A. Kris (personal communication) suggests that "instructions are designed to reduce *reluctances,* but to highlight *resistances,* not to circumvent them." This will not solve the problem of what Gray (1982) has called analysts' resistances to resistance analysis, but it is an attempt to correct what Apfelbaum and Gill (1989) note as the difficulty for many analysts to integrate the structural model into clinical technique.

SELF-REFLECTION AND FREE ASSOCIATION

The role of the analysand's interest in and capacity for thinking about his own thought processes has been confounded from the beginning of the method of free association. Freud's (1900) stated view was that *reflecting* on one's thoughts, in contrast to *observing* them (i.e., like a passenger on a train), was antithetical to the method of free association.

> I have noticed in my psycho-analytical work that the whole frame of mind of a man who is reflecting is totally different from that of a man who is observing his own psychical processes. In reflection there is one more psychical activity at work than in the most attentive self-observation, and this is shown amongst other things by the tense looks and wrinkled forehead of a person pursuing his reflections as compared with the restful expression of a self-observer. In both cases attention must be concentrated, but the man who is reflecting is also exercising his *critical* faculty; this leads him to reject some of the ideas that occur to him after perceiving them, to cut short others without following the trains of thought which they would open up to him. . . . [pp. 101–102]

Yet shortly after rejecting a reflective mode of thought as an interference to free association, Freud (1900) in quoting the writer Schiller, supports the necessity of self-reflection in order to make sense of associations.

> Looked at in isolation, a thought may seem very trivial or very fantastic; but it may be made important by another thought that comes after it, and, in conjunction with thoughts that may seem equally absurd, it may turn out to form a most effective link. *Reason cannot form any opinion upon all this unless it retains the thought long enough to look at it in connection with the others.* On the other hand, where there is a creative mind, Reason—so it seems to me—relaxes its watch upon the gates, and the ideas rush in pellmell, *and only then does it look them through and examine them in a mass.* [p. 103, emphasis added]

Here Freud is saying that observation of one's thoughts is really not enough. In order to make anything of one's observations, the observations need to be observed. Freud's concern over the critical component of reflection is regarding the first level of observations (i.e., free associations), not the further reflections on the observations. Yet, given Freud's theoretical views and clinical experience at the time, it is not surprising that he would come to focus on the freedom of the free associations as the key to symptom removal. Thus, his instructions to patients were geared toward as little self-reflection as possible. Even though Freud (1917) recognized there were patients who could associate perfectly well, yet nothing ever came of it.

While Freud championed the importance of the analysand's associations, the significance of the analysand's contemplation, reflection, or observation of his associations remained in murkier territory—where it still remains. As mentioned elsewhere (Busch 1992), the primary model for many analyses is that the analysand associates, and the analyst *observes* and interprets. The analysand's interest and ability to reflect back upon his thoughts, or his resistance to doing so, seems not to be a common part of the analytic field.[1] Yet, as we shall see, the capacity of the analysand to observe his thoughts is seen as an important, yet neglected, part of the outcome of psychoanalytic treatment.

Sterba's (1934) classic paper on the fate of the ego in psychoanalysis brought analysts' attention to the significance of the analysand's observations of the ongoing analytic pro-

---

[1] While I agree with the thrust of Spacal's (1990) article on free association, I believe his description of the method as one of self-observation has its limitations. The method is designed to help patients become aware they are having thoughts (and resistances to these thoughts), and, as A. Kris (1982) notes, one of the goals of psychoanalysis is to increase the freedom of associations. In this sense it is designed to increase observation of a part of the self (i.e., thoughts). This is only a beginning step in a larger process of seeing thoughts as having a coherent meaning. I believe it is this second process that fits the spirit of the term self-observation.

cess. He describes what he calls a "dissociation" in the ego, which develops during the analytic process and becomes the *sine qua non* of the success of the analysis. Freud (1932) had already suggested this when he described the ego's capacity to take itself as an object and observe itself, while also characterizing the goal of psychoanalysis as widening the ego's field of perception. Sterba states that the "dissociation" occurs when, via the analyst's interpretations, an alliance is formed with the ego that helps dissociate it from instinctual and repressive forces. The fate of the analysis is seen as resting with experiences where "the subject's consciousness shifts from the center of affective experience to that of intellectual contemplation" (p. 121). According to Friedman (1992), "Sterba saw it as a variant of the normal, characteristically human capacity of reflection, the sort of thing a Piagetian might describe as operating upon one's operations, or a philosopher might refer to as abstracting from one's abstractions, or a man in the street might say amounts to looking hard at oneself" (p. 3). It is a process whereby the analysand steps back from his experience of the analysis (i.e., his thoughts and feelings), and reflects upon it—just the type of analytic experience Freud seemed ambivalent about.

Surprisingly, Sterba's concept remains "dissociated" from the theory of the psychoanalytic process. It is one of those concepts that, while generally accepted as a necessary component of the process, is not fully integrated into our theory. Friedman (personal communication) calls it "an unscrutinized presupposition of the psychoanalytic procedure." The centrality of the concept is captured poetically by Gardner (1983) when he states, "Every patient and every psychoanalyst, the first and each after, has struggled and will struggle between aims to advance self inquiry and aims to obstruct it" (p. 8). While Friedman (1992) points out that it is often confused with the "therapeutic alliance," there seems to be a generally accepted developmental line from self-reflection to self-analysis. The essence of this perspective is caught in the statement by Kantrowitz and her colleagues (1990), "We define self-analysis as the capacity to *observe and reflect* upon one's own behaviors, feelings, or fantasy life in a manner that leads to understanding the meaning of that phenomenon in a new light" (pp. 639–640, italics added). Others have seen this capacity as an important one that develops during the analysis, and as a criterion for termination (Gaskill 1980, Novick 1982). Yet, for the most part, comments in the literature on the significance of patients' capacity to reflect on their association are presented as sidelights to other issues, and not addressed head-on. For example, Loewenstein (1963) notes, "Not only does the analyst pay equal attention to id, ego, and superego manifestations, but even the patient is expected to *observe and express* his emerging thoughts as well as his reluctance to perceive or verbalize them" (p. 178, italics added). Later (1972) he writes, "What the patient learns from his analyst is to allow certain thoughts to become available to himself, and to look at them from a point of view acquired from the analyst" (p. 221). Similar thoughts (i.e., on the significance of a split-off ego for the success of the analytic process) have been expressed by others (A. Freud 1936, Fenichel 1941, Greenson 1967, E. Kris 1956, Nunberg 1955). Weinshel (1984) highlights the significance of the development of self-reflection to the analytic process in this way: "I would suggest that this organization and these structures—the psychoanalytic process—remain as permanent products of the reasonably successful analysis and that their presence is reflected most immediately and most tangentially in the operation of a more effective and more 'objective' capacity for self-observation" (p. 82). He bolsters his argument for the importance of this development (as do Kantrowitz et al. 1990) by citing data on followups of successfully completed analyses which indicate the importance of the internalization of an observing function. Sonnenberg's (1991) description of his ongoing analysis supports this view. However, for Weinshel, as for those analysts who have considered the subject before him, the development of the observing capacity is not so much a part of the analysis as a *side effect*. It is most frequently written about as a function of identification with the analyst, or the work of the analysis, but not as an integral part of the analytic work.

The significance of self-observation *as part of* the analytic process has been most clearly articulated by Gray (1973, 1986, 1990, 1992). In elaborating on Sterba's early views Gray (1986) stated:

> I believe we can move beyond the implications of the word *fate* by thinking of the changes in the self-observing ego as more than a kind of inevitable byproduct of the analysis. Systematic attention to self-observation, when clinically appropriate, can become a more explicit aim of analysis of the neuroses. [p. 260]

Gray sees self-observation not only as an important goal of analysis, but as the focus of the analysis. Following the work of Anna Freud (1936), he treats the ego as the seat of observation. He reminds us that the ego is under the sway of various forces that influence how an analysand thinks about himself. The primary focus of his technique is helping analysands observe their unconscious defensive activity designed to keep thoughts out of awareness. By staying closely attuned to conflicts in action that are observable to the patient, Gray works toward strengthening and giving greater autonomy to those ego functions involved with observation and thought. This is in contrast to techniques that rely primarily on the analyst's empathic or intuitive reading of the unconscious, bypassing the ego's participation in the process except as admirer of the analyst's observational capacities. He deplores that "as a result, the ego's often highly detailed role in enforcing the repression is less likely to be subject to the important perception, examination, and exploration of its history" (Gray 1990, p. 1092).

Using Freud's later model of the mind, Gray has shown the significance of the ego's self-observation capacities for the analytic process in resistance analysis, and the growth of autonomy via strengthening those observational abilities. The resistances Gray highlights are those seen in the moment-to-moment observation of the patient's associations. A typical example cited by Gray is when there is a break in the associative narrative after the emergence of a disturbing thought. Gray then helps analysands to observe the resistances in action, while helping them to understand the causes for the resistances. This is one form of expanding the ego's observational capacities.

Important, also, is the analysis of resistances to thoughts as meaningful (i.e., self-observation as a method for self-analysis). Analysts have long been aware of the dynamic significance of resistances to self-analysis (e.g., self-analysis as a dangerous challenge to the analyst, or as a capitulation; thoughts representing feces that can be presented but not touched, or are presented to the analyst for admiration). However, there is a way of thinking, characteristic of an ego caught in conflict, which ensures that the analysand remains oblivious to thoughts about his thoughts. This thinking, which is descriptively unconscious, leads to resistance to the analysis of thoughts, and becomes a crucial determinant of whether self-analysis is possible. At these times, the patient may be accepting of the analyst, seeing meaning in his thoughts, but the patient remains descriptively resistant to engaging in this aspect of the analytic work for himself. Unless one keeps the analysand's capacity for self-observation as an active component of the free association method, an important impediment to self-analysis may not be analyzed. An analysand's acceptance of the analyst's interpretation of meaning is a limited method of judging analytic change.

Increasing understanding of the role of the ego in the psychoanalytic process allows us to understand the changes in orientation of the analysand in relation to his thoughts, as aspects of conflict are brought into awareness. While data from followup studies indicate the importance of the development of self-analysis, Loewald (1971, 1975) suggests that what one sees in successful analyses in areas of conflict is the move from lower- to higher-level ego functioning. Descriptively, we see this in the way patients can move from total immersion in the affective truth of a transference reaction, to the capacity to step back from it momentarily and wonder why they might be feeling the way they are. In this one sees a movement from thinking based on what Piaget (Inhelder and Piaget 1958) called "preoperational" thought to that based more on "formal" operations. Developmentally, it is in adolescence that the capacity for thinking back upon one's thoughts, using a variety of perspectives, becomes possible. A patient under the influence of preoperational thought "feels neither the compunction to justify his reasonings to others nor to look for possible contradictions in his logic. He is, for example, unable to reconstruct a chain of reasoning which he has just passed through; he thinks but he cannot think about his thinking (Flavell 1963, p. 156).

Thus, in the early stages of treatment, one would not expect reflective thought in areas of conflict. The ego in a regressive state is not capable of looking back upon itself, while in nonconflictual areas self-reflection may be highly developed. As more components of the conflicts are brought into awareness, there is a move from actions and thoughts being closely intertwined—as they are in preoperational thought (see Busch 1989)—to the capacity for objectifying thoughts and reflecting back upon them. Thought now has, "through this new orientation, the potentiality of imagining all that might be there—both the very obvious and the very subtle—and thereby of much better insuring the finding of all that is there" (Flavell 1963, p. 205).

From this perspective, movement toward increasing self-observation is a developmental step in thinking which then enhances the self-analytic process. Self-analysis without self-observation seems a contradiction in terms. How conscious this process need be, however, is not yet clear. Seeing the capacity to reflect as a developmental step in the analytic process, then, changes the view of the free association method. Observing one's thoughts as they are occurring is one developmental step, being able to then think about what one is thinking, is still another developmental step.

In contrast to Freud's initial view of reflection and observation, we now see them as vital for continuing self-analysis. Without the ability to observe thoughts along with the resistances to thoughts in action, it is difficult to see how an analysand may find meaning in them. It is, after all, a major analytic accomplishment when a patient recognizes there is something in his thoughts or actions to understand, and that it can be helpful to understand. This whole process can be seen most dramatically with patients whom we see in a second analysis. These patients will frequently show the capacity for reflective observation, except in areas of unanalyzed conflict where they remain "blind" to the possibility there is something to be observed.

CONCLUDING THOUGHTS

For a variety of historical reasons, our method of instructing patients in "free association," as first explicated by Freud, is designed to circumvent resistances and keep the *analyst's* ability to understand the associations at the forefront of analytic technique. This is not surprising as Freud's views on the method of free association were developed at a time when his understanding of the psychoanalytic task was very different from our current views. Furthermore, "Freud repeated himself on this important topic, and though he came back to it again and again throughout his life, he never got far beyond some early core ideas" (Mahony 1979, p. 163). Based on a particular patient population, which contributed to a theory of anxiety and the unconscious heavily influenced by nineteenth-century views of energic principles, Freud's view of cure was the verbalization of unconscious ideation. Furthermore, his great discovery of "meaning" behind seemingly random thoughts and actions ultimately led to a view of the analyst's role as a type of psychic cryptographer. In conjunction, these two perspectives led to the model of the analysand as provider of primary data on his unconscious fantasy life, while the analyst became the reader of these data. As has been pointed out, Freud never fully integrated his ego psychology with technique (Busch 1992, 1993, Gray 1982). Furthermore, later forays into ego psychology tended toward understanding normal development, and not the role of the ego in the clinical process. This has hampered our understanding of the ego in the psychoanalytic process, as exemplified in our uncritical (for the most part) acceptance of the method of free association as first described by Freud.

It seems clear that analysts need to reorient themselves to the method of free association. This would include taking into account Freud's second theory of anxiety, and the growing body of data on what is essentially psychoanalytic in the psychoanalytic process (i.e., followup studies showing the significance of self-analysis in successful analyses). Whereas Freud's first theory of anxiety explained symptom formation as due to dammed-up libido, his second theory emphasized danger to the ego as the basis of the sense of threat. What is significant is that Freud's second theory of anxiety seems only to have been episodically grasped in our written history. An analyst's orientation toward resistances to free associations will differ dramatically based upon his stance regarding the source of anxiety.

One important component of the lag in evaluating the method of free association is the tension that exists between psychoanalysis as the understanding of meaning in memory, and psychoanalysis as the understanding of meaning in process. There is considerable disagreement on the appropriate stance of the analyst when listening to a patient's masturbatory fantasy told with a great many pauses. The psychoanalytic stance from the position of memory is to try and understand the meaning of the fantasy in the context of the general transferential ambiance as a repetition of the past. The psychoanalytic process stance would be interested in the meaning of the pauses, especially within the understanding of ongoing, demonstrable ego resistances. Psychoanalysis, from its very beginning, has been the study of memory. While Freud was well aware of the clinical importance of the psychoanalytic process, this understanding became lost in the ill-fated theoretical link between repetitions in action, the repetition compulsion, and the death instinct. Traditionally, the analysand has been viewed as the purveyor of associations. We have been much slower to integrate the associative *process* into our work, especially the ego's role in it as seen in surface manifestations of conflict.

Currently differences exist in how free associations are viewed not only by obviously divergent schools, but by those who might be considered similar in persuasion. There are subtle but important differences in the nature of what the analyst is looking for as seen in the work of Arlow and Brenner (1990), and that of Gray (1992).

> In doing so [demonstrating transference], the analyst helps the patient to distinguish between fantasy and reality, between past and present. It becomes possible to

> demonstrate to the patient how much his or her thought and behavior are determined by unconscious conflicts and fantasies deriving from the past. [Arlow and Brenner, pp. 681–682]

> My aim is a consistent approach to *all* of the patient's words, with priority given to what is going on with and within those productions as they make their appearance, not with attempts to theorize about what was in mind at some other time and place. [Gray, p. 324]

Protestations aside about the many similarities in outlook between these analysts, there is a subtle but significant difference between them in their views of the associative process. Arlow and Brenner are geared more toward the elucidation of the *meaning* of the associations and their echoes from the past, while Gray is focused more on the immediate conflict as seen in the *process* of associating. This difference in emphasis reflects continuing tensions between unintegrated components of the topographic model, especially the role of consciousness, that linger in limbo in the structural model. While few analysts would disagree with the importance of elucidating unconscious fantasies, it remains cloudy as to how this is best accomplished in the face of ongoing unconscious resistances, which themselves may become the repository of wishes that are then defended against. Proponents champion one side of the conflict, and tend to finesse this issue. I believe this is one factor in why Freud's view of the method of free association has not been sharply contrasted with an approach consistent with his later views on the resistances. That is, we blend these two approaches as we attempt to accommodate clinically to a thorny technical problem. B. Landau (this volume) suggests the concepts *ego syntonicity/dystonicity* are more at the core of the structural theory than consciousness. This promising line of thought orients the psychoanalytic clinician to the analysand's associations from the perspective of the ego, a perspective that has been missing in our conceptual understanding of the method of free association. It orients the clinician to the ego in the defense/drive oscillation typical in associations, while providing a new dimension for examining the analysand's view of his own thoughts.

In essence, then, this chapter is not so much about the words the analyst uses to describe the method of free association to his patients (although I do not consider the words insignificant), but about the orientation of the two participants toward the process. Our heritage has been geared toward using the method to bypass the ego's participation. Taking advantage of our increased understanding of the role of the ego as mediator of psychic threat, as well as the seat of the observation of conflict, analytic interest in the patient's free associations could most fruitfully be turned (again) toward the ego. Other orientations to the process of free association have the potential to collude with the patient's wish to avoid threats by circumventing the resistances.

References

Apfelbaum, B., and Gill, M. M. (1989). Ego analysis and the relativity of defense: technical implications of the structural theory. *Journal of the American Psychoanalytic Association* 37:1071–1096.

Arlow, J., and Brenner, C. (1990). The psychoanalytic process. *Psychoanalytic Quarterly* 59:678–692.

Blum, H. P. (1981). The forbidden guest and the analytic ideal: the superego and insight. *Psychoanalytic Quarterly* 50:535–556.

Breuer, J., and Freud, S. (1895). Studies on hysteria. *Standard Edition* 2.

Busch, F. (1989). The compulsion to repeat in action: a developmental perspective. *International Journal of Psycho-Analysis* 70: 535–544.

—— (1992). Recurring thoughts on the unconscious ego resistances. *Journal of the American Psychoanalytic Association* 40:1089–1115.

—— (1993). In the neighborhood: aspects of a good interpretation and its relationship to a "developmental lag" in ego psychology. *Journal of the American Psychoanalytic Association* 41:151–178.

Epstein, G. (1976). A note on the semantic confusion in the fundamental rule of psychoanalysis. *Journal of the Philadelphia Association of Psychoanalysis* 3:54–57.

Fenichel, O. (1941). *Problems of Psychoanalytic Technique.* New York: Psychoanalytic Quarterly.

Flavell, J. H. (1963). *The Developmental Psychology of Jean Piaget.* Princeton, NJ: Van Nostrand.

Freud, A. (1936). *The Ego and the Mechanisms of Defense. Writings,* 2. New York: International Universities Press, 1966.

Freud, S. (1900). The interpretation of dreams. *Standard Edition* 4, 5.

—— (1912). Recommendations to physicians practising psychoanalysis. *Standard Edition* 12.

—— (1913). On beginning the treatment. *Standard Edition* 12.

—— (1917). Resistance and repression. *Standard Edition* 16.

—— (1923). The ego and the id. *Standard Edition* 19.

—— (1926). Inhibitions, symptoms and anxiety. *Standard Edition* 20.

—— (1932). New introductory lectures on psychoanalysis. *Standard Edition* 22.

Friedman, L. (1992). How and why patients become more objective: Sterba compared with Strachey. *Psychoanalytic Quarterly* 61:1–17.

Gardner, M. R. (1983). *Self Inquiry.* Boston: Little, Brown.

Gaskill, H. S. (1980). The closing phase of the psychoanalytic treatment of adults and the goals of psychoanalysis: "the myth of perfectibility." *International Journal of Psycho-Analysis* 61:11–23.

Gray, P. (1973). Psychoanalytic technique and the ego's capacity for viewing intrapsychic conflict. *Journal of the American Psychoanalytic Association* 21:474–494.

—— (1982). "Developmental lag" in the evolution of technique for psychoanalysis of neurotic conflict. *Journal of the American Psychoanalytic Association* 30:621–655.

—— (1986). On helping analysands observe intrapsychic activity. In *Psychoanalysis: The Science of Mental Conflict. Essays in Honor*

of Charles Brenner, ed. A. D. Richards and M. S. Willick. Hillsdale, NJ: Analytic Press.
—— (1990). The nature of therapeutic action in psychoanalysis. *Journal of the American Psychoanalytic Association* 38:1083–1097.
—— (1992). Memory as resistance and the telling of a dream. *Journal of the American Psychoanalytic Association* 40:307–326.
Greenson, R. R. (1967). *The Technique and Practice of Psychoanalysis.* New York: International Universities Press.
Inhelder, B., and Piaget, J. (1958). *The Growth of Logical Thinking from Childhood to Adolescence.* New York: Basic Books.
Kantrowitz, J., Katz, A. L., and Paolitto, F. (1990). Follow-up of psychoanalysis five to ten years after termination: development of the self-analytic function. *Journal of the American Psychoanalytic Association* 38:605–636.
Kanzer, M. (1972). Superego aspects of free association and the fundamental rule. *Journal of the American Psychoanalytic Association* 20:246–266.
Kris, A. O. (1982). *Free Association: Method and Process.* New Haven, CT: Yale University Press.
—— (1983). The analyst's conceptual freedom in the method of free association. *International Journal of Psycho-Analysis* 64:407–411.
—— (1990a). Helping patients by analyzing self-criticism. *Journal of the American Psychoanalytic Association* 38:605–636.
—— (1990b). The analyst's stance and the method of free association. *Psychoanalytic Study of the Child* 45:25–41. New Haven, CT: Yale University Press.
—— (1992). Interpretation and the method of free association. *Psychoanalytic Inquiry* 12:208–224.
Kris, E. (1956). On some vicissitudes of insight in psychoanalysis. *International Journal of Psycho-Analysis* 37:445–455.
Lichtenberg, J. D., and Galler, F. B. (1987). The fundamental rule: a study of current usage. *Journal of the American Psychoanalytic Association* 35:47–76.
Loewald, H. W. (1971). Some considerations on repetition and repetition compulsion. *International Journal of Psycho-Analysis* 52:59–66.
—— (1975). Psychoanalysis as an art and the fantasy character of

the psychoanalytic situation. *Journal of the American Psychoanalytic Association* 23:277-299.
Loewenstein, R. M. (1963). Some considerations on free association. *Journal of the American Psychoanalytic Association* 11:451-473.
—— (1972). Ego autonomy and psychoanalytic technique. *Psychoanalytic Quarterly* 41:1-22.
Mahony, P. (1979). The boundaries of free association. *Psychoanalytic Contemporary Thought* 2:151-198.
Moore, B. E., and Fine, B. D. (1990). *Psychoanalytic Terms and Concepts.* New Haven, CT: Yale University Press.
Novick, J. (1982). Termination: themes and issues. *Psychoanalytic Inquiry* 2:329-365.
Nunberg, H. (1955). *Principles of Psychoanalysis.* New York: International Universities Press.
Panel. (1971). The basic rule: free association—a reconsideration. H. Seidman, reporter. *Journal of the American Psychoanalytic Association* 19:98-109.
Searl, M. N. (1936). Some queries on principles of technique. *International Journal of Psycho-Analysis* 17:471-493.
Sonnenberg, S. M. (1991). The analyst's self-analysis and its impact on clinical work: a comment on the sources and importance of personal insight. *Journal of the American Psychoanalytic Association* 39:687-704.
Spacal, S. (1990). Free association as a method of self-observation in relation to other methodological principles of psychoanalysis. *Psychoanalytic Quarterly* 59:420-436.
Sterba, R. (1934). The fate of the ego in psychoanalytic therapy. *International Journal of Psycho-Analysis* 15:117-126.
Weinshel, E. M. (1984). Some observations on the psychoanalytic process. *Psychoanalytic Quarterly* 53:63-92.

4

Use of the Close Process Attention Technique in Patients with Impulse Disorders

JAMES H. HUTCHINSON, M.D.

INTRODUCTION

In his seminal papers and teaching, Gray integrates theory and technique. His clear view of the ego and of therapeutic process offers an orientation and suggests interventions for a wide range of analytic and psychotherapeutic situations.

Like most important advances, his views can be simply stated. He would have us stay acutely aware of the analytic situation. Two people, one troubled and one trained, meet in quiet, private circumstances on a frequent basis to study the thoughts and feelings of the former as they are put into words to the latter. The focus of study is the pattern of the analysand's thoughts and feelings as he tells them to the analyst—not his troubles, or relationships, or life history as it could be known through his narrative. During the period of study, the analysand is asked to put his awareness into words as freely as he can. Action is relinquished during treatment hours. The analyst tries to minimize his influence on the direction of the analysand's thoughts. In addition, the analyst listens to the analysand in a unique way. The analyst suspends part of the cognitive processes that operate almost automatically in everyday life to focus more acutely on the information to be found *in the sequence or flow* of the analysand's words. Like a painter who translates a three-dimensional world into a two-dimensional array of pigments, the analyst maintains a consistent attention to the precise details of the two-dimensional array—the moment-to-moment flow of communication from analysand to analyst. The analyst does not fall into the easy habit of feeling he is hearing about a reality of some other time or location.

The analysand is informed early in treatment that candor in describing his mental contents furthers the treatment and that the usual social constraints on verbal expression of sexual or aggressive thoughts do not apply. In this setting, appetites of a sexual or aggressive nature become active and seek expression in both parties.

When these appetites achieve a certain intensity, or clarity of representation, or mode of proposed expression in the analysand's thoughts, they induce anxiety in the analysand, who then finds ways to distort his expression or suppress awareness of the now troubling idea; that is, the analysand invokes a defense. An important part of the analysand's motivation to defend and an important determinant of the *mode* of defense is his picture of the analyst as a source of danger to the analysand (shaming, punishing, or abandoning, for example) if he should continue to communicate his thoughts freely.

Some defenses, such as the isolation of affect of the obsessional, are always present. Others operate in the blink of an eye. Fluctuating psychic events are more easily demonstrated to an analysand.

The analyst's purpose is to help the analysand become more fully aware of:

1. His means of distorting his thoughts and feelings and of disguising them from himself and the analyst.
2. The analysand's pictures of himself and the analyst at such moments of distortion.
3. The wishes toward the analyst or others that need to be warded off at such moments of distortion.

The analyst is opposed in his attempt to broaden the analysand's self-awareness by the following:

1. The analysand, during a moment of defense, is limiting his capacity to think and feel in some manner, thus limiting his capacity to fully consider what the analyst is saying.
2. The analyst, in his intervention, is attempting to redirect the analysand's attention to a moment in which the analysand experienced the analyst as dangerous. Thus, the analysand's motivation for defense increases as the intervention proceeds.

This view of the analytic process has the following technical ramifications.

Gray attends to moment-to-moment defensive shifts in the analysand's awareness as manifested in the hour. This is a very different style of listening from that of most analysts. Even ego psychoanalysts who are quite interested in defense usually listen to a body of material from an analysand and then comment on what the analysand is "doing defensively" over the time of the listening. Such interventions direct the analysand's attention to persistent modes of thought, which serve chronic defensive purposes. Thus, such interventions are comments on the analysand's character. Gray, in contrast, addresses brief specific moments of thought and feeling.

Gray's recommendations as to how and when to interpret are precise. Interventions are made at moments when defensive shifts can be *demonstrated* to the analysand. Massive anxiety invokes massive defense that can interfere with recall or consideration of the analyst's words. Chronic characterological defense may suppress a drive derivative so much that there is little feeling and, thus, no convincing demonstration of defense. Brief but distinct moments when a drive derivative appears, followed by a clear defensive shift, are Gray's choice for intervention. To enlighten an analysand about his characterological defenses or defenses that invoke regression, Gray suggests finding brief transient manifestations of the defense and exploring these in a progressive manner with the analysand.

Gray educates analysands early in analysis about the process of psychoanalysis. He finds moments to explain the concept of defense, the manner in which defenses interfere with the capacity to think clearly and how analysts can modify a defense by offering a greater awareness of how it operates and what it operates against. But, in addition, *his interventions themselves are carefully crafted to assist the analysand in developing self-analytic skills.*

The intervention has several components:

1. The intervention starts with the analyst empathically aligning himself with what was last conscious in the analysand's mind, the moment before the analyst began to speak.
2. The analyst describes the defense to the analysand.
3. The analyst directs the analysand's attention back to the moment of expression of the conflicted drive derivative (just past) that invoked the defense.

4. The analyst describes this moment as open-endedly as possible and questions the analysand as non-directively as possible as to what he senses in terms of internal conditions or his experience of the analyst that made the defense necessary.

The description of the surface[1] is usually a relatively comfortable moment for the analysand. The analysand has just invoked a defense, which lessens anxiety. The analyst's accurate description of the analysand's thoughts at that moment conveys understanding, which usually evokes a transference with positive feeling toward a competent figure. Because this transference carries with it the danger of compliance with the analyst's ideas, it is very important that the analyst be non-directive. When passive analysands accept the analyst's ideas, it hampers their active pursuit of self-knowledge. When analysands are trying to grapple with conflicted drive derivatives, they are all too willing to accept suggestions from their analyst, whether correct or not, and make defensive use of them.

An elaboration of this moment of relative comfort can take place if the evocation of a positive transference is useful at a particular time—that is, if the analysand is in the midst of a painful or counterproductive regression and such a transference would help in re-organization.

If the patient is engaged in a defensive operation that may preclude his capacity to consider the analyst's observations, Gray may start his intervention with a preamble, which allows the patient's ego a chance to disengage from the defenses it has invoked. Such a preamble may also serve to

---

[1]The "surface" for Gray is what is consciously available in the patient's mind at the moment the analyst begins his intervention. His concept is similar to that of Fenichel. For a useful description of several variations of this concept see Levy and Inderbitzin 1990.

counter defensive transference distortions that would interfere with the patient's thinking about the intervention.

For instance, to a patient who is regressing in the hour and becoming overwhelmed with affect: "You seem to be feeling kind of flooded right now. I wonder if we can take a moment and step back and look at what you were just telling us."

Or, to a masochistic patient who is prepared to feel the analyst is not sympathetic to the problems he faces in his life and uses the irritation of feeling misunderstood to obscure what the analyst is trying to tell him: "I realize that one of the things you want me to understand is just how difficult things are for you right now in your life. It is an added burden to try to do analysis when struggling with the kind of things you describe in your life, but I wonder if, in addition to that, we can notice that. . . ." The analyst's description of defense takes place at a level of detail and sophistication that matches the level of analytic sophistication and current self-observing capacity of the analysand. The analyst's characterization of the moment when the drive derivative appears is gauged to match the analysand's capacity to tolerate the intensity of drive derivative that this description re-evokes.

Interventions early in analysis might begin with a simple description of the sequence of the thoughts. For example, "You called yourself mean just after you were telling me of observing your father in your memory." Such an intervention demonstrates to the analysand the manner in which the analyst is noticing sequences of thoughts in which shifts of feeling take place. The "telling me" introduces the analysand to the idea that it is what he tells the analyst that is being noticed, and "observing your father in your memory" is a reminder of the analytic situation—that he and the analyst are observing his thoughts of father, not dealing with father himself.

At a later point in the analysis, it might be possible to add detail to the description of the defense and to add affective temperature to the characterization of the conflicted drive derivative. Such graded use of complexity and directness of description assists the analysand in seeing the more subtle, complex workings of his mind and in being able to bear more direct representation of drive derivative.

The same material might be interpreted as follows: "You called yourself 'mean like your father,' just after you were telling me of the anger you felt as you remembered him slapping you." The wording of the intervention reminds the analysand of another aspect of the analytic situation. He is putting thoughts and feelings into words to a professional listener in a setting of absolute confidentiality. This realistic picture of the analyst is in contrast to the transference that invoked the defense and may assist the analysand in seeing the transference more clearly.

For example, a minimal allusion to transference in the first intervention is the part "telling me" and "in your memory," which allude to the analytic situation. A more explicit inquiry into the transference of defense is, "It seems hard to tell me these thoughts and feelings about your father. Can you sense anything about that?"

After sufficient details of the transference of defense[2] have emerged, the analysand, spontaneously or in response to inquiry from the analyst, may note that the developing picture of the analyst is familiar. Such recognition often permits analysands to link transference feelings to memories of experiences with significant figures in their life. Data of this kind offers deepening insight *into the conditions that led to the adoption of specific defenses.*

---

[2]This concept comes from Anna Freud (1936). She suggested that not only are feelings toward past figures reawakened and directed toward the analyst, but defenses that had their origin in contending with the anxiety of these early relationships are repeated as well. Defense within an analytic hour is resistance. The focus on the transference that gives rise to resistance is the transference of defense.

The analyst slowly increases the analysand's recognition of the way he avoids awareness of anything (including the analyst) and allows the analysand to accumulate data on what is being warded off and the analysand's views of the analyst that necessitate the warding off.

Interventions in close process attention remain very close to the analysand's experience. Open-ended inquiry about the moment of defense lessens the risk of the analyst imposing his views on the analysand. Analysts who tell analysands things that the analysands formerly did not know, but subsequently see as true, seem to possess secret knowledge and power. Such interventions invoke transferences that can heighten resistance. For example, the analysand may turn from self-analytic activity to trying to get the analyst to speak *ex cathedra* again. In close process attention, on the other hand, the analyst presents himself as a careful observer, but there is nothing magical about him.

Gray's method encourages analysands, in their subsequent self- analysis, to keep close to the data and tolerate the ambiguity of not knowing, with confidence that steady application of the analytic method will, over time, provide reliable and useful insight.

Close process attention strives for a gentleness with analysands so as not to compromise their self-observing capacity. The following elements contribute to that gentleness:

1. the timing of the intervention which directs the analysand's attention to moments of transient, bearable drive derivative;
2. the meticulous approach to the defense through the surface of the patient's consciousness;
3. the approach to the moment of just-suppressed drive derivative through a description of the defense;
4. the characterization of the defense at a level of detail that can be easily grasped by the analysand;

5. the description of drive derivative at a level that can be tolerated; and finally,
6. the steady clarification of transference at a depth determined by the analysand's capacity to examine transference at the moment of intervention.

These elements of technique encourage subsequent self-analysis to take place at a level of affect that permits sustained inquiry.

The way in which close process attention addresses transference is worth emphasizing. Transference usually has deeply unconscious components. Thus, transference *interpretations* run the risk of bypassing defense. Deep interpretations carry the risk of regression with the invocation of new and uninterpretable defenses or shifts in the transference. On the other hand, an analysis can be stalemated by a failure to address a transference that is the source of a powerful resistance.

Close process attention actively addresses transferential issues from the first intervention. (The technique addresses transference specifically at the point of resistance.) Looking for transference of defense offers the analyst a non-disruptive window on transference. This lessens the destructive potential of the uninterpreted transference.

Close process attention helps analysands in their post-analytic self-analysis to consider the nature of their imaginary audience at the moment they notice their use of a defense.

APPLICATIONS OF CLOSE PROCESS MONITORING TO IMPULSIVE PATIENTS

Gray's recommendations were intended for highly functioning neurotics in classical analysis. This paper describes the technical problem of offering insight to more disturbed patients. The issue with this second group of patients has been to approach them carefully enough so that insight does not disrupt needed defenses, yet forcefully enough to influence entrenched maladaptive defense. Gray's entire focus is to understand the defensive needs and methods of the ego in its moment-to-moment struggle in the therapeutic situation, and to find the moments and methods to make carefully dosed insight available to the patient. This frame of reference finds immediate productive application to the "wider scope of analysis."[3]

More disturbed patients in insight-oriented psychotherapy often need supportive measures to safely sustain the work. Gray's precise formulation of the ego and its defensive operations allows for a more precise tailoring of supportive measures. This precise formulation permits a psychological "cost benefit analysis" for making some estimate of the likely benefit to a specific patient of a given supportive measure and the likely cost of that measure to insight-oriented work.

The remainder of this paper considers applications of close process attention technique to patients subject to primitive mental states, with a special emphasis on analytic responses to patients subject to impulsive action.

---

[3] Just how wide a scope can be illustrated by a vignette. A 20-year-old schizophrenic adolescent described how he freed himself from command hallucinations. He had been subject to hallucinations in spite of several years of neuroleptic use. He began by trying to predict the moment in which he would hear hallucinations. After some practice, he was able to do so. He then practiced predicting the content of the hallucination. After a time, he was able to do this as well. He then began to predict the exact words of the hallucination. When he could do this, the hallucinations were recognizable to him as appearing in his own voice—he was hearing his thoughts out loud. Shortly after this, he recognized that the thoughts that appeared to him out loud were the thoughts of his own conscience. With this recognition the hallucinations stopped. At that point, the young man appeared moderately neurotically ill—not schizophrenic.

Impulsive action can be understood as a moment in which the drives overwhelm the combined forces of the ego and superego. A person subject to impulsive action may be subject to any combination of the following conditions.

1. The sudden eruption of drive usually accompanied by urgent feeling. Action is on a continuum between discharge of the drive and defense. Action as defense introduces thoughts or bodily sensations that distract away from impulses or thoughts that feel more dangerous to the patient. For example, "I will think about drinking or about having predatory sex with this woman rather than think about attacking her."
2. Sudden regressions of the ego. These regressions can take several forms.
    A. Cognitive regressions where there is a loss of accurate perception of the situation. The "impulsive" behavior occurs when the patient responds to only part of the obviously available data, for example, regressions in which splitting and denial are prominent. The cognitive regression may have been initiated in the hopes of containing the drive. For example, "If I let myself see how demeaning and manipulative this salesman is, I will want to kill him on the spot." On the other hand, in the case cited, such a blurring of perception might lead to impulsive spending of money.
    B. Regressions that impair access to memory. The "impulsive" behavior occurs when the patient is unable to think of more adaptive alternatives. An example is a person panicked by fire who leaps out of a second story window when he could leave through a door and down a fire escape. He can't use the door because panic erases the memory of which key works the lock.

C. Regressions that impair self-perception. Many regressions are accompanied by a feeling of being younger, weaker, etc. This self-perception may make libidinal or aggressive thoughts seem less dangerous. There can also be regression to a grandiose fantasy of the self.

> One physically powerful 14-year-old, a victim of childhood beatings, said, "When I'm angry I am so powerful bullets can't stop me." He was arrested shortly after this statement after he had fought four armed police officers to a standstill. [The fifth and sixth managed to subdue him without use of deadly force, which several of the original four were about to resort to].

The impairment of self-perception can also assist in disarming the ego, or the superego, in ways permissive to the id. For example, "I can't let myself do what I want to do unless I keep myself confused about what I am doing. If I am clear, I will be ashamed or think I am crazy or be too frightened of the possible outcomes."

D. Regressions that impair the capacity to anticipate the future, estimate odds, or maintain a disciplined course of action. In some cases this is a product of massive defenses such as denial, repression, depersonalization, active-into-passive, or passive-into-active. These defenses may so compromise assessments of reality or so preoccupy the patient with carrying out and then coping with the results of urgent defensive needs that he would not be able to plan and carry through disciplined sequential thought. At other times, however, the patient may be too frightened to permit himself such planning due to fear of the heightened sense of

power that such thinking gives to aggressive or libidinal wishes. The patient cannot permit *thoughts* along the line, "Revenge is a dish best savored cold."
3. Regression of the superego.
   A. The patient may have a partial turning of aggression on the self, where he suspends his usual self-protective functions. "When I'm angry I don't think bullets can't stop me; I just don't care if they do."
   B. The superego may be so harsh in its regression that the ego is subject to regression. Impulsive action takes place in the face of this weakening of the ego.
   C. The superego may become so harsh that the ego has devised methods of total evasion. Wurmser (1974) wrote of the manner in which patients susceptible to severe states of shame or guilt learned to simply disconnect superego function. Such patients present as sociopaths.
   D. There may be regressions of the superego to a state in which values are externalized and, as part of the projective state, the target of the projection is seen as dangerously hostile. For example, the patient thinks, "You are the one who thinks I am bad and dangerous. You hate me and will hurt me." The impulsive action is in response to the perceived threat. The grandiose 14-year-old displayed this pattern.
   E. There may, at the same time, be a regression to a more primitive superego state in which projection labels some prospective victim as evil and having "asked for it." The grandiose 14-year-old also displayed this pattern.

GRAY'S APPROACH WITH IMPULSIVE PATIENTS

The application of Gray's approach to impulsive patients can be considered in eight parts.

1. Analytic responses to powerful drive states.
2. Using words to replace action.
3. Analytic responses to the transference in those subject to primitive mental states.
4. Understanding the symbolic meanings of action.
5. Analyzing ego tendencies (defenses or regressions) that promote or permit impulsive action.
6. Ego splinting.
7. Modifying the harshness of the superego without weakening its necessary role in control of the drives and self protection.
8. Establishing needed auxiliary modalities of treatment with a minimum of disruption to insight-oriented work.

Analytic responses to powerful drive states

The first priority in patients subject to imbalance between drive and restraint is not to provoke the drives. Many standard technical recommendations are directed toward this end. Fenichel's (1941) recommendation of analyzing defense before drive and of beginning interpretations at the surface, and Anna Freud's (1936) emphasis on the need for the analyst to remain equidistant from the ego, superego, and id, are examples. A child case illustrates how the failure to speak to both sides of a conflict can generate immediate defensive and transferential adjustments in a patient, which leads to action.

> A six-year-old, referred for problems with fears, impulsiveness, aggressiveness, and poor peer relations, was play-

ing out a theme in the playroom in which figures were barely able to stay inside a toy car that was driving all over the floor and walls. This play was reminiscent of the history the analyst had of the youngster being taken for rides at 120 mph in his father's racing car. In his first intervention, the inexperienced analyst suggested, in a somewhat moralistic tone, that the people in the car were having a scary ride. The patient said defiantly, "They are not scared," and threw a block at the analyst's head. [The analyst had lined up with the superego in this comment. The child was assisted in his tendencies for externalization and rebelled.] The analyst's second try with similar material was to suggest that the people in the car were having an exciting ride. The child repeated, "Exciting, yes exciting," and with mounting excitement was soon climbing on all of the furniture of the office, including the desk and bookshelf. [The analyst, by naming the drive and speaking to its strength, had enhanced its expression.] At the next opportunity, after supervision, the analyst commented on the scary *and* exciting ride the people were having. The boy then said, "Yes, scary and exciting. Scary and exciting," while having the car gently come in for a landing. He then shifted themes in the play to two small children who went to a circus and were frightened by the clowns and the wild animals. [This was reminiscent of the history of another early overstimulating experience.] Subsequent associations permitted the analyst to clarify to the patient his use of action as a defense against the fear and helplessness he felt in the unfamiliar and frightening analytic situation.

Close process attention is a refinement of Fenichel's (1941) and A. Freud's (1936) widely accepted technical recommendations. The analyst's interventions describe the patient's defensive surface and return his attention to the moment when the unacceptable drive derivative appeared. Gray places great importance on the analyst's accurate characterization of the surface of the patient's mind at the moment of intervention. A lengthy description of the surface (clarification of the sources of conflict after invocation of the defense) can allow the analyst to serve as an auxiliary ego by helping the patient put his feelings into words. As mentioned earlier, this elaboration can evoke a transference to a competent, helpful person. Such a transference can help contain a drive that stems from fear by evoking the presence of a powerful and well-disposed helper.

An example of such an intervention follows:

> Analyst: You seem to feel flooded and helpless at the moment. The flooded feeling seemed to start as you were telling me of the combination of anger at the memory of your boss's comment and fear that you would leave here after remembering this comment and go to him and say something that would get you in trouble. You also have talked of liking your boss at other times. To the extent you like him, you don't want to think of hurting his feelings.

The analyst here chose to leave the patient at a moment of conflict over anger when the anger and wishes for control were both conscious elements, rather than take the patient all the way back to the moment when the patient was permitting himself pure anger uninhibited by any conflicting emotions. The regression in the hour suggested to the analyst that the latter moment was too intense for the patient's ego to handle at this time. Using empathic intervention in a supportive fashion is elaborated in the section on regression.

Gray gives careful attention to the affective temperature of the words used to describe the patient's drive derivatives. The more direct the description of the drive derivative, the more powerfully the drive is re-invoked. These words are carefully selected on the basis of how intense a drive derivative the analyst feels the patient can hold in awareness.

For example, if a patient said, "I hate my father," the analyst might describe the drive derivative as, "your thoughts of your father . . . looking at your father in your thoughts . . . , evaluating your father . . . , judging your father . . . , remembering annoyance at your father . . . , remembering anger at your father . . . , remembering fury at your father . . . ," and so on.

For the sexual drive derivative, "I wanted to kiss her," the analyst might speak of "your thoughts of . . . interest in . . . affectionate feelings . . . tender feelings . . . sensual feelings . . . loving feelings . . . sexual feelings . . . erotic feelings," or "your thoughts of wishes to make love with your mouth."

The analyst picks a moment to intervene when the defense invoked is against a drive derivative that is sufficiently intense to be demonstrable to the patient but not so intense as to require immediate formation of a rigid defense. A regression of the id, ego, or superego after a well-phrased defense interpretation suggests the drive derivative selected for interpretation (or its characterization) may have been too intense for the patient to handle at this point in the work. Gray likens the repeated exposure of the patient's ego to gradually incremental levels of drive derivative to weight lifting. He sees one aspect of "working through" as the ego's accumulation of experience and capacity in contending with ever clearer, and more intense, levels of drive derivative without regression.

The analyst's observations are focused exclusively on the patient's words in the analytic situation so that the analyst's words appear as non-judgmental as possible. Observations are limited to the immediate expressed associations of the patient; they are not pronouncements on character. Thus, they have less potential for narcissistic injury.

The analyst's observations are directed toward what is immediately conscious to the patient. Thus, the patient is in the position to *immediately evaluate* the analyst's accuracy. The patient is on an even cognitive footing with the analyst so there is less chance for tilting the transference in the direction of someone with secret knowledge and power. The iatrogenic longings and disappointments of such transferences that can stimulate eruptions of drive in more disturbed patients are thus avoided.

As with a child, it is useful to clarify the urgency of the patient's driven states. The analyst starts at the surface of the patient's thought and returns him to the moment when the thought expressed intense drive. The analyst empathizes with the urgency of the patient's feelings at such moments *and how difficult this makes it for the patient, given his natural wish for self-control.* This intervention departs from Gray's usual recommendations in several ways. Naming the drive and addressing its strength both tend to reduce the drive. Thus, it is important to use marked care when describing the drive derivatives. The analyst should make such an intervention at a moment when the patient can remember the feeling of urgency, but is not in the grip of it. The defense of displacement in time may be ignored or even encouraged. In addition, the analyst tries to assist the ego in maintaining control by addressing the ego-based and the superego-based desire for control. If the patient can begin to think about such moments, it is often possible to clarify fantasies that contribute to the sense of urgency. For example, "If I don't get this now, I will never get it," and "If I don't get this now, something terrible will happen."

Using words to replace action

Another aspect of Gray's approach, which has not been spelled out directly in his papers but is very much a part of his practice and supervision, is the meticulous establishment of the analytic field. The privacy and quiet of the setting, meticulous regard for confidentiality, punctuality in starting and stopping sessions, general attitude of courtesy and respect, accuracy and timeliness of billing, and general consistency of manner are all important aspects of the analyst's work. Many patients prone to action have had important figures in their past who used action in preference to words for communication. Such patients tend to be even more reactive than usual to the analyst's actions. The analyst's behavioral consistency means his actions tend to drop into the background and the patient looks to the analyst's words for communication. Langs (1974), although using a very different therapeutic approach, reports a series of vignettes that illustrate the need for a well-established analytic field.

Some patients have had to deal with important figures who used words to disguise and distort rather than to convey the truth, or to hurt or manipulate rather than to help. Such patients often quietly discount what the analyst says. For the therapy to proceed, it may be important to clarify the patient's experience of the analyst's words.

> A young professional in a low-fee analysis would barely listen to interventions and would often go on as if the analyst had made no comment. There were frequent expressions of a feeling of hopelessness about the analysis—a process that was, after all, "just talk." Early in the evaluation, this patient had told of the almost routine use of words for manipulation, deceit, and harm by multiple family members. The patient had a change in circumstances that required an adjustment of the fee, but was unwilling to describe in detail the nature of the financial change. The analyst stated that the fee could be adjusted either up or down according to circumstances, but that it was important to look at both the reality of the patient's circumstances and the thoughts and feelings that might come to mind about a change

in the fee. At another point, the analyst remarked that people often had difficulty in thinking clearly about issues of money and that a clarification of thoughts and feelings about money in the analysis might help with some of the difficulties the patient was having thinking clearly about money. The patient reacted to the analyst's words as if it were obvious to both of them that the analyst's comments were completely disingenuous and were designed to put the patient at a disadvantage while the analyst negotiated for as high a fee as possible. The analyst noted that the patient seemed to see his [the analyst's] words as being used for manipulation and had discounted them completely. The analyst added that such discounting seemed to take the analyst's lying as a matter of course and avoided the vulnerability that might come from being taken in by the analyst's words. Such a stance also guarded against the possibility of a sudden disappointment with the analyst. If there was no hope for the analyst's honesty, then catching him in a lie or manipulation would not be a disappointment. Developing such a protection would make a great deal of sense, given the fact that the patient had consistently talked of several members of his family who used words to disguise rather than convey the truth. The intervention led to a series of recollections of manipulation and lies by family members and a greater awareness of moments of discounting the analyst's words. In subsequent sessions, the patient attended and responded to what the analyst said and expressed increased hope about the possibility of help from the analysis.

While abreactive therapies do not aim for insight, it is possible to analytically explore the resistances a patient might have to making use of the abreactive potential of the analytic situation. Using abreaction in the safe analytic setting can provide a safety valve to patients to assist in the control of impulse in their lives. This would be a component of what others have called the holding environment of therapy.

A 26-year-old male with problems with aggressive impulse control, in about the third month of therapy said:

> *Patient:* I hate that guy [supervisor]. But it was really stupid of me to mouth off at him like that at work. [The memory of the "mouthing off" is primarily painful as it is presented. Remembering the incident constitutes a turning on the self within the hour. Highlighting this aspect of the patient's use of memories of action allows the analyst to bring the patient's reality testing to bear on one self-destructive aspect of the action in a neutral way—neither seductive nor condemning.]
>
> *Analyst:* You and I both know that for you to mouth off at work might have all sorts of consequences that would be undesirable for you. [This area can be elaborated to the extent that the analyst needs to serve as an auxiliary ego for the patient, but it will be at a cost of distracting attention from the main point, which is the use of the memory of the impulsive action within the hour as a source of embarrassment or guilt to turn aggressive impulse on the self. Such elaboration may offer a point of purchase for any need the patient has for turning the analyst into a superego figure.] The thought of yourself as stupid comes up here as you are talking to me about this boss, and interrupts the feeling of safety you were experiencing just a moment or two ago to tell me just how angry you were at him. Can you sense anything about what feeling of tension might have started to intrude on that safety?
>
> *Patient:* Well, I don't want to get all steamed up. I don't want to go out of here and maybe hit him. When I get started. . . . [The patient is unable to include any

view of the analyst in his awareness of difficulty in speaking freely. He sees the tension as a one-person phenomenon. There may be transference close to the surface, such as the idea that the analyst would be unable or perhaps have no interest in assisting the patient to get control of himself before leaving the hour. It is important to get a clearer idea of what the defenses are that keep the patient from including the analyst in his view of the analytic situation].

Analyst: It seems as though there is a picture of yourself as just getting madder and madder here until you have to act on it. It makes sense that with that picture of yourself you wouldn't want to go on talking to me about angry feelings. It is very difficult at a moment like that to have the feeling you were talking about earlier in the week—that because you were able to get angry in here, you were kind of blowing off steam and not feeling so out of control at home and at work. It's very far from the feeling, "I'll keep talking about it so I *don't* go out and deck the guy." [Offers the potential of abreactive relief from the therapy as a legitimate byproduct of the search for insight.]

Interventions on the same issue at other times allowed the patient to elaborate some of the dangers that prevented his use of the therapy situation for abreaction. He knew from experience that anger above a certain intensity led him inevitably to turn on himself and become ashamed, depressed, or regressed. It was only after much work that he could start to consider the transferential implications of his tension in experiencing anger in the hours. He recognized that he created several transferential constellations in such a setting. These included figures who disapproved of his anger at authorities, who were sadistically gratified by his turning on himself, who narcissistically thought his anger was "really" directed toward them, or who had a tendency to identify with the people he was angry at and would retaliate. As the therapy progressed, he became much freer in his expression of anger in the hours.

Analytic responses to the transference in those subject to primitive mental states

Patients susceptible to primitive mental states have urgent defensive needs at the moments of regression. These needs can call forth rapidly formed transferences that are difficult to interpret. A major technical consideration is how to respond to such primitive transferences in analytic treatment. Such transference tendencies can be exacerbated if the analyst ignores the dictum "defense before drive" or comments too deeply on drive derivatives. As with children, drive derivatives may be obvious to the analyst and obscure to the patient. The analyst may fail to appreciate subtle forms of isolation of affect or denial in fantasy. Patients may put their thoughts into words, but be shocked on hearing them repeated by the analyst.

Even meticulous respect of defenses does not eliminate upsurges of transference in patients subject to primitive mental states. Gray's approach offers assistance in bringing issues of transference into therapeutic consideration. His focus is on the transference of defense. The following vignette illustrates how this focus allows a continuous access to transference at a level that does not stimulate the patient to engage in profound defensive maneuvers and thus leaves the patient able to continue to think.

> A professional man in his mid-thirties sought help for anxiety attacks, depression, and fear that co-workers were plotting against him. He was seen in three-times-a-week intensive psychotherapy. He immediately formed an

idealizing transference and seemed to need this to overcome his fear of treatment. In spite of what he consciously felt was a uniformly positive attitude toward the analyst, he would become silent when his thoughts moved in the direction of the details of his fears of co-workers. He also began to miss sessions. Interventions were made along the lines: "You became silent just after you were starting to tell me of your fears of your co-workers."

After the patient's awareness of the sequence was established, interventions of the sequence included follow-up inquiries seeking clarification of his picture of the analyst *at the moment of the silence*. Approaches along these lines helped develop the following sequence of transference pictures.

The patient could not continue talking at these moments because to do so might lead to overwhelming depression and anxiety (he feared the painful states of shame or guilt he would use to defend against his anger at the memories of his co-workers' behavior). The transference at such moments was that the analyst would not be able to help him with his feelings within the hour and he would leave overwhelmed and alone. These transference feelings were linked in his associations to experiences with his mother who had not protected him, recognized his distress, or even believed him when he was subjected to sexual abuse by a socially powerful neighbor.

He could not become angry in his hour because he believed that displays of these feelings would not be acceptable to the analyst. These transference pictures were linked in his associations to the repressive, nondemonstrative style insisted on by the patient's father.

He could not be angry in his hour because the angry feelings might spill out of the hour and into the workplace, where they would evoke retaliation from his fellow workers. The analyst would be completely ineffective in helping him contain himself. These transference pictures were later linked in his associations to his mother's incapacity to set limits on the father or older siblings in their conduct toward the patient.

He could not have thoughts of vengeance. He assumed these thoughts were not acceptable to the analyst who would assume he was on the verge of carrying out his fantasies. The transferences here were from the religious figures in his early life who insisted that the thought equals the deed.

The patient maintained his generally idealized idea of the analyst but was able to incorporate the view that at the moments in which he found it difficult to speak, the fears he had of people, based on past experiences, had intruded into his therapy hours. His capacity to speak in the hours and his attendance improved significantly.

Patients often develop transferences in which the analyst is seen as permissive or even encouraging of drive expression outside of the analysis. Close process attention consistently focuses the patients on the fact that the analyst and the patient are in a special situation, with special safeguards and special purposes. Such focus forestalls much of this kind of misunderstanding of therapy. But patients with special needs or particular experiences are not immune from misunderstanding even the most carefully phrased interventions. Prior experience with an abreactive therapy can predispose a patient to see his analyst as encouraging sexual or aggressive expressions outside the analysis. It is not unusual for people to have had childhood experiences with adults who encouraged sexual or aggressive action in the child to meet their own needs. Patients who need the fantasy of a permissive transference to be free to talk about sexual or aggressive fantasies have not truly worked through their inhibition to such thoughts. The usual difficulties that result from patients adopting the approach of "letting out their feelings" in their lives can then be used as resistances to thinking about or putting sexual or aggressive feeling into words in the therapy. In addition, seductive figures have usually failed to protect or have even actually exploited the patient. If the analyst is not attuned to the possibility of permissive transference, these aspects of the transference are less likely to be explored.

A 28-year-old woman was in psychotherapy for depression, difficulty in keeping jobs, and an inability to terminate a highly unsatisfactory love relationship. In the hour following a session in which her turning on the self had been demonstrated to her, she said:

> *Patient:* You would have been proud of me. I really told the creep [boss] off.
>
> *Analyst:* If I mentioned in the last session in here that you seemed to be having some difficulty feeling free to express an angry feeling in these special circumstances where you are talking in a soundproof room to a professional who has suspended all social mores so the two of us can get a clearer picture of your thoughts, would it have felt like I was encouraging you to be free putting angry thoughts or feelings into words in your life in general—a kind of principle of mental hygiene?
>
> *Patient:* You mean you think I shouldn't?
>
> *Analyst:* Well, I don't know actually. I suppose there might be circumstances where the best thing might be to tell someone off. I suppose some people might not understand what you were saying unless you said it in a very forceful way. I suppose in some situations it would be a disaster to tell a boss off. I know so little about your boss and your job. You could talk to me here for hours about it and I would still know only

1/1000th of what you know about the situation. [Because this is early in therapy and the patient was coming from a therapy in which there was a good deal of advice, the therapist offers an educational comment on why he is not offering advice.] It seems like one part of the picture you had of me is that in the picture I felt like I knew better than you how to act in that situation even though you had been in it and I hadn't. Is there anything about that, that seems familiar?
Patient: Well, yes it does. Dr. X felt I let myself get pushed around. And there was my father. He used to tell me that you can't be a wimp. He used to say people will walk all over you if you let them.

Understanding the symbolic meanings of action

Impulsive action can be considered as existing on a continuum. At one extreme is "acting out" or "acting in," where the action is a symbolic representation of a conflict. An example is Freud's case (1893–1899) of the sexually abused, obsessional child who carefully arranged the pillows at the foot of his bed each night before sleep. At the other extreme is defensive action that is largely devoid of symbolic content. An example is an overstimulated child who runs chaotically around the playroom to generate bodily sensations that keep dystonic sexual thoughts and sensations at bay.

Many acts lie between these extremes. An example is taking a drink of alcohol. The act of drinking might have a symbolic meaning, whereas the sensation of the alcohol might also be sought for defensive purposes.

An analyst who did not use the close process attention technique might listen to a patient's description of impulsive action outside the hour and then present the patient with a suggestion as to a possible meaning of that behavior. The interpretation of the action might be informed by the themes of conflict under consideration in the patient's recent hours. If the action were self-destructive or impulsive the analyst might include some characterization of the impulsive or self-destructive quality of the action to try to clarify the patient's thought on the matter. These situations often present the analyst with a dilemma. Impulsive patients, by definition, have found ways to overcome their superegos. Externalization followed by avoidance or defeat of the person representing the externalized trends is a common tactic. The more standard analytic approach to impulsive action (particularly if a negative judgment on the adaptiveness of the action is made) lends itself to defensive externalization of the superego onto the analyst in a way in which its transferential features are hard to demonstrate.

The manner in which close process attention explicitly keeps the psychoanalytic process in focus, including the safety of the psychoanalytic setting, offers advantages because the focus is on *thoughts or memories* of action. It is not necessary to pass judgments or to serve as an auxiliary superego in the psychoanalytic setting. The setting implies an implicit agreement between patient and analyst to suspend action for the hour. The patient and analyst are addressing *memories* of action, or *thoughts* of action, perhaps even the formation of a plan of action where the patient's intent is to carry out the action, but not action itself. This means that both the patient and the analyst do not need to evaluate the adaptive or maladaptive qualities of the action (except possibly in the last case, if the thought of action clearly portends action and the action is obviously out of touch with reality). By observing the moment at which the thought of action appears in the stream of associations and the effect the thought of action has on that stream, there is a potential for developing reliable insight into the *range of meanings* of thoughts of specific actions. If the patient says, "I'm going to leave here then go hit my boss," the analyst is in a good position to clarify what defensive operations contribute to the patients's failure to consider consequences.

An action that often complicates treatment is the use of psychoactive substances.

A 28-year-old business executive with a strong family history of substance abuse had talked in previous hours of drinking to intoxication several times a month. There had been no job loss, no medical complications from drinking, and no accidents or injuries, but several relationships had foundered because of fights while the patient was under the influence of alcohol. The patient's use of alcohol seemed to be increasing. More than one analytic hour had been compromised by the effects of a hangover.

> *Patient:* We won. After we closed the deal a couple of us went out last night and . . . well, we weren't exactly drunk [smiling].
>
> *Analyst:* Your thoughts seemed to go to the effects of the alcohol—the relaxing quality of it. [Patient nods yes.] It was almost as if the thought of alcohol's relaxing quality helped with some tension in telling me of being out with your friends, celebrating winning and closing the deal.

Subsequent associations in the hour led to a clarification of the sense of tension that the patient felt in the presence of friends. The fear was of becoming exhibitionistic and then alienating a friend. Similar sequences, interpreted in subsequent hours, led to clarification of fears experienced in the transference that the analyst would say disparaging things and attempt to disrupt the patient's friendships, just as his siblings and father had done in earlier years. There was another series of hours in which thoughts of the use of alcohol appeared in association to memories of lovemaking. A number of anxieties were soothed by the thought of the alcohol in this situation. These included fears defending against exhibitionistic wishes, fears of revealing himself as a sexual being to the analyst, and fears of the analyst's competitive feelings in regard to the sexual partner. During the course of this analytic work the patient described drinking less. Reports of drinking or of the disruptive effects of drinking subsided.

Analyzing ego tendencies (defenses or regressions) that promote or permit impulsive action

A number of defenses predispose a patient to impulsive action. The most obvious is changing passive into active, followed closely by those defenses that would grossly compromise the patient's capacity to assess inner and outer reality, or remember sequences of cause and effect. Such defenses interfere with the capacity to predict the future and think of alternative approaches to a situation. Massive repression, denial, derealization, depersonalization, devaluation, marked isolation of affect, or affective flooding could operate singly or in combination to predispose to impulsive action. The patient may give a history that suggests massive overwhelming defense at the time of action in his life and demonstrate intense manifestations of such defenses during the hour. The therapist looks for minor manifestations of the defense to interpret, knowing that the *forme fruste* of the defense is easier for the patient to tolerate.

A 25-year-old woman, subject to massive states of confusion during regressions, described her anger at her lover:

> *Patient:* I'm going to throw his God-damned tools out in the rain. No I won't. I'm going to loan them out. We have some neighbors who never return anything—except in pieces. I'm going to . . . Oh. I don't know . . . I can't . . . [voice falling] I'll never be able to get the key.

Analyst: You seemed to start feeling helpless about the key just after you were telling me thoughts of a plan of revenge. It was almost as if it were dangerous to reveal to me anger and a capacity to plan at the same time. Can you sense anything about that? [The tirade resumed with opportunities in subsequent associations to pick up on the "I don't know . . . I can't," which actually ushered in a very mild state of confusion or helplessness in the patient's thinking.]

Ego splinting

Those who work with children clearly see the wishes for a supportive figure that is part of regression. This issue can also be usefully addressed with adults—how in the face of the stress associated with such thoughts one could even wish to be younger so there would have to be someone there to help out, or wish to be younger so the distressing details would just be going over one's head. But, as mentioned, the analyst can invoke the transference of a competent understanding figure, if such a figure is needed to foster reintegration. The empathic elaboration of the defensive surface is one way of invoking such a figure. Tone of voice can be quite important in inducing a supportive transference. Timing is another important factor. The analyst's capacity to intervene early, before overwhelming pain sets in, is very important in those patients who have been left to struggle in overwhelming circumstances. The many opportunities to intervene that are available through the close process attention technique offer a distinct advantage in countering disorganization caused by the too-early appearance of such disappointed feelings toward the analyst. Extreme states of anxiety, depression, or fear that rage will be put into action carry with them the transferential picture that the analyst is absent, indifferent, or impotent. Clarifications of such implicit transferential feelings can be useful during moments of extreme regression.

Clarifying the specific losses of cognitive capacity that occur during regression can leave a patient feeling understood by a competent listener, but, in addition, the analyst is in the position to quietly supply needed soothing thoughts, if necessary, as part of a relatively neutral interpretation. The analyst can gently clarify the kinds of thoughts the patient is *not* able to have at certain moments of regression. This serves as an ego splinting activity but is less disruptive to therapy than taking over and doing something for the patient. For example:

Memory:

When you feel flooded and overwhelmed and alone like this it gets so hard for you to remember that you are an adult who knows how to drive a car, can use a telephone, has friends, has money in the bank, etc. You feel totally helpless and without resources.

Time sense:

When you start to feel depressed, you feel as though the sense of depression will go on forever. You know in your head that these moods only last for a day or two but it feels like they won't ever end.

Access to language:

You started to struggle to find the word just a moment or two ago. It seems when the feelings reach a certain level of intensity you have a hard time finding the words. This seems to add to the burden of worry you have at such moments, the extra burden of thinking that you won't be able to make yourself understood.

Capacity to sequence:

You seemed to become confused about the order in which events took place, and that made you frustrated with yourself just at the point when you were starting to feel irritated by your employee.

Mode of representation of thought:

Your thoughts shifted from words to images and it was hard to put the images into words. It seems that without the words the meaning of your thoughts was much harder to sort out. That occurred just after you were observing your spouse in your memory. [This led to more detailed description of disappointing aspects of the spouse.]

Sense of self:

You seemed to get sleepy just after you were starting to translate the images into words. [This yielded a clearer description of the images over time beginning with fragments of words and later leading to rather full descriptions.]

You thought of the way in which you lose minutes from your experience and I think it distracted you here, just after you were starting to tell me what your mother said to you at the dinner after the funeral. [This led to recall of detail of provocations by the patient's mother.]

These interventions lend the analyst to the patient as a soothing transference figure and as an auxiliary ego to help with immediate reintegration. They contribute to the patient's sense of hope, but they are confined to comments on the patient's thoughts and feelings in the hour. (These interventions include details of how the regression is used defensively, the kind of conflict that precipitates the regression in the hour, and the transferential aspects of such moments. The analyst *has not* stepped out of role. Clinical observation suggests that it is insight—the patient's observing the details of the regression—that is correlated with permanent lessening of regressive potential. In a session with a 28-year-old professional:

> *Analyst*: As you started to feel flooded with feeling, you lost your usual facility with words and began to struggle to find the words you wanted. This came up just as you were telling me about wanting to tell your mother off. Can you sense anything about how it would feel to be telling me about your anger at your mother and feel in full command of your usual capacities for language?

In this last vignette, the patient's thoughts went to my interrupting and criticizing the patient for being critical of a parent. The patient later identified this as a maternal transference. In subsequent material, the patient's perception of me interrupting and criticizing included the view of me striking first because I was vulnerable to harsh words. The patient was worried that if he had full command of language, he might devastate me as he had learned to worry in childhood about a potentially lethal effect of accurate hostile words on his depressed, often suicidal, mother.

Modifying the harshness of the superego without weakening its necessary role in control of the drives and self-protection

Certain superego functions operate in a manner similar to the self-protective and adaptive functions of the ego and powerfully influence the self-protective functions of the ego. Obviously, self-love is an essential component of self-protection and is powerfully influenced by superego forces. There are many ways in which the higher executive functions of the ego function like the superego. Both attempt to anticipate the future, choose from a hierarchy of possible responses, and stay focused on a distant goal, in spite of distractions and frustrations. Both ego and superego can rapidly incorporate into the psyche complex pictures of another human. The superego may identify with the values of the early parents and incorporate their punishing capacities as a way of controlling drive; the ego may incorporate ego traits of a parent (without fully understanding these ego traits) for the purpose of obtaining a wise and powerful way of understanding and addressing the world. These ego traits may include the parent's synthesis of a large amount of experience on how the world works, what it is important to attend to, react to, strive for, how to behave, and so on. In the healthy personality, these trial identifications in the ego serve as templates for trial action. The ego freely modifies these templates through experience. To the extent that a new template violates the rules of the superego, the child must endure self-inflicted pain to gain the benefit of trial identification. To the extent that the superego forbids the examination of a template, the person is precluded from "metabolizing" trial identification by testing it against experience.

Close process attention analysis continually encourages the detailed re-examination of identifications as they are externalized onto the analyst and used by the patient for resistance. Thus, it holds the promise of returning to the patient the free use of two ego functions vital for wise living—trial incorporation of new and apparently successful approaches used by others and the modifying of trial incorporation through experience.

Ego psychoanalysis strives to free the ego from inappropriate and harsh restriction of *verbally* represented thought and feeling. The action-prone patient has moments when his ego is dangerously overpowered by his drives, usually interspersed with longer periods of inappropriate superego harshness and inhibition of both thought and action. In the course of therapy, the technical task with such patients is to help them be less vulnerable to inappropriate superego constriction without weakening the superego in its vital function of appropriately assisting the ego to control drives in the patient's life. The vignettes involving the man and woman who were having outbursts at work are examples of the way in which the analyst might clarify such a distinction to a patient.

Many patients equate the harshness of states of shame or guilt with effective self-control. Wurmser's (1994) data clearly demonstrate the fallacy of this view. In addition to total disengagement of the superego, harshness also often leads to regressions that result in losses of control. A vignette illustrates this process.

> A generally calm and generous man entered treatment with complaints of marital conflict. He reported memories of eruption towards his wife, with open verbal aggression, usually followed by turning on himself. After the turning on the self was clarified, it was possible to see more clearly in the sessions that the memory of the anger at his wife came up at moments when he was feeling guilty. When the analyst noted that the memories of eruption followed moments in which he was cruel to himself, the patient rapidly got the idea. He added that for things to get better with his wife, he would need to feel less guilty about her accusations and remembered several explosions at home that had followed her touching on areas in which he was highly critical of himself.

When turning on the self is severe, the ego may relinquish its protective functions. With more disturbed patients, the inexperienced analyst is tempted to become an auxiliary ego. The experienced analyst is less tempted because he or she understands how such interventions can lend themselves to projection of superego trends onto the analyst and externalization of the conflict. Approaches like this are usually ineffective in altering conduct, and often disrupt therapy. For example, unmodulated action can follow externalization because the patient becomes frightened of the analyst and impulsive under the influence of the defense of identification with the aggressor. Impulsive aggression is a way of defending against the anxiety of the analyst's expected attack. The first child vignette, in which the child threw a block at the analyst's head, illustrates such a moment.

Impulsive patients are deficient in protecting themselves. Analysis of the superego can help strengthen the function of the ego in the ego's self-protective function. There may be a fantasy of invulnerability that allows such patients to disregard their own safety.

A 22-year-old woman several years into twice-a-week psychotherapy for the first time told of her pattern of engaging in casual sexual intercourse with a series of older substance-abusing males. It should be noted that there was no mention during the preceding material about whether her partner was using condoms. This patient had already demonstrated in therapy a ready capacity for externalization.

> *Patient:* Yeah. It was fun. I don't think I will see him again. But we had a really good time. [Patient is relaxed, smiling.]

The intervention that follows illustrates several aspects of Gray's technical recommendations. It is an attempt to focus on the presentation of the patient's thoughts within the hour with a specific view towards the defenses demonstrated at that moment, in spite of the lure of treating the patient's revelation as a clinically important piece of history. It makes use of a rather lengthy preamble in the hope of helping to lift the patient out of the regression of the moment and allow her to hear the intervention and think about it. It also minimizes the possibility that the patient will dismiss the analyst as a moralist.

Analyst: When you were remembering and telling me of the last night's love making, it seemed to me that you were thinking of it a certain way.

Patient: Um?

Analyst: Yes it seems that the feeling was generally one of relaxed pleasure—is that right?

Patient: That's right [smiling, seductive, and provocative tone of voice].

Analyst: I wonder if you could help me understand a little better an aspect of that pleasure. Can you sense what it is that contributes to the sense of safety of the moment that seems to be a part of the pleasure?

Patient: I don't understand what you mean.

Analyst: You are a generally well-informed person. You are aware of current conditions that make thoughts of sexual activity anxiety-provoking for many people [deliberately phrased in a somewhat intellectual and disguised manner hoping to avoid the ego needing to contend with the affect that would be generated by a more graphic description of the dangers of AIDS].

Patient: [She begins to look a little anxious]

Analyst: For a person to have a fantasy of sexual activity in complete comfort, particularly if they are well informed and living in the last few years, they usually have to weave some element into the fantasy to provide the sense of safety. For instance, one person might never have a sexual fantasy without thinking at the same time of some means of providing protection for herself [looks more anxious], another person might have a kind of fantasy of herself as a super-hero who couldn't be hurt [a deepening of concern], a third person might think that no matter what

kind of trouble she was in there would be someone around strong or wise enough to help her out. I suppose it might be a religious figure for some, or a sense of fate. The list could be almost endless. Do you have a sense in these last thoughts what provides the feeling of safety?
Patient: I think it's number two and three.

The patient, in a halting manner, went on to talk of a pattern of counterphobic behavior extending back into early adolescence, including roaming dangerous areas of San Francisco alone and intoxicated, engaging in high-risk sports without instruction or adequate equipment, and traveling in wartorn areas of the world where Americans had been killed. In her subsequent associations, the initial memory was accompanied by significant anxiety followed by hypomanic counterphobic defensive associations. Exploration of these shifts led to clarification of her belief in herself as special to God. Subsequent associations to her feeling unique led to memories in which she recalled her parents as loving, protective, but grossly overindulgent and failing to set protective limits.

Establishing needed auxiliary modalities of treatment with a minimum of disruption to insight-oriented work

Many therapeutic approaches to impulsive patients do not rely on insight. The therapist can lessen or deflect drive, or can serve as, or help to establish, an auxiliary ego or superego for the patient. The use of the hospital, medication, mobilization of social structure (involving family or AA, for instance), education, advice, confrontation with consequences, and prohibition are all approaches that have widespread use and utility. Approaches that are not designed for assisting the development of insight carry the risk of being used for resistance against insight. When the therapist helps the patient avoid the burden of his conflict by assuming some portion of it, the therapist increases the likelihood that the patient will bend his effort toward trying to put the analyst in such a role again.

Gray understands that clinical conditions may require the full range of both analytic and non-analytic interventions. However, his approach helps to select interventions so as to minimize the cost to an ongoing insight-oriented therapy.

In general, those approaches in which the analyst assumes the role of superego are more costly to insight-oriented work than are those approaches in which the analyst assumes the role of the ego. If the analyst behaves in reality as a superego, he increases the difficulty of demonstrating the transferential nature of the patient's view of the analyst as a moral force. Such interventions make it harder to delineate to the patient the transferences that contribute to resistance.

Interventions that require repeated non-analytic action on the part of the analyst are also more susceptible to being used for resistance. For example, administering medication oneself, and periodically inquiring about side effects, is probably more disruptive than sending the patient to a colleague for medication. Referral to a colleague for medical or psychopharmacological treatment is probably more disruptive than dealing with the resistances to thinking about and pursuing a consultation for additional treatment. The analyst should do the minimal amount of thinking for the patient consistent with preserving sufficient comfort and safety of the patient and analyst for the work to continue. Whenever possible, interventions should stay on the side of, "Why have you not permitted yourself to think of such and such?"

Supplemental therapies that depend on charismatic transference for results would generally not be actively encouraged unless there were some overriding consideration or benefit, such as an alcoholic who might die without AA, or a fundamentalist patient with religious orientation working on a focal issue in psychotherapy who maintains a relationship with a charismatic religious leader. (Such a patient might swamp his psychotherapy with charismatic transference if his needs for such transference were not met in another setting.) In general, the coexistence of a charismatic therapy along with an insight-oriented one tends to dim the possibilities of clear transference pictures emerging in therapy. Because charismatic therapies depend on transference for cure, they do not encourage the examination of transference. Thus, the two therapies are fundamentally working at cross-purposes.

There are times when therapists suggest supplemental measures in psychotherapy that encourage the patient to use the healthiest of their repertoire of defenses (see Fenichel 1945). A therapist encouraging a patient to address his depression with obsessional self-care is one example. A therapist encouraging the shift of a paranoid conflict from worries about the CIA to worries about food additives is another. In general, the defense picked for such manipulations is the most adaptive defense available to the patient and one that the therapist has decided *not* to approach in his insight-oriented therapeutic work.

SUMMARY

This chapter offers a picture of the ego psychoanalytic technique developed by Dr. Paul Gray and the manner in which this technique can be of assistance in approaching the technical difficulties of impulsiveness. An important advantage of this method is that it preserves the possibility of insight as a curative force in the therapy.

The benefits of the technique fall into several categories:

1. Analytic responses to powerful drive states.
2. Using words to replace action.

3. Analytic responses to the transference in those subject to primitive mental states.
4. Understanding the symbolic meanings of action.
5. Analyzing ego tendencies (defenses or regressions) that promote or permit impulsive action.
6. Ego splinting.
7. Approaching the harsh and inhibiting functioning of the superego without weakening its necessary role in control of the drives and in self-protection.
8. Establishing needed auxiliary modalities of treatment with a minimum of disruption of insight-oriented work.

References

Fenichel, O. (1941). *Problems of Psychoanalytic Technique*. New York: The Psychoanalytic Quarterly.

—— (1945). *The Psychoanalytic Theory of Neuroses*. New York: Norton.

Freud, A. (1936). *The Ego and the Mechanisms of Defense*. New York: International Universities Press.

Freud, S. (1953). The neuropsychosis of defense. *Standard Edition* 2:172–173.

Gray, P. (1994). *The Ego and the Analysis of Defense*. Northvale, NJ: Jason Aronson.

Langs, R. (1973). The ground rules of psychotherapy. In *Psychoanalytic Psychotherapy*, vol. I, pp. 89–215. New York: Jason Aronson.

Levy, S. T., and Inderbitzin, L. B. (1990). The analytic surface and the theory of technique. *Journal of the American Psychoanalytic Association* 38:371–392.

Wurmser, L. (1974). Psychoanalytic considerations of compulsive drug use. *Journal of the American Psychoanalytic Association* 22:820–843.

5
The Importance of Facial Expressions in Dreams

MARIANNE GOLDBERGER, M.D.

In a discussion focused on analyzing defenses in dreams, I described the use of superego derivatives as defenses (Goldberger 1989). I said, "Very important references to the superego are often contained in the facial expression . . . of a person in a dream" (p. 410). At that time I did not elaborate more fully on either the phenomenon itself or how to help make it useful to a patient in analysis. The purpose of this brief chapter is to do so.

I want to emphasize the fundamental importance of the visual sphere in the formation of the superego functions of the ego. Facial expressions in dreams provide a unique opportunity to study the vivid re-externalization of various kinds of authority. For this reason, facial expressions in dreams can be extremely useful for the analysis of the superego. This is in keeping with Gray's view of the technical advantage of approaching superego manifestations from the point of view of hierarchical functions of the ego (1987, p. 152). The re-externalization of authority can be more convincing in a dream than when one studies a patient's "reading" of the facial expression of another person in waking life, because the dreamer is both interpreter *and creator* of the dreamed facial expressions.*

I have been impressed by the frequency with which patients make only casual reference to someone's facial expression in a dream. A patient may not return to this consciously available detail unless the analyst draws his or her attention to the "passing over" of the image. In other words, the superego reference is very often warded off, and by subtle means. In my experience, once the analyst simply points to the inattention, patients often discover richly affective experiences having to do with early signals of approval or prohibition from important authorities. I emphasize the visual aspects because these communications from authorities can be extremely powerful yet may *never* have been verbalized. Their re-emergence in the telling of a dream is often warded off exactly because of the nonverbal, powerful, but unpleasurable feelings that might be stirred up.

Dreams from the analyses of two patients illustrate the initially vague but ultimately richly detailed and very significant superego derivatives represented in facial expressions.

A man dreamt about an encounter with a woman in which they were discussing some plans regarding work that he was supposed to complete. "She had some kind of look on her face and was doing most of the talking. She showed me pieces of paper that listed what needed to be done, and I thought there was an awful lot and wondered whether I'd be able to do it all." His associations were that he had felt

---

*This is not to minimize the importance of patients' reactions to the facial expressions of others in waking life, especially those of the analyst. For example, it was almost three years before an analytic patient revealed that each day as she passed me on entering my office, she glanced at my face "to see what the weather was."

overwhelmed at his job the day before, that he had left the office late and still had a great deal to do. He dislikes women who are too bossy. That reminded him that his secretary had not been her usual cooperative self yesterday and he had kept wondering if something was the matter. He mentioned that he could usually discern his secretary's mood because of her mobile face. The analyst mentioned that he had been vague regarding the expression on the face of the woman in the dream. At first the patient demurred, saying he had been vague because he could not describe the expression. On second thought, he realized she had a slight resemblance to his sister. With palpable hesitation he then began an attempt to "get hold" of her look. It was mostly in her eyes, a sense of reproach in her eyes. After a deep sigh, he said,

> This is something I never like to think about . . . how she feels about my having gotten further in life. I always did better than her in school, and the worst was when they sent me to a better college. My father was for it, but I could tell from my mother's eyes that she was unhappy about it.

Reading this material, many potential latent themes will spring to the mind of any analyst, but I only want to highlight the defenses that needed analytic attention before the patient could become more free from the constraint of "never liking to think about this." Initially, the reproachful look *itself* was warded off, as if the patient were trying to shield himself from it. The look represented the re-externalized authority, and when he finally did experience the painful feelings evoked by that look, he had nothing but painful thoughts and feelings about his capabilities and achievements. In this way, any aggressiveness toward his sister was kept far away from his awareness.

The second dream comes from the analysis of a young woman who was raised in a rigid, strongly authoritarian household where the children's upbringing was in the hands of a kind but firm German nanny. The patient dreamed that "a woman was showing me around an apartment. I followed her from room to room until we stopped in one room. She had a funny look. I began to rearrange objects in the room the way I like them to be." She said that the dream was just like real life and she sounded as if she were ready to dismiss it on that account. She had been apartment hunting and had looked at lots of different places with her real estate agent. The last part was just like the way she often goes around her own apartment when someone else has been there—that is, she touches various objects to make sure each one is in its right place.

The analyst wondered if the patient could describe the "funny look" of the woman. She responded, "Now that you mention it, it wasn't so funny. It was a stern look. It was the look of my old nanny when she didn't like something we were doing. We would know just from one of those looks that we had to stop whatever it was. But I wasn't doing anything bad in the dream." She became silent. The analyst pointed out her protest about "not doing anything bad," as if her nanny were right now putting a stop to all bad thoughts. Then there were further associations and the patient was able to talk about various kinds of touching that had indeed been strongly prohibited in her early years.

When the patient first related her dream, the nature of the look had *itself* been kept out of full awareness by maintaining its vagueness. Once her attention had been drawn to the look, she could describe it without difficulty, but then her thoughts came to a stop. Finally, she was able to experience the old prohibition during the hour.

Observational studies of young children give ample evidence supporting the importance of preverbal communication between children and parents. Studies of "social referencing" point to the significance of nonverbal signals on specific aspects of ego development—for example, infants discern the safety of a physical activity, such as crossing a "visual cliff," by examining their mothers' facial expressions. Emde and his colleagues (see, for example, Buchsbaum and Emde 1990) have been particularly interested in observing early moral development in young children. They found the tendency toward fairness and reciprocity beginning to develop during the latter part of the second year. They described the process of social referencing during which the child checks with significant others for guidance by means of various signs of prohibition or approval. A whole set of affective consequences are already apparent at the end of the second and third years of life as language is just beginning to become coherent. Although data from infant and child observation are not comparable to data derived from the analysis of adults, I mention them here because they illustrate the importance of emotional expression in the early development of moral inhibitions.

In summary, I have used two clinical examples to demonstrate how the vividness of the re-externalization of authority in dreams can often enhance a patient's emotional conviction about the specific ways that prohibitions are used to interfere with free verbal expression in the analytic situation. Over the years I have come to recognize that the phenomenon of vague reference to facial expressions in dreams is encountered in analysis with considerable frequency. Drawing the patient's attention to the vagueness has been remarkably useful for me and a number of colleagues in eliciting new material. I hope that readers of this report will also find the technique helpful.

References

Buchsbaum, H. K., and Emde, R. N. (1990). Play narratives in 36-month-old children: early moral development and family relationships. *Psychoanalytic Study of the Child* 45:129–155. New Haven: Yale University Press.

Goldberger, M. (1989). The analysis of defenses in dreams. *Psychoanalytic Quarterly* 58:396–418.

Gray, P. (1987). On the technique of analysis of the superego—an introduction. *Psychoanalytic Quarterly* 56:130–154.

6
The Clinical Use of Daydreams in Analysis*

MARIANNE GOLDBERGER, M.D.

I am going to focus on a particular kind of daydream occurring during analysis, which I call a *transference daydream* because it involves a patient's thoughts and feelings about the analyst. Such daydreams can be created outside analytic sessions, or might be newly elaborated during an analytic hour. When they happen during an hour, the analyst has a special opportunity to observe in detail an individual's defenses at work. Daydreams, just like night dreams, can be studied as compromise formations. My emphasis is on one aspect of the compromise, the defense aspect, which automatically involves superego functions as well. The self-critic and editor is importantly motivated by superego demands.

---

* This chapter was presented at the December 22, 1993, meeting of the American Psychoanalytic Association as part of a panel on the clinical use of daydreams.

Here I am borrowing some words from the title of one of Martin Stein's papers: "Critic, Editor, and Plagiarizer" (1989). He used those words to refer to the process of secondary revision in dreams, but in a way they apply even more perfectly to daydreams. Naturally, people edit their daydreams in any case, but when they have to be spoken out loud in the presence of the analyst, the transference spin is likely to be stronger, even if the content of the daydream does not actually include the analyst.

Clinical illustrations of daydreams occurring during analysis will demonstrate how they can enhance our understanding of the patient's defenses. The defenses on which I will focus are the criticisms and editing that go on as the daydream is being created. Since daydreams are much more under the author's conscious control than are dreams during sleep, the process of the ego's editing is more accessible. At the same time, all clinicians are aware that patients are usually more hesitant to tell their daydreams, as compared to night dreams. Most people feel more responsible for them, and the ego's defensive function can be revealed by following carefully a patient's difficulties in relating a daydream.

Before the specific illustrations, an example which can serve as a paradigm may be helpful. A patient is late for an analytic hour and starts talking about the analyst having looked annoyed when he came in. He is almost never late and he goes on to describe the events that led to his lateness today. He doesn't think there was any "unconscious" motive making him late, but he speculates about some possibilities. Then his thoughts go back to the real adversities encountered en route today, emphasizing that they made him late despite the ample time he had given himself. The analyst comments that he sounds as if he is defending himself against an unspoken accusation. The patient agrees, and again mentions the annoyed expression he saw on the analyst's face. The analyst wonders if perhaps he has some ideas about what might be annoying about his lateness. After protesting that he "knows" this is probably not true, the patient speculates that since the analyst is almost always on time, punctuality must be important to her, and therefore she might think he doesn't take his analysis seriously enough if he's late. He says, "It's not so much that you dislike being kept waiting; it's the implied insult that's irritating, that it'll seem as if I don't think you're important enough."

That is the paradigm. Fantasies about the analyst, such as that one, can be viewed as daydreams that are formulated during the analytic session itself and can lead to further elaboration.

My first illustration comes from the analysis of Mrs. A., a biochemist, who had an obsessional character with marked isolation of affect. Her inhibitions were particularly apparent in her fears of any manifestation of aggression. Here I need to describe my former Washington office. A freestanding, three-car garage had been converted into an office which was reached by a different street from the one on which the front of my residence was located. It was situated in such a way that patients could remain unsure about which of two houses belonged to the office. In the course of Mrs. A.'s analysis, some construction work, including several days of bulldozer activity, was done on the back yard which patients passed en route to the office parking area, so the construction was unavoidably conspicuous.

Mrs. A. began having a daydream that I was building a swimming pool, and she had considerable difficulty telling me about it. One reason for the difficulty was her awareness that her thoughts were accompanied by a sense of annoyance, and the idea that I was building it with her money. She was troubled that her feelings were distinctly "not nice," since her sense of worth was heavily dependent on thinking of herself as a nice person. After some analytic work on this issue, she was able to become aware of her resentment about the idea that I made more money than she. For some time, the pool issue remained on the level of thoughts of this kind, usually experienced as intrusive and alien.

One day, during an analytic session, she was a little surprised to find herself picturing people playing in and around a pool. As soon as she realized that this daydream had to do with my pool, she slowed down and finally fell silent. She had become silent because of the annoyed feeling towards me that always made her uneasy. Although she knew better intellectually, she still felt that I would dislike her if she expressed direct criticism of me. All the people in her family, her mother in particular, were touchy about criticism. The next day, the pool fantasy recurred, this time with children in it, playing and using a diving board. She fell silent, and toward the end of the hour said that her thoughts had taken "such a horrible turn" and were so "unspeakable" that she could not bring herself to tell me.

In the next session, she did not remember the daydream until halfway into the hour. She forced herself to tell me her rejected thought, knowing that this was expected in analysis, but accompanied her confession by repeated assertions that this was the most terrible thing she could possibly tell me. She said she had thought about those children around the pool as my children, and after insisting that she did not even know if I had any children, she said,

> And I pictured that one of them got killed by diving into the pool. [After a pause she continued.] And that isn't even the worst of it. The thought that passed through my mind that I can't stand to tell you is: it serves her right! That's the worst thing anybody can say to a mother. That means that I'm wanting one of your children to die. I can't stand it that I'm a person who's capable of even thinking such a thing.

This session was actually a turning point in the analysis. Mrs. A. had told the daydream only under duress; she forced herself to say it out loud. This meant that she maintained a certain defensive distance from the thoughts even as she said them—she disavowed them in a particular way. Her insistence on the vileness of her thoughts meant that she was still honoring her strong prohibitions against aggression. As long as she was in pain she demonstrated to herself and to me that she knew these thoughts were wrong, that she was suffering as a result of thinking them, and that she would try not to allow this to happen again. The intensity of the coercive tone with which she forced herself to talk about these thoughts made it clear to me that more analysis of her inability to own her aggression was necessary before she would be able to integrate the murderous content of the daydream.

The imperative need to keep her archaic prohibitions unchanged began to be understood when she experienced her fears that I would be extremely hurt by her striking me in a highly vulnerable spot, and that I would abandon her by removing myself from her emotionally. Her fantasies about the "worst things one could say to a mother" led to a new awareness of her capacity to entertain cruel thoughts, at the same time as she realized how thoroughly she had learned to inhibit such a capacity. During this period of analysis, she first made meaningful connections with the time when her younger brother was born.

When I was still living in Washington, D. C., I worked with an analytic patient from an affluent and elegant diplomatic family, who "almost never" had thoughts about me. Since she was a sophisticated reader, she was aware that analysis had a lot to do with transference, but she said I was simply never on her mind, and, besides, she did not know anything about me. After several years of analysis, it became clear that she feared saying anything that would suggest that she was superior to me. With trepidation she admitted that she had noted what I was wearing at the beginning of every session, but had never commented, since it was "none of [her] business." It took some time before she could tell me that her hesitation stemmed from her feeling that her clothes were much more fashionable and of better quality than mine.

A couple of years after she had begun to talk about clothes, she was able to tell me that she sometimes had thoughts about the linen napkin on the pillow of my analytic couch. That napkin somehow gave her an unpleasant feeling; she knew she did not want to talk about it, but had no idea why. This remained a puzzle until she revealed her distress about the fact that I did not live in one of the more elegant neighborhoods, as did she. Now she realized that she had had a persistent picture of me as "down-scale," an idea which troubled her so much that she was hardly able to admit it to herself. She thought of me as the main source of income for my family and this meant I would have little money left for myself. That is how she explained why my clothes were not nicer. Then she connected her down-scale view of me with the linen napkins, but could not say any more. I wondered about her initial hesitation to tell me her feelings about the napkins, but she had only the vague feeling of wanting to avoid the subject.

After many months of analytic work dealing with her considerable fears about saying anything that might be hurtful to me, she ultimately remembered that during her childhood, refugees had come peddling at her family's back door, showing a suitcase filled with linens from the old country. She had not thought of this memory since she was a child (though it had been consciously available), and she could not bear to connect that memory to me.

This patient's fixed daydream about me as down-scale served important defensive purposes. It kept out of awareness any competitive feelings toward me, and allowed her feelings of sympathy for me to remain in the foreground. Only after the fantasy was finally explored could she entertain the possibility that there were areas in which she was more capable. She spoke cautiously about her superior sense of color and fabric. Although our ages were identical, she had always imagined that I was younger. Now she was able to mention, and then later enjoy, the fact that she had maintained a more youthful figure than I.

My next example comes from a colleague who has kindly allowed me to use detailed process notes from his analysis of an anxious and depressed woman writer in her twenties.

The patient had been talking about her upset after a telephone conversation with her sister the day before. Her sister had brushed her off, saying this wasn't a good time to talk, and the patient felt she really had to talk to her about a particular issue. She said,

> There's no use in playing this phone game that we always get into, and getting hurt and angry and guilty, all the same things over and over again without talking about the issue itself. It's hard for me to talk to her about this because I'm so neurotic and such a spaz and Lisa is really laid back, and I'm scared she's gonna say "there's no problem."

After a long pause, the analyst inquired about the silence. The patient shrugged the matter off, saying "I don't know ... It's not really important ... I just don't wanna get into it ... it's something I want to say to *Lisa* so why should I say it to *you?*"

The analyst said, "Maybe you're making it unimportant because you don't want to say it in front of me," and the patient said, "Well, I relate differently to Lisa from the way I relate to you."

Silence again. Then she went on.

Okay, I'll just tell you and then it'll be over, and we don't need to discuss it. I'd just been thinking about what I'd say to Lisa when I do call her again. I'd apologize for . . . you know . . . for what a jerk I am about this kind of thing. This is what I'd say to her: "I'm sorry I'm this way, such a spaz. I'm sorry I'm so neurotic and so hyper, but there's this thing that bothers me and I know it's not your fault, it's all me, I'm sorry, but this really bothers me and I wanna talk to you so it won't happen any more, so we won't have a problem when we talk on the phone."

Now I wanna call her. I know what I want to say. The reason I didn't tell you is that I don't want you to think I'm a wimp. I talked to you about what I claim to be valid feelings, and then I diminish them when I plan my talk to Lisa. I want you to take me seriously. You see, that's why I didn't want to tell you because I was afraid you wouldn't take me seriously and then you'd be disapproving. [Pause] I wanna please you, I want to be a *good* patient, quote unquote, so I wanna do the good patient things . . . which is to stick with what I talked about in analysis. You stick with it, have some integrity.

Analyst: If you do it differently you think I'm not going to like it. Apparently I want you to do it just how we talked about it.

Patient: Yeah, you'll look down on me. You'll say, "Oh, you're so good in analysis but when you get out in the real world you suck." Also I'm disappointing you . . . you're helping me, you're thinking you're helping me, and then when I go backwards it's a disappointment, I'm letting you down, I'm failing you.

Analyst: So I have certain expectations of you.

Patient: Yeah, don't you consider this your job? Don't you want to be successful at your job? [Pause] I have two things in my analysis I have to do: I have to come in with something interesting to say, hopefully a dream, and I have to go away improved in some way.

Analyst: A dream is interesting and a daydream about what you plan to say to Lisa isn't.
Patient: Well, daydreams are boring, they don't mean anything. Night dreams . . . well, I like my visual images. I think of myself as a creative dreamer, and I always find a lot to talk about in my dreams that I didn't know about, and also whenever I say I had a dream last night you perk right up. You don't care about daydreams. What's important about daydreams? They're intentional . . . they sort of reflect what I say to you . . . but in this case it didn't . . . I mean this daydream that I just had was inspired by our talk, so it didn't seem relevant at first. I thought it was exactly what we'd been talking about, until you actually made me say it, and then I realized that it *wasn't* what we'd talked about, it was different, it was a new version that was less scary to use; it was modified.
Analyst: It's the new version you didn't want to say, because I don't want you to make new versions.
Patient: Yeah, I should stick to what you say, you're the analyst, you know more than I do. [Pause] Sometimes, if we discuss something about Jay [the patient's boyfriend] and then I talk to him, I say what we talked about, rather than being spontaneous. You know, I'll think back, now what did we say. 'Cause I know it's right. [Pause] Actually, I guess I was kind of lying then, too, I *do* modify it for Jay. [Laughing] Now that I think about it, I totally modify it for him. I water it down. Yeah, you and me talk about X and what I talk to other people about is watered down X. I'll try to bring it up 'cause if it's relevant in my life, if I have a realization about something in analysis I want to talk with the person involved, but I don't think they can take the concentrated version. I have to water it down and make it more palatable for them.

This vignette illustrates several aspects of the use of daydreams in analysis. Initially, the patient was ready to delete the daydream altogether—a common occurrence. Sometimes patients do not realize they are actually having a daydream; only through the process of analysis do they become aware of their frequency. Once the patient was able to tell the daydream, her need for revision became clearer. The ever-present tendency to edit gave access to the patient's hesitations in speaking, and of course the analysis of those defenses yielded more information—about the transference, in particular.

In this example, the patient initially was aware only of her reluctance to tell her daydream. But as she did tell it, she realized she was troubled by having to reveal to her analyst that she had edited it, because this made her think she had revealed a weakness. She was certain this weakness would make the analyst lose respect for her. Exploration of her concern actually led to the expression of another daydream, and this other daydream was about the analyst's expectations of her. It had characteristics that one often sees in such transference daydreams—that is, some elements had already been formed at an earlier time, but were only now brought into the analysis, and, if the defense analysis has been adequate, spontaneous elaboration is possible.

Looking at the first daydream we can learn something about the patient's defenses. She said to her sister, "I know it's not your fault, it's all me." We see the aggression turned on herself. Another way of warding off aggression was demonstrated when she said she had "watered down" the original version—she had taken all the sting out of it. Similarly, in the transference the patient was convinced that the analyst would approve of her only if she bowed to his authority, and renounced assertions of her own.

My last example comes from the supervised analysis of a man in his 30s, the oldest of several children born in quick succession, who came to analysis because of his severe sexual inhibitions. He was referred through a psychoanalytic clinic and was aware from the outset that his analyst was a candidate in training. During the third year of analysis, his analyst became pregnant, and although he had previously been very hesitant to give voice to any thoughts or curiosity about her, at this point he was increasingly able to talk about his fantasies, or rather his daydreams, about her.

The sequence I would like to describe contains old daydreams about the analyst, never spoken about before, as well as a new daydream spawned during an analytic hour. As already mentioned, this phenomenon is not uncommon in fantasies about the analyst—that is, they are often present for a long time before the patient can risk talking about them. After analysis of defenses against verbalization of such daydreams, which have been preconscious or conscious all along, the patient also feels freer to have new, spontaneous elaborations.

When the patient first talked about the analyst's pregnancy, his upset feelings were dominated by envy, expressed primarily in terms of the analyst "having her life in order," in contrast to himself. He was concerned about her being away when the baby came, and even more concerned that she might be away for a long time, or even permanently. During this period he was starting to earn more money through free-lancing. On one occasion he was elaborating on his difficulties charging by the hour for his free-lance work, and his reluctance to charge for all the hours he had worked for fear that his client would leave him. The material seemed to parallel so closely the situation of his analytic fee that the analyst suggested such a connection. The patient had not been aware of this but he understood and was made uneasy by it. He soon mused, "What makes a person announce what they're usually paid," consciously referring to his free-lance fee. The analyst recalled that during the consultation she had told him what her usual fee was. The patient had probably had thoughts about this subject at that earlier time, but had been unable to talk about them, and he might be close to recalling these thoughts now.

During the very next analytic hour the patient said he had been wondering why the analyst brought up the fee since he himself had not been aware of the fee issue. He said, "You don't usually just bring up something I haven't talked about at all." He described a number of fantasies. He thought first that the analyst wondered how he handles his money, and why he apportions money as he does. He thought that she was "just curious," not critical or intrusive. He emphasized that he uses his free-lance income for "extras" and does not count on it as part of his regular income. He also fantasied reasons why the analyst might need money, and said, "You've a right to say, 'What about me?'" (The analyst had recently moved into a new office.) Then he confessed that he'd often wondered about the reason why she charged him a low fee. Maybe in the beginning she took him for educational reasons, but now that she was out of her student phase she would drop patients like him. Perhaps he should come only twice a week, and step aside for high-fee patients.

Then he talked about the time the analyst had told him she was pregnant. He was pretty sure she had told him only because she had had to, that she would have avoided it if she could. He said he felt the analyst was angry about this, and then he became silent. He did not know what more to say. After the analyst had addressed his difficulty in elaborating his picture of her being angry, the patient went on. The analyst had not answered his few personal questions about her, but tried to analyze them, so he *now* said he had concluded that she strongly prefers to be anonymous. As he entered the office today his brief glance at her face had made him think that perhaps she was angry. Now he felt sure that this was the case, and that the reason was that she had been forced to tell more about herself than she wanted to.

He returned to his image of her preferring to keep her pregnancy hidden from him. His thoughts now went to his mother's secretive ways. He had previously described his mother's furtive manner in regard to her affair with the man who was later to become his stepfather. He described in greater detail than before the forceful ways in which he felt she indicated that his curiosity was entirely unacceptable. He also mentioned that at the same time his mother would leave visible traces of her lover's presence in the house.

This example illustrates that interpreting the defense in a daydream may allow the patient to remember more details and even a whole forgotten segment of the daydream. It also demonstrates how a patient's increasing ability to elaborate a transference daydream may facilitate understanding inhibitions, as well as the genetic origins of those inhibitions. This patient spontaneously made the connection to the genetic origins (thereby documenting the transference of defense).

In conclusion, I have shown that patients are commonly reluctant, even fearful, about revealing daydreams about their analysts. A frequent fear has to do with sounding foolish, in case they are "wrong" in their fantasy. Most patients are embarrassed about the possibility of saying something about their analysts that is "way off." A considerable amount of analysis is required before they are willing to mention their speculations out loud. After all, transference daydreams are invented pictures of the analyst. If we can create an analytic atmosphere in which these fantasy views of the analyst are taken as a unique source of information, transference daydreams will become more available.

The analysis of defense allows a patient to make the unattended background into a daydream. And I use the term *unattended background* to refer to thoughts available to consciousness that are nevertheless not put into words. It refers to Fenichel's (1941) famous advice about interpretation: an interpretation is at the right level if the preconscious derivative can be recognized as such by the patient, *merely by turning his attention to it.* As the defense imagery of daydreams is analyzed, images of the analyst gradually shift from a restrictive authority to an object of sexual and aggressive drives.

References

Fenichel, O. (1941). *Problems of Psychoanalytic Technique.* New York: Psychoanalytic Quarterly.

Stein, M. H. (1989). How dreams are told: secondary revision—critic, editor, plagiarist. *Journal of the American Psychoanalytic Association* 37:65–88.

7

External Reality as Defense

LAWRENCE B. INDERBITZIN, M.D.
STEVEN T. LEVY, M.D.

> He too wants to experience realities and despises everything that is merely imaginary.
>
> Sigmund Freud

Our purpose is to examine the relation between external reality and the work of clinical psychoanalysis. In doing so, we have chosen the frequently used phrase "grist for the mill" as a point of departure, because we believe that a change in its usage in relation to psychoanalytic technique highlights many of the issues we wish to explore. This change can be described as follows. Originally, "grist for the mill" referred to the need to analyze any unanticipated intrusion of external reality into the analytic work. Such intrusions were to be treated as grist for the mill of analytic exploration. In some quarters, "grist for the mill" is now used to indicate that everything is analyzable. In our view, this shift from "analyzing everything" to "everything is analyzable" represents a change in the way some analysts regard external reality in terms of its role in clinical work and clinical technique. In the extreme, this means that it makes little or no difference how much or what kind of reality enters into the psychoanalytic situation, including interactions between analyst and analysand, because everything is analyzable. We shall emphasize external reality used in the service of defense by analysands and by analysts, the latter often obscuring this defensive activity by assuming a position about reality epitomized by the second meaning of "grist for the mill."

In the past, most analysts would have agreed that the central subject of psychoanalytic exploration is the analysand's unconscious intrapsychic activity. Invariably, during the course of analytic treatment there occur instances in which some piece of external reality intrudes noticeably, and sometimes dramatically, into the analytic situation. Examples include interactions around appointments, schedule changes, bill paying, insurance, unavoidable extra-analytic contacts between analyst and patient, and a host of similar phenomena, all involving some piece of external reality that becomes "grist for the mill." By this we mean that the analyst helps the patient to explore how an external event is elaborated intrapsychically and becomes the subject of mental processes that reveal similarities to those conflicts and compromises that have been the focus of the day-to-day analytic scrutiny. Such grist for the mill becomes a means of demonstrating to the patient the unity and connectedness of mental life, at times providing the analysand with concrete and vivid examples that enhance his or her conviction about previous interpretive work. Adoption of the "grist for the mill" metaphor is an indicator of psychoanalysts' search for ways to make interpretive use of external reality when it intrudes into the analytic situation. Many have emphasized that extra-analytic contacts and other reality events stir up important material and can enliven the analytic process. Analysts have also recognized that external reality factors can disrupt the analytic work and make certain problems more difficult to analyze.

ON REALITY

Psychoanalytic investigators, including Freud, have written extensively about the issue of reality and its place in mental functioning. While it is beyond our scope to review these many psychoanalytic contributions to a theory of reality, it would be fair to say that Freud's efforts, as well as those of many who followed him, can be viewed as centering on two related themes: (1) psychic (as opposed to external) reality, to which we could attach contributions that focus on the many different views of reality and its highly subjective nature; and (2) the reality principle and its relation to the pleasure principle in normal and pathological mental functioning. The first of these themes emphasizes the role of mental processes in creating what is for each person a highly subjective and ever-changing view of inner and outer worlds. Freud and all psychoanalysts after him recognize that what exists as a person's private version of reality is heavily influenced by wishes, fears, and fantasies, both conscious and unconscious. It is this private or psychic reality, not any objectively and externally corroborated reality, that plays a crucial role in the outcome of intrapsychic processes. From the technical side, it becomes one of the central tasks of the analyst to help the analysand become as fully conscious of this psychic reality as possible so that its subjective and usually highly distorting[1] nature can be explored and modified in relation

---

[1] As Hoffman (1983) pointed out, "distortion" can, and we believe should, refer primarily "to selective inattention to and sensitivity to certain facets" (p. 409).

to the analysand's mature efforts at self-examination, perception of the analyst, and adaptation.

Freud developed the reality principle as a second principle of mental functioning to represent the ego's attempts to achieve gratification of drives by turning to reality rather than to hallucinatory wish fulfillment. Hartmann (1956) filled in our knowledge of the way the ego's activities are governed by both pleasure and reality concerns, and how the reality principle extends beyond merely following the pleasure principle in relation to external reality. The reality principle means "that uncertain pleasure is renounced" (Hartmann 1956, p. 32), that postponement, delay, anticipation, and other ego functions come to "wrest our activities from the immediate need for discharge inherent in the pleasure principle" (p. 33). Hartmann noted that reality can be said to make its own demands, although it is not correct to consider reality or the reality principle as opposed to the pleasure principle. The interactions are complex, and, in relation to our main theme, we can recognize the possibilities reality considerations afford in regard to the ego's defense against the pleasure demands of the drives.

We wish to mention here Rapaport's (1958) contribution to a theory of ego autonomy in which he explored the complex relationships among the psychic structures. Specifically, he described the way the ego, in order to maintain the independence of its activities from impingement both by reality concerns and by the demands of drive forces, balances inner and outer pressures. He referred to this independence as *autonomy*, noting that such autonomy is only relative, the ego always being vulnerable to having its activities or functions co-opted by drive or environmental influences. Especially pertinent to our interest is his idea that "the ultimate guarantees of the ego's autonomy from the id are man's constitutionally given apparatuses of reality relatedness" (p. 18). He (along with Freud and Hartmann [1956]) referred to the obsessional's exaggeration of reality relatedness, "reasonableness," and elaboration of the secondary process as a means of defending the ego against what are perceived to be drive demands that would compromise the ego's autonomy. Rapaport (1958) noted that while such defense "thus maximizes the ego's autonomy from the id," it is at the cost of "ever-increasing impairment of the ego's autonomy from the environment" (p. 23). Such a theoretical matrix serves as a means of conceptualizing the way in which reality can be viewed as balanced against the pressures of hidden unconscious wishes, fantasies, and prohibitions in the psychoanalytic situation. We are especially interested in the use to which both analyst and analysand put reality to defend against full awareness of unconscious drive elements in the treatment setting, recognizing that such a use of reality can enhance as well as impair analytic treatment. We wish to show how analysands make use of reality factors to help them manage both the oscillation between experiencing and contemplation during sessions and the shifts into and out of an analytic mode which they require in order to fit analytic work, with its sometimes intense emotional upheavals, into their everyday lives.

It is surprising how little has been written about the role of external reality in neurotic conflict and its effect on psychoanalytic technique. Fenichel (1945) emphasized that the external world shapes defenses and that it is only when a conflict originating between the id and the external world has been "transformed into a conflict between the id and the ego" that "a neurotic conflict can develop" (p. 130). In addition to stressing that the external world can ward off impulses through the ego *only*, Fenichel reminded us that external reality can also be defended against when it is a threatening stimulus. Focusing on extra-analytic contacts, Ganzarain (1991) wrote about reality in the psychoanalytic situation, emphasizing the dynamic balance between reality and fantasy. Gray

(1973, 1986) pointed out the importance of focusing on the analysand's thinking *processes* in the here-and-now rather than on the content of the thoughts as they apply to external reality.

DEFENSE

Although Freud first used the term *defense* as early as 1894, it is Anna Freud's (1936) landmark treatise, *The Ego and the Mechanisms of Defense*, that has most influenced our views on defense. Her lucid description of ten specific and repetitive modes of defensive ego functioning initiated in response to signal anxiety is familiar to most analysts. Despite the clinical utility of these formulations in understanding psychic conflict, to consider defense only in terms of specific mechanisms is misleading (Schafer 1968). It implies that only certain ego functions are used for purposes of defense. In fact, the entire range of ego functioning, including those ego activities most closely associated with external reality (perception, motility, reality testing), can be used for defensive purposes.

Brenner (1982) argued that a given mental content or function is a defense if its function is to reduce unpleasure. Apfelbaum and Gill (1989) pursued a similar line of reasoning, emphasizing the relativity of defense. They noted that any mental content or function can be either defense or wish, depending on its relation *at the moment* to some other given content or function. In most instances, multiple defenses operate synergistically rather than in a unitary or isolated manner. These important revisions of the theory of defense and psychic conflict provide the foundation for our ideas about the use of external reality as defense.

There are many clinical examples described in the literature of the ego altering its perception of reality in the service of defense, including fainting, negative hallucinations, and *déjà vu* phenomena, to mention but a few. However, these all represent attempts at denial of external reality for defensive purposes. The emphasis, enhancement, or exaggeration of external reality in the service of defense has received far less attention and is central to the position we take here. The impetus for this exploration derives, in part, from certain points of view prominent in current trends within psychoanalysis, specifically the reality of traumatic events in the causation of psychopathology and the focus on aspects of the "real" relationship in the theory of the therapeutic action of psychoanalysis.

We suspect that for many analysts the concept of the use of external reality to defend against psychic reality is so obvious that no further explanation seems necessary. This is probably particularly true for analysts who view psychopathology as the result of infantile sexual and aggressive conflicts as they are embodied in unconscious fantasies. For them, the understanding and resolution of pathological compromise formations is the central analytic task. They regularly pursue the infantile origins of instinctual conflicts via the analysis of resistance to effect greater freedom in mental life. These analysts probably could find common examples of reality as defense in almost every analytic hour. For instance, they might describe the patient who comes to sessions late over months, or even years, and each time cites a reality reason in order to avoid thinking about the pattern of lateness and the conflicts motivating it. Another patient doggedly recites in minute detail everything that has happened "out there in real life," either without affect or with exaggerated affect in order to prevent frightening feelings about the analyst from emerging in the sessions. Other examples are patients who manage to keep something stirred up in reality at all times in order to avoid facing their inner experience in the analytic situation. Still other patients use memories of "real" traumas, such as physical and sexual abuse, in order to defensively deny or obscure their own active aggressive and sexual impulses.

We suspect that some analysts with a narrative or subjectivist theoretical orientation would consider a further exploration of external reality as defense to be outmoded, irrelevant, and even erroneous. They might argue, for instance, that consideration of external reality as defense inevitably installs the analyst in the position of arbiter of what is real and important.

It is reasonable to inquire what it is about the compelling nature of reality that contributes to its extensive involvement in defensive processes. Perhaps the most obvious factor is the easy visibility of reality, as compared with the inferential nature of inner life. This not only means that reality can be consensually validated but also that it can be used easily to muster corroborating allies, including the analyst. Second, what actually occurs in reality is in the vast majority of instances relatively socialized and tempered when compared to the raw content of unconscious fantasies. Social pressures that emphasize reality events, such as current interest in child abuse, may make it more difficult for analyst and analysand to get beyond external reality.

Developmental factors are important in understanding the ego's pervasive use of reality as defense. Freud (1923) emphasized "that the character of the ego is a precipitate of abandoned object-cathexes and that it contains the history of those object-choices" (p. 29). The developing ego, via identification, internalizes adaptive functions formerly carried out by important external objects. Prominent among these are controls which serve essential defensive purposes.

Various neurotic constellations tend to utilize reality in multiple ways for defensive purposes. We have already noted this in regard to obsessional patients. Gray (1982, 1986) referred to patients who manifest narcissistic personality problems as being "reality bound." Phobic patients use reality magically for defensive purposes. They often seek out the phobic object, and one can frequently observe phobic and counterphobic attitudes occurring together in ways that result in defensive uses of reality. For instance, Allen (1974) described phobic patients who are afraid of looking at the analyst, including the analyst's possessions, thought processes, and feelings. In exploring scopophilic and exhibitionistic conflicts in these patients, Allen noted, "I believe that the patient who is fearful of turning his scopophilia on the analyst, the analytic setting, and the analytic process—the entertaining and vividly verbal patient who invites the analyst to look *with* him at his life and dreams but who does not look *at* the analyst, literally and figuratively—is actually preventing the analyst from looking at him in a more deeply perceiving, more emotionally intimate way" (pp. 106–107). He emphasized that it may be difficult for either patient or analyst to detect the scopophilic–exhibitionistic anxiety, particularly if the analyst is fascinated by the patient's life or threatened by the patient's curiosity about and scrutiny of the analyst. In such cases, the patient's exhibitionistic focus on some piece of reality is also often itself part of a counterphobic attitude. If undetected, the underlying anxieties remain unanalyzed, and one of the patient's autonomous ego functions (perception) remains significantly compromised. In these situations the patient is using reality to defend against phobic anxieties about looking at the real analyst. This is the converse of using the reality of the analyst as a defense, a subject we shall discuss below.

We believe that the use of external reality as defense poses a formidable obstacle for the analyst and that its specific use is determined by each patient's unique conflicts and compromises. Furthermore, this may go unrecognized, partly because of the exceedingly complex melding of the use of external reality with other defenses. In addition to repression and denial, one regularly observes that defensive displacements, a variety of reversals, and sometimes actions are combined with the defensive use of external reality. Transference as defense or resistance is usually at the center of the processes we are describing.

TRANSFERENCE

Most analysts agree that the analysis of transference is of central importance to the psychoanalytic endeavor. However, as Bird (1972) pointed out more than two decades ago, this does not mean that transference is easily or well understood. Freud wrote only a few papers on the subject, and his ideas about it were grounded in the topographic theory. As with many of his key discoveries, he made no systematic attempt to incorporate or integrate transference into his structural theory. A comprehensive review of transference is beyond the scope of this discussion. Instead, we shall focus on transference as a defense, and its relation to reality.

Transference creates a current interpersonal reality to defend against awareness of troublesome internal wishes and fears. As Arlow (1987) pointed out, transference is not only resistance to recollection, as originally discussed by Freud, but also functions as defense against the current emergence of conflicted, infantile drive derivatives and affects. Careful attention to the process of the patient's associations often reveals that transference as a defensive compromise formation appears just at the moment when the patient's associations are close enough to derivatives of unconscious wishes toward the original object to stimulate signal anxiety. This is the most familiar manifestation of transference. Such instances are usually described in the literature as "transference resistances," and interpretations of them are so common that they are at times almost formulaic. Sometimes, in addition to the displacement, a reversal takes place, so that the impulses and feelings experienced and expressed toward the analyst are the opposite of those originally experienced toward important figures in childhood. Although the latter is a somewhat more complicated situation, it nevertheless still involves primarily the displacement of impulses and can be relatively easily recognized by the analyst.

Very often, especially in the early stages of analysis, another defensive structure, sometimes referred to as "displacement of the transference" or "resistance to the awareness of the transference" (Gill 1982), complicates the situation further. This displacement can involve either the transference of impulses toward the analyst or the more difficult to recognize transference of defense.

Transference of defense, in contrast to transference of impulse, was first made explicit by Anna Freud (1936), who emphasized that sometimes "the instinctual impulse itself never enters into the transference at all, but only the specific defense adopted by the ego" (p. 20). Furthermore, in regard to technique, she advocated a change in the focus of the analyst's attention from instinctual derivatives to defenses against them, stating, "The interpretation of the second type of transference [defense] is more fruitful than that of the first type, but it is responsible for most of the technical difficulties which arise between the analyst and the patient" (p. 21). She pointed out that the reason for this is that the defense transference is not experienced by the patient as a foreign body; rather, it is ego syntonic. In discussing the nature of personality disorders, Fenichel (1945) elaborated on the same points in regard to transference of defense. More recently, Brenner (1982) has emphasized that transference is always a compromise formation containing drive, defense, and superego elements. Nevertheless, as Gill (1982) and Gray (1973) pointed out, transference of defense is emphasized much less than transference of impulse in analytic practice and in the literature.

Gray (1987, 1991) described two types of transference of defense in his papers on superego analysis as well as a rationale and methodology for analyzing them. Both represent externalized superego manifestations that are repeated in the transference in order to defend against emerging conflicted drive derivatives, especially aggression. In one version, the analyst is cast as the authoritarian inhibitor, controller, and even critic in order to achieve auxiliary protection. In the other, the analyst is experienced as an affectionate, approving, and protecting authority for the same purpose. In emphasizing that transferences such as these are under-recognized in analysis, Gill (1982) considered all "defense transferences" (p. 30) as resistances to the awareness of transference, and transference of defense as a defense against transference of wish.

We emphasize that these transferences of defense are not limited to wider-scope patients and in fact are ubiquitous among neurotic, analyzable patients. Because transferences of defense tend to be more silent and ego syntonic than transferences of impulses and also represent an additional level of complexity, they are in general more difficult to recognize. There is yet an additional reason why the second type of transference of defense described by Gray (1991) (the permissive, affectionate, approving protector) is difficult to recognize and analyze. All analysts want to be helpful and see themselves as such. As Bird (1972) pointed out, "One of the most serious problems of analysis is the very substantial help which the patient receives directly from the analyst in the analytic situation" (p. 285). He went on to describe and give examples of the many ways that the analyst and the analytic situation may be of current real value to the patient, while at the same time this "intrusion of reality into the analysis" (p. 286) interferes with the analytic task. Bird went so far as to assert that "this kind of usefulness may be one of the major reasons why analysis fails" (p. 286).

In his clinical examples of common "reality-caused" problems, Bird stated, "In none of these patients did any significant transference relationship develop" (p. 286). Bird was referring to the fact that the patient's underlying infantile instinctual conflicts did not manifest themselves in the analysis in a way in which they could be analyzed. Bird brought us to the heart of a problem that still plagues analysts: a misleading division between transference and reality. Reality does not prevent transference from developing because of some inherent antagonism between transference and reality. In fact, when Bird said, "They clung to their actual dependence upon the analyst in the analytic situation" (p. 286), he was describing an important aspect of transference—namely, utilizing the imago of the helpful, supportive, protective parent to ward off other conflicts. The reality of the analyst's helpfulness is used defensively to reinforce this transference of defense. Transference always attaches itself to and exploits some reality. This occurs not only with the transference of impulses *but also transference of defense.* We do not wish to imply that a better understanding of transference of defense, and in particular the way it exploits external reality in the service of defense, will render patients such as those described by Bird easily analyzable. This depends on many factors within both analysand and analyst, especially the strength of the resistances and counter-resistances. However, to the extent that the analyst needs to maintain an image of himself as a helpful, supportive protector, the patient's transference of defense is likely to move the analyst into a co-enactment that precludes interpretive resolution.

INTERACTION

Contemporary psychoanalysts such as Gill (1983), Hoffman (1983), Jacobs (1973, 1986), Mitchell (1992), and others have called our attention to the complexity of the interaction between analyst and patient. While it is certain that previous generations of analysts were aware of both the complexity of the analytic relationship and of the many-layered contributions made to it by each participant in the analytic dyad, some modern analysts have focused increasing attention on acknowledging the role the analyst plays in determining how and why the patient experiences and interacts with the analyst in the unique ways we usually refer to as "the transference." Many analysts call for a recasting of our technical theory in interactional terms, moving away from an analysand-centered, intrapsychic focus. We believe this movement reflects, at least in part, the impact of interest in object relations theory; the increasing recognition of and wish to incorporate the wide diversity in technical approaches among different psychoanalytic schools; and emphasis on the here-and-now, viewed as meaning all that occurs between patient and analyst during analytic sessions; and especially, viewing the analyst–patient relationship as having a "real" component with an underscoring of the significant impact of the analyst's "real" personality traits.

What, from a psychoanalytic perspective, is meant by interaction? We believe the term should be and is used clinically to refer to instances when psychological processes in either patient or analyst affect the psychological processes of the other in some observable or potentially observable way. Psychoanalysis as a therapeutic endeavor can be seen as a series of interactions, set in motion by the analyst, that are designed to influence the analysand. It is argued that our older intrapsychic language ignores the interactive perspective, obscures the biases, positive and negative, introduced by the analyst, and underestimates the analysand's capacity accurately to recognize and respond to the analyst as a real and often conflicted participant (Hoffman 1983).

Many of these issues are raised in a slightly different context in the expanding literature on transference–countertransference phenomena, often described as interaction. Mutual influence is certainly at the center of such thinking, frequently delineated in terms of projective and introjective identification, role responsiveness (Sandler 1976), and related processes.

We wish to note two central points in support of our view that an interactive technical emphasis has the potential for and sometimes serves defensive purposes in its focus on the reality of the analytic relationship. One concerns self-observation; the other, the difference between intrapsychic and interpersonal perspectives. It is paradoxical that many who emphasize an interactive focus point critically to the traditional way of describing the analyst as a blank screen (Hoffman 1983) whose commentary on the analysand's distortions of the analyst in the transference represents a mistaken and defensive belief in a single, objective reality (Mitchell 1992). Yet these same interactionists emphasize the reality of the therapeutic encounter, the "real" contribution of the analyst to what becomes transference, and build a case that these "real" interactions should occupy center stage in the interpretive process. Thus, on the one hand, there is no "independent, unmediated, objective reality" (Mitchell 1992); on the other, real interactions are the most appropriate data for interpretive intervention. While we believe this apparent paradox rests on an either/or, polarized and polarizing premise, it is a premise characteristic of the psychoanalytic literature on interaction. This premise holds that the analyst must choose between reality as totally objectively discoverable, and reality as relative, subjective, and unknowable. We believe there is a broad middle ground that acknowledges the importance of subjectivity *and* the possibility of a consensually validatable "objective" reality.

TECHNICAL ISSUES

It is our contention that the analytic situation is deliberately structured to diminish the role of external reality in mental functioning in the service of changing the balance of forces so that the analysand's and analyst's ability to observe intrapsychic processes is enhanced. In an extension of Rapaport's (1958) theoretical view to technical issues, the psychoanalytic situation is designed to bring about a diminution of reality input by virtue of the analyst's anonymity, relative silence, and focus on the analysand's inner experiences rather than outside life. The use of the couch reduces "reality feedback." Safety from "outside" influences is provided by the strictly managed "boundaries" of the analytic situation (including privacy, confidentiality, and time considerations) in order to facilitate observation of the influences of id and superego pressures on the ego. This decrease in the analysand's relative autonomy from id and superego is what is often referred to as "therapeutic regression" or "regression in the service of the ego," although we believe regression is not the best or most approriate term to describe what occurs clinically. Intrusions of reality, whether extra-analytic or occurring within the hour, interfere with the analysand's capacity for observation of himself, especially of his id and superego pressures. It is our clinical impression that analysands turn to these interactive realities, whether "outside grist" concerns, "real" interactions, or transference, in order to defend themselves against observing and fully experiencing intrapsychic pressures. It is here that the analyst intervenes to examine why the analysand considers such defense to be necessary. Even transference represents a turning to reality in the sense of attempting to establish or enact in reality what is unconsciously experienced as too painful or otherwise conflictual intrapsychically.

Derivatives of id and superego pressures are invariably represented in the therapeutic interaction. We believe these real derivatives, which certainly merit analytic scrutiny, represent tamed or socialized versions of their intrapsychic counterparts. Long ago, Hartmann (1948) noted that the singularly human capacity for repression and unconscious containment of instincts desocializes them, increasing their dangerousness.

This is especially true for aggression, which is difficult fully to enact in reality except under exceptional circumstances. Analysands and analysts alike seek protection from the full and primitive impact of unconscious forces by emphasizing their interactive representation in reality. Thus, the analysand's "cruelty" toward the analyst in disregarding the latter's interpretive efforts, or in calling attention to the analyst's obvious or not-so-obvious shortcomings, is tame when compared to unconscious, destructive aims. We recognize that it is often via interactions that the presence of such aims is inferred and initially made observable. Our point is that the analyst must create a balance between attention to the interactive and to the intrapsychic. We believe that tilting toward the interactive, which is emphasized increasingly in the current psychoanalytic literature on technique, may be motivated by analysts wishing to avoid the full and frightening impact of unconscious derivatives in their fantastic, neurotogenic (rather than socially realized) forms. When patients emphasize the analyst's "real" contribution to interaction, this is often recognized as avoidant. When analysts do it, it may be disguised under a cloak of self-revelatory honesty, pseudo-egalitarianism, and supposedly appropriate focus on transference–countertransference. This is sometimes defensive in origin, even if it seems to capture the here-and-now moment of greatest affectivity of the analytic process, a long-cherished criterion for correctness of focus of intervention. "Here-and-now" likewise can refer to events observable in the patient's associations, reflecting manifestations of intrapsychic conflict that may include interactions as content. In structural terms, free association provides an opportunity to observe the ego managing intrapsychic forces rather than a way of discovering unconscious content as in the topographic point of view. This allows for a better way of thinking about psychoanalytic technique that addresses the balance between intrapsychic and interactive emphases. When an analysand's associations turn to the analyst, whether as source of excitation, gratification, protection, or punishment, one can see the ego pursuing its aims of managing intrapsychic equilibrium. Thus, one might comment, "You think of me at this moment in your thoughts, disapproving of your wish to outsmart everyone, in order to shore up your ability to control your worries about your competitiveness getting out of hand," instead of "You remind yourself of my comment yesterday about who is in the know in here as an example of how we compete with each other." One is not more "correct" than the other, but the analyst makes choices on the basis of where the patient's attention is best directed, where the dangers lie, strategies for therapeutic enhancement of the ego's autonomous capacity of self-observation and management of intrapsychic pressures and anxieties.

EXTRA-ANALYTIC CONTACTS AND REALITY

In a paper on extra-analytic contacts, Ganzarain (1991) pointed out how little has been written about this subject. The idea that reality prevents, distorts, or dilutes the transference is challenged by those who assert that transference will prevail (Strean 1981, Tarnower 1966, Weiss 1975). Although potential hazards to analysis are acknowledged, the main emphasis is that extra-analytic contacts can and should be analyzed. They are compared implicitly and explicitly to dreams with regard to their technical handling and their positive impact on the analytic process. "The 'special event' triggers off intense feelings and fantasies about the analyst and like the dream can lead directly to the unconscious" (Weiss 1975, p. 74).

Scopophilic and exhibitionistic conflicts, as well as primal-scene material, often become manifest in response to extra-analytic contacts. Patients often do not mention these "special events" during the analysis (Weiss 1975). Tarnower (1966) suggested that patients respond to outside meetings with unusually strong feelings because they are off-guard. He and Ganzarain (1991) noted that both analysand and analyst may respond symptomatically, particularly phobically.

We have stated previously that reality does not prevent transference. The important issue concerns which transference will prevail and whether or not it will be analyzable, something that is not predictable. The clinical examples cited in the extra-analytic contact literature focus almost exclusively on instances of transference of impulses stimulated by extra-analytic contacts, and only secondarily on the defenses that these impulses stir up. Undoubtedly, such instances do occur, but in our experience, not exclusively or primarily. Instances are more likely to occur with unexpected extra-analytic contacts and when some aspect of reality coincides with an unconscious fantasy in a manner that results in a breakdown of defenses and subsequent confusion and symptom formation. This can create a fault in the analytic work because the logical line of interpretation based on gradually accumulated understanding of a patient's central conflicts is disrupted. The fault can be widened by the analyst's premature interpretation of the id eruption. This sometimes represents a special instance of interpreting everything observed, which can lead to a chaotic analytic situation. A principle of relevance should be applied that gives priority to interpretation of the important determinants of the patient's thoughts and feelings that are close enough to the surface to be observed by the analysand. Interpretation of transference impulses before exploration of associated fantasied dangers that stimulate defense leads to defensive flight, often manifest in the form of an intellectualized agreement with the analyst.

Patients sometimes respond to an extra-analytic contact by some version of, "It wasn't as bad as I thought it would be." In doing so, they emphasize that the imagined dangers are both outside the analytic situation and not as bad as expected. A *fantasy* of safety prevails in the here-and-now, and the external reality occurrences are used to reinforce this transference of defense. We have commonly noted such a constellation, which is similar to those alluded to by Weiss (1975). He hypothesized that patients who do not bring up extra-analytic contacts in their analytic sessions "wish to return rapidly, without analytic scrutiny, to the safety and regression of the analytic situation and to the silent gratification of the transference" (p. 75). We would emphasize *fantasy* of safety. Whether patients mention the extra-analytic contacts spontaneously, or whether the analyst points out the avoidance and thus brings up the topic, patients emphasize their anxiety "out there." They noisily point to the dangers out there that they have survived. The content of this material is usually concerned with scopophilic and exhibitionistic conflicts. However, a counterphobic attitude prevails in the analysand, and sometimes in the analyst, in the service of avoiding the very same issues within the analytic situation. This defensive structure becomes even clearer in those not infrequent instances when extra-analytic contacts are sought in repeated, active attempts to overcome an unconscious infantile conflict situation. Fenichel (1953) referred to this as a "flight to reality" (p. 170) and stated, "The experience that imaginary ideas connected with a certain situation actually do not prove true, is precisely the basis of most counterphobic attitudes." The situation must be sought repeatedly because no amount of reassurance is sufficient proof that the feared fantasy will never occur. The essence of the most familiar counterphobic mechanism involves a reversal, turning passive into active. When actively sought, the feared situation can actually be pleasurable, but when the feared situation is experienced passively, as often occurs with extra-analytic contacts, the old fears emerge.

In other instances, the counterphobic individual remains

passive, depending on the omnipotent protection and permission of someone of importance, such as the analyst. Sometimes patients state this directly in some form of, "I was scared, but you didn't look scared, and I knew you wouldn't let anything bad happen." We believe that the "hundreds of varieties of this mechanism" to which Fenichel referred (1953, p. 169) have been somewhat overlooked, especially with regard to extra-analytic contacts.

Certain realities within the analytic situation cannot and should not be avoided. Similarly, all extra-analytic contacts cannot be avoided, particularly within psychoanalytic institutes. Furthermore, occasional professional contacts are not the same as extensive social contacts. We agree with those who have emphasized that when these contacts do occur, attempts should be made to analyze them. However, there are vast differences in the way different analysts approach this task. Arlow (1987) pointed out that an analyst's theoretical model inevitably influences technique. Clinical vignettes are difficult to assess and can often be misleading, but it is our impression that the technical approaches to reality in the extra-analytic contact literature are rooted in the topographic model. The multiple ways that transference operates defensively, and reality is used synergistically and collaboratively to reinforce it, have not been explored and described. This is a striking example of the "developmental lag" in technique described by Gray (1982).

Every analyst knows of instances in which the reality of the analyst in the present and some usually unknown transference paradigm from the past combine in a way that results in a failed analysis. When experiences in reality coincide closely with aspects of inner conflicts, analysis of these conflicts inevitably becomes more complicated and difficult, if not impossible. "Experiences in reality" refers here not only to extra-analytic contacts, but also to the analyst's "real" behavior within the analytic sessions, and "real" traumas in the past. It is worth noting here that even the most radical critics of the "blank screen" concept, such as Hoffman (1983), advise against self-disclosure by the analyst because it "is likely to pull the therapist's total personality into the exchange *in the same manner that it would be involved in other intimate social relationships*" (emphasis added, p. 417). Hoffman pointed out, as did Freud, that analysts can assume they are immune from being drawn into reciprocal enactments that compromise their objectivity only if they assume their mental health is vastly superior to that of their patients.

The analytic situation is constructed to facilitate the exploration of the inner realities underlying crippling neurotic conflicts. When analyst and analysand meet outside the analytic situation, nothing *fantastic* occurs. It is the fact of this reality that allows these events to strengthen transferences of defense, which if unanalyzed will obscure the emerging anxieties stemming from the infantile, the instinctual, and the irrational.

LIFE CRISES AND THE ANALYTIC SITUATION

We use the term "life crisis" to mean a stressful event that affects a person during the course of analysis and requires an adaptive response (Inderbitzin 1988–1989). Although field studies of normal populations have led to hierarchical ratings of life events based on the amount of stress generated, individuals vary greatly in their responses to any given event, depending on its personal conscious and unconscious meanings. It is important to distinguish life crises from analytic crises, situations that threaten the analytic situation. Certainly some life crises, such as medical or psychiatric emergencies, can disrupt an analysis and even require a departure from a neutral analytic stance. However, such instances are infrequent and generally pose no technical dilemma for the analyst. In other instances, analysands may handle stressful external events well, and because such stresses are not related significantly to the analysand's central conflicts, they do not enter prominently into the analytic work (Dewald and Dick 1987).

The most difficult and interesting situations for the analyst lie between these two extremes and result from an almost endless variety of events such as threatened divorce, death of a family member, or financial crises. These events are often highly charged with affect and imbued with a sense of urgency. A crisis atmosphere draws the attention of analysand and analyst to both the "outside" event and the responses generated by it, regardless of their relation and relevance to the current analytic focus.

Life crises offer many opportunities for the analysand to use reality as a defense. In this section we shall highlight the analyst's unconscious participation in the defensive process. We wish to emphasize that because the analyst's reactions to a major event in the analysand's life will be multiply determined in much the same way as the analysand's, the potential for countertransference enactments is significant. Most likely, in our experience, is the tendency to abandon analytic neutrality and respond as a benign, "helpful," or authoritarian parent. Such responses, which may also represent failures of empathy if they do not take into account the analysand's often hidden and conflicted adaptive potential, are usually referred to as "transference gratifications." Although certain drive derivatives certainly are satisfied, we think the more important and often overlooked possibility is the analyst's contribution to the strengthening of a specific transference of defense, that of benign protector, utilized by the analysand especially against aggressive transference wishes and impulses. A variety of factors can predispose an analyst to unknowingly "fall in" with this transference disposition, including the strong pull of the analysand's transference (Sandler 1976) and an identification with the patient as victim, due in part to the particular unconscious meaning of the reality event *to the analyst*. The analyst who feels anxious and vulnerable in such instances is more likely to exaggerate the analysand's vulnerability and therefore assume a protective and supportive role *for the patient*. Raphling (1992) explored an issue related to this predilection. Some analysts experience the assertiveness necessary to be interpretive as assaultive and, therefore, dangerous, especially when the analysand presents as overwhelmed, at a loss, or otherwise desperate for assistance. Raphling (1992) said, "Aggression called forth by the interpretive act is problematic for analysts and is, I believe, largely responsible for the persistent trends in psychoanalysis that have aimed at reducing the importance of interpretation for analytic technique" (p. 352).

In focusing primarily on how external reality in the form of a crisis in an analysand's life can affect *the analyst* and contribute to counterresistances, it is not our intention to deemphasize the analysand's use of these realities defensively, as described in earlier sections of this chapter. Neither are we advocating avoiding efforts to draw the patient's reactions to such events into the analytic process. We believe that a better understanding of the complicated, multiple ways these events can enter into and strengthen defenses and resistances in both analyst and analysand is essential to their successful management.

CONCLUSION

We have consistently emphasized the many ways reality concerns enter into mental conflict during analysis and serve the purpose of defensive aims. Reality is especially well suited for purposes of defense against unconscious instinctual and moral pressures because of its compelling visibility, because it often engages both analyst and analysand experientially (as in interaction), and because of its here-and-now quality, its "socializing" nature, and its many other attributes that contrast with the confusing, slippery, and often fantastic quality of what can be inferred about unconscious drive and superego forces during analysis. Some contemporary analysts, in focusing on the complexity of the analyst's contributions to the analytic interaction, advocating a two-person psychology and emphasizing the potential value as analytic data of enactments, extra-analytic contacts and other "real" events during analysis, have shifted toward what we view as the belief that, as grist for the mill, such realities in general enrich the analytic process rather than interfere with it.

We do not mean to imply that the value of exploring current realities, life crises, extra-analytic contacts, enactments, and other interactions is illusory, invariably defensive, or otherwise not worthwhile. In fact, in keeping with what we feel is the first meaning of "grist for the mill," we would insist that all such phenomena be analyzed. We are emphasizing here what we hope is a balancing perspective, that one should not lose sight of the defensive use of such "grist," that reality can be falsely and counterphobically reassuring and often draws the analyst into a similarly reassuring posture, frequently outside of his or her awareness. We have not tackled a difficult question raised in considering critically the idea that everything is analyzable, the second meaning of grist for the mill we described at the beginning of this chapter—namely, the question of what makes something *un*analyzable. We have described in detail many of the ways "grist" can be used defensively, interfering with analytic insight and making its accomplishment more difficult. Whether specific instances of reality used for defense can lead to inherently insurmountable resistances, whether it is a matter of the extent and sheer number of such instances, whether it is a matter of failure to recognize their often subtle defensive functions, or whether, as we suspect, it is some confluence of several of these factors, we believe calling for a more cautious and balanced view concerning the role of reality in defensive processes occurring during analytic treatment is warranted. It is our sense that the phrase "grist for the mill" became a familiar piece of psychoanalytic jargon as a means by which analysts reassured themselves. It meant that certain problems they faced when reality concerns intruded on the protection usually afforded by the analytic situation were, in fact, surmountable. They used the metaphor to indicate to themselves that such problems might even be useful if properly handled. We wish to caution against losing sight of the considerable potential for defense afforded by those reality phenomena occurring during analysis we have come to refer to as "grist for the mill."

References

Allen, D. (1974). *The Fear of Looking*. Charlottesville, VA: University Press of Virginia.

Apfelbaum, B., and Gill, M. M. (1989). Ego analysis and the relativity of defense: technical implications of the structural theory. *Journal of the American Psychoanalytic Association* 37:1071–1096.

Arlow, J. A. (1987). The dynamics of interpretation. *Psychoanalytic Quarterly* 56:68–87.

Bird, B. (1972). Notes on transference: universal phenomenon and hardest part of analysis. *Journal of the American Psychoanalytic Association* 20:267–301.

Brenner, C. (1982). *The Mind in Conflict*. New York: International Universities Press.

Dewald, P. A., and Dick, M. M. (1987). *Learning Process in Psychoanalytic Supervision*. Madison, CT: International Universities Press.

Fenichel, O. (1945). *The Psychoanalytic Theory of Neurosis*. New York: Norton.

—— (1953). Counter-phobic attitude. In *The Collected Papers of Otto Fenichel, Second Series*, pp. 163–173. New York: Norton.

Freud, A. (1936). *The Ego and the Mechanisms of Defense. Writings*, 2. New York: International Universities Press, 1966.
Freud, S. (1894). The neuro-psychoses of defence. *Standard Edition* 3.
—— (1917). The paths to the formation of symptoms. *Standard Edition* 16.
—— (1923). The ego and the super-ego (ego ideal). *Standard Edition* 19.
Ganzarain, R. (1991). Extra-analytic contacts: fantasy and reality. *International Journal of Psycho-Analysis* 72:131–140.
Gill, M. (1982). *Analysis of Transference, vol. I. Psychological Issues*. New York: International Universities Press.
—— (1983). The distinction between the interpersonal paradigm and the degree of the therapist's involvement. *Contemporary Psychoanalysis* 19:200–237.
Gray, P. (1973). Psychoanalytic technique and the ego's capacity for viewing intrapsychic conflict. *Journal of the American Psychoanalytic Association* 21:474–494.
—— (1982). "Developmental lag" in the evolution of technique for psychoanalysis of neurotic conflict. *Journal of the American Psychoanalytic Association* 30:621–656.
—— (1986). On helping analysands observe intrapsychic activity. In *Psychoanalysis: The Science of Mental Conflict–Essays in Honor of Charles Brenner*, ed. A. D. Richards and M. S. Willick, pp. 245–262. Hillsdale, NJ: Analytic Press.
—— (1987). On the technique of analysis of the superego: an introduction. *Psychoanalytic Quarterly* 56:130–154.
—— (1991). On transferred permissive or approving superego fantasies: the analysis of the ego's superego activities. *Psychoanalytic Quarterly* 60:1–33.
Hartmann, H. (1948). Comments on the psychoanalytic theory of instinctual drives. *Psychoanalytic Quarterly* 17:368–388.
—— (1956). Notes on the reality principle. *Psychoanalytic Study of the Child* 11:31–53. New York: International Universities Press.
Hoffman, I. (1983). The patient as interpreter of the analyst's experience. *Contemporary Psychoanalysis* 19:389–422.
Inderbitzin, L. (1988–1989). Life crises, neutrality, and caring. *Bulletin of the Association for Psychoanalytic Medicine* 28:107–110.

Jacobs, T. J. (1973). Posture, gesture, and movement in the analyst: cues to interpretation and countertransference. *Journal of the American Psychoanalytic Association* 21:77–92.
—— (1986). On countertransference enactments. *Journal of the American Psychoanalytic Association* 34:289–308.
Mitchell, S. (1992). *Relational Concepts in Psychoanalysis: An Integration.* Cambridge, MA: Harvard University Press.
Rapaport, D. (1958). The theory of ego autonomy. *Bulletin of the Menninger Clinic* 22:13–35.
Raphling, D. L. (1992). Some vicissitudes of aggression in the interpretive process. *Psychoanalytic Quarterly* 61:352–369.
Sandler, J. (1976). Countertransference and role-responsiveness. *International Review of Psycho-Analysis* 3:43–48.
Schafer, R. (1968). The mechanisms of defense. *International Journal of Psycho-Analysis* 49:4–62.
Strean, H. (1981). Extra-analytic contacts: theoretical and clinical considerations. *Psychoanalytic Quarterly* 50:238–259.
Tarnower, W. (1966). Extra-analytic contacts between the psychoanalyst and the patient. *Psychoanalytic Quarterly* 35:399–413.
Weiss, S. (1975). The effect on the transference of "special events" occurring during psychoanalysis. *International Journal of Psycho-Analysis* 56:69–75.

8

The Envy Complex: Its Recognition and Analysis

PEGGY B. HUTSON, M.D.

Envy is an ego state, a complex feeling and attitudinal state, which is ubiquitous. At its best, envy may evolve into ambition. In a more conflicted form it may evoke the ego's defense activity, resulting in denigration, prejudice, drive for success without conscience or without a lasting sense of accomplishment, fear of success, and other compromise formations. At its most primitive level, it leads to the taking of that which is envied.

In this chapter, envy is approached as a complex. Its components include complicated comparisons, a narcissistic wound or drop in self-esteem accompanied by shame, and wishes in the form of covetous fantasies. The covetous wishes in the envy complex are compromise formations due to ego defense activity signaled by shame. Although the covetous wish, which is usually aggressive, is a result of defense activity, it often is itself conflictual. Again, defense activity is engendered. Thus, problems with envy often present through complex defense activity.

The goals of this chapter are to better understand, recognize, and analyze the components of the envy complex and the subsequent compromise formations developed through the defense activity of the ego. I focus on the application of defense analysis because the envy complex manifests itself mostly through defense activity by the ego.

There have been differences of opinion about the time during development when envy originates. Freud's interest in envy centered on the child's rivalry with parents and siblings in the oedipal complex, where it was felt to be drive linked, and on penis envy in women (Joffe 1989). Klein (1957) saw envy as a primary motivating force or drive, operating from birth. Frankel and Sherick (1977) wrote that envy proper occurs after object constancy. Joffe (1989), referring to psychoanalytic and neurological research, pointed out that the reaction of envy requires that the child be capable of distinguishing between the self and the object, and be able to have fantasies of the end state of the wish. Perhaps the earlier states can be looked at as precursors of envy.

Frankel and Sherick (1977) confronted envy from the developmental point of view. They used direct observation of nursery school children to outline such a developmental approach. The observations ran from years one to five and emphasized the affective and the ideational content of envy, along with the differing orders of organization of this complex at different ages. The covetous responses in children ranged from the earliest form of simply taking that which was envied without regard for the object, to modifying the covetous wish through imitation or identification. This article noted the importance of object constancy and of evocative memory and language development to the development of envy. Knowing of the changing forms of envy along its developmental line may alert the analyst to the assorted and often primitive covetous fantasies to be found during analysis.

To define envy clearly has long been an academic challenge. Klein (1957) defined envy as "the angry feeling that another person possesses and enjoys something desirable." She clearly differentiated it from jealousy. Spielman (1971) approached envy as a complex affect. He listed emulation, narcissistic wound with its affect, covetousness or longing for the desired possession, and anger at the possessor as the affects in the envy complex. Frankel and Sherick (1977) wrote of envy as "the wish to experience the good feelings that one imagines are being felt by another person due to the possession of a valued attribute or thing" (p. 277).

Rosenblatt (1988) asserted that envy may be more accurately conceptualized as the consequence of the frustration of a wish. It may range from a simple wish to possess some tangible item to the more complex wishes to have certain attributes or good feelings, as described by Frankel and Sherick. In *Psychoanalytic Terms and Concepts* (Moore and Fine 1990), envy is defined as discontent over another's possession of what one would like for oneself. "It is characterized by a sense of uneasiness about the other's good fortune, animosity toward that person, chagrin or mortification over one's own presumed deficiency, and longing for the missing attribute" (p. 68).

Relatively resolved envy is a powerful motivational factor and its fantasy can spur one to an adaptive ambition and achievement. But early and unresolved conflicts involving components in the envy complex can skew subsequent development.

As aggression plays a major role in the covetous fantasy and in some other aspects of the envy complex, significant difficulties result when it is conflictual and prompts strong defense activity. Accordingly, use of defense analysis is crucial when working with problems of envy.

COMPONENTS OF THE ENVY COMPLEX

The envy complex is made up of four components. The covetous fantasy, the only component engendered by defense activity, is examined apart from the other three below.

Comparisons, narcissistic injury, and shame

A narcissistic wound or drop in self-esteem with its accompanying shame is always present in the envy complex. Self-esteem is usually not clearly conscious; it is noticed mainly when it is diminished. When the value judgment is positive, the affective response is characterized by heightened confidence. Deflated self-esteem may be more keenly experienced as the affect of shame. It may operate unconsciously, influencing decision-making and mood. This will be considered below under shame anxiety.

But what may lead to a drop in self-esteem? Sandler (1963) advanced the concept of the ideal self and the notion that shame arose when discrepancies appeared between the ideal self and the currently perceived self. Morrison (1989) wrote that for envy of the powerful object to flourish, the object must be compared with the shame-ridden, incompetent self. In this way of viewing envy, object relations are dyadic, and not triadic as found with problems of jealousy, an observation made by earlier writers.

Moore and Fine (1990) defined self-esteem as the end result of two comparisons. One is the comparison in which current self-appraisals are related to ideal self-concepts, ambitions for the self, and one's set of values. The other is a comparison of the result of the first to concepts of important others. This process of comparison is usually not fully conscious, and self-esteem is usually not fully experienced, as mentioned earlier.

Ordinarily, self-esteem vacillates somewhat with the ups and downs of life. But what causes self-esteem to drop regularly, resulting in shame in some individuals? What makes an individual more susceptible to developing shame and painfully sensing real and imagined slights? Those individuals with a significant discrepancy between the current and ideal representations of the self, which is mostly unconscious, have a sensitivity to and vulnerability for shame.

The importance of the unconscious sense of self, including the ideal self, should not be underestimated in any analysis involving self-esteem problems. The sense of self has both conscious and unconscious aspects. When self is used as a common-sense term, it includes and overlaps more technical aspects of self-concept, self-image, self-schema and identity (Moore and Fine 1990). Analysis of individuals with a particular vulnerability to shame calls for the fullest possible recovery from the unconscious of material related to the sense of self. This includes the ideal self, from its earliest components, the body components of self (S. Freud 1923, Roiphe 1968), to all other mental components including the gender messages so extensively added during the dyadic preoedipal period (Tyson 1980, Tyson and Tyson 1990). By using such a broad understanding of self, all ideas of worthlessness of any type are included.

Shame has often been called the most powerful affect. Patients may express it in terms of mortification, chagrin, humiliation, disgrace, despair, remorse, apathy, embarrassment, and lowered self-esteem. And even when shame may not seem a prominent experience of a given individual, it is implicitly involved when envy of another occurs (Morrison 1969). How is it that shame may not seem a prominent experience of a given individual? Shame is an affect just as anxiety is an affect. And like signal anxiety, shame may unconsciously signal the ego's defense activity to avoid pain. Thus, the shame might never reach consciousness (A. Freud 1936, Jacobson 1994). Shame anxiety (Moore and Fine 1990), the unconscious signal of the affect associated with a sense of impending failure and defectiveness, sets into action defensive activity resulting in new compromise formations.

Morrison (1969) noted there may be a multitude of defensive activities set off by the signal affect of shame. When the defensive maneuvers are successful, self-esteem is heightened and shame averted. Some of the common defenses and subsequent compromise formations are listed here. The development of the covetous fantasy necessary for the envy complex is the most important one for the purposes of this chapter. The envy complex, now complete with its covetous fantasy, usually involves some aggressive aspect which may necessarily call again on the defense activity of the ego. This is illustrated in the case material (see below).

Another compromise formation is contempt, which involves projecting the shame onto another. It is a more structured way to deal with shame than is rage (Morrison 1989). Denigration is also included here. A reaction formation against the shame may be an attitude of haughtiness, arrogance, and withdrawal. The inner sense of shame may be externalized, mostly by inviting debasement from the outside instead of suffering shame from within. Another manifestation of projected shame is seen in ideas of reference. Shamelessness, the negative therapeutic reaction (Horney 1936), and hypochondriasis may also be attempts to deal with shame. Another very common result of defensive activity to avoid the painful experience of shame is anger and rage (Rochlin 1973, Kohut 1972).

Covetous fantasy

A covetous fantasy develops because of defense activity and resultant compromise formation called into action by the drop in self-esteem, and by shame based on a feeling of deficiency. The envier usually feels some degree of entitlement in order to have a sense that he or she is entitled to have that which is felt to be missing (Rosenblatt 1988). The covetous fantasy is most often aggressive concerning getting that which is missing. Very frequently it is unconscious and conflictual. And now a new set of defense maneuvers must begin, and one of several compromise formations may evolve to avoid that which is feared in the unconscious covetous wish. Thus, the envy is often not obvious; only the result of the defense is observed. Careful defense analysis is called for if the individual is to be able to bring into conscious awareness the covetous wish with its aggressive components.

Recalling the developmental line of envy, the covetous fantasy might be in keeping with any one of several different developmental levels. One example of an early fantasy may be to simply take that which is imagined to be needed. It is important to remember that the covetous fantasy evolves because of a disturbance in self-esteem. If this is corrected through analysis, the compromise formation in the form of the covetous fantasy may also change.

DEFENSE ACTIVITY DUE TO
THE CONFLICTUAL ENVY COMPLEX

The conflictual covetous fantasy, and thus the envy complex, usually presents in a form secondary to ego defense activity (Rosenblatt 1988, Spillius 1993). When the individual is not free to have conscious aggressive thoughts, which are strong components in the covetous fantasies, the fears of aggression must be analyzed before the covetous fantasy can surface.

As the ego's defenses against the envy complex result in numerous compromise formations, the analyst can be alerted to their manifestations, some of which are noted below.

Denial

Denial of the desired object and repression may evolve. The classic example of this is the early denial by girl or boy that the opposite gender possesses anything different from her or his own genital equipment. The adaptive value of this denial is limited.

Denigration

The desired object or attribute, or the possessor thereof, is denigrated. This removes the need for envy. It is the sour grapes attitude. Denigration may occur through ego defense activity when self-esteem has fallen and shame ensues, alone or when the covetous wish is conflictual. Only the unfolding of the analysis will reveal what components of the envy complex the denigration defends. Denigration is an aggressive activity. It may be considered, in a way, a mini-narcissistic rage in order to raise self-esteem to a better level (Kohut 1972, Rochlin 1973).

Driven to succeed

The escape from the unconscious covetous fantasy occurs through being driven to succeed, but no success is ever enough. As long as the unconscious sense of deficit remains unconscious, it will remain disconnected from adult experience. Therefore the success does not "seep" into one's sense of self. Even when someone has obtained the envied object, the vulnerability to shame and proclivity for covetousness will remain if the early sense of deficiency is still unconscious. Individuals with poor self-esteem often have little empathy for others and thus may be callous to the needs of others as they pursue their ambitions.

Identification

The necessity for envy is obviated through identification, as the desired attribute is now vicariously possessed. Rosenblatt (1988) described a partial identification leading to a sense of being proud of a son, a daughter, being an American, and so on. In this way envy is diminished.

Destruction of the envied

Often the envious one, unaware of the shame and covetous wish, begins a campaign to disqualify the envied one. The envier may use rationalizations to explain this campaign. Destruction may range from disqualifying to, in the worst cases, actual death of the person.

Projection

The unconscious envious feelings and fantasies may be projected. This contributes to fear of success from a preoedipal origin (Hutson 1994, Rosenblatt 1988). Freud (1914–1916) reported cases of individuals wrecked by success. In these cases "forces of conscience which forbid the subject to gain the long hoped for advantages" (p. 318) were connected with oedipal-level connotations. In the cases referred to in this paper, the unconscious covetous fantasy to appropriate that which is envied is projected. Now the unconscious and sometimes conscious fear is that the original envier, when in a state of "more," is in danger. This is central to "evil eye" beliefs around the world. Tragically, it may lead to a patient's need to fail in treatment, part of the so-called negative therapeutic reaction (Horney 1936, Olinick 1964).

TREATMENT

The components of the envy complex are comparisons, self-esteem drop with subsequent shame, and covetous fantasies. The drop in self-esteem accompanied by shame is so painful and the covetous fantasy so conflictual that they usually present as compromise formations resulting from the ego's defense activity. Observations of the minute-by-minute associations, whether they are of dreams, the transference, or any other perceptions or associations to them, reveal the signs of defense activity and thus the areas of conflict. Through this close process monitoring and the subsequent use of defense analysis (Gray 1994), the range of conscious thought in these patients should widen. At this point, these patients are no longer led by their unconscious conflicts, but are free to apply adult thinking and make conscious decisions based on conscious considerations. The certainty that conscious thinking need have no limitation, as one has a choice of action or no action, is a very significant gain in analysis and therapy.

In these cases, thorough work must be done to unearth the extensive unconscious sense of the self which has resulted in vulnerable self-esteem. Parallel work is to recover unconscious fears of aggression. This facilitates the recovery of aggressive covetous fantasies.

It is noteworthy that the most primitive covetous fantasies often involve some change of the body, frequently through a fantasy of oral incorporation. One usually recovers unconscious verbal self-messages (such as a belief that one's gender limits one's capacity), body-image misconceptions, and other relevant notions. Such messages seem to interfere with optimal evolution of the self-representation. Primitive aggressive and mutative fantasies, produced by primary process condensation, are often used to correct the perceived deficiency. I think this accounts for the frequent finding of primitive, covetous body-part fantasies in those with a strong sense of deficiency.

CASE MATERIAL

The following case material depicts the conflictual envy complex, its defenses, and its compromise formations. As is usually the case, the early material portrays not envy, but problems of self-esteem, shame, and anger.

Mrs. Z., a 30-year-old married mother of three, presented with complaints of frequent bouts of anger. "I'm so ready to be insulted, I can't get out of it." She felt distant from her husband, whom she loved. "I don't want to open up to him. He'll see the awful truth and leave me." She was at a loss as to what the awful truth was.

Worries about her competence in the work world drove her to get a master's degree in business. Although she did very well, she was afraid to try to look for a job for fear of failure. She prided herself on her cleanliness, neatness, and punctuality. Her clothes were sporty and her demeanor was quite feminine. Ample time was spent on self-grooming and positive responses to her appearance were extremely important to her. Exhibiting for admiration, described by Edgecumbe and Burgner (1975) as frequent in the phallic-narcissistic stage of development and now more accurately called the infantile-genital phase (Tyson and Tyson 1990), had persisted into the adult period. She would remember what clothes she had worn to various gatherings and the responses to them as far back as her high school years.

During the evaluation, she reported that a seamstress took a dress that did not fit and made it perfect. "That's what I want here. Something is very wrong. I'm so angry and sometimes so sad." This demonstrated her early transference wish for my cure, wanting an "alteration" of her body and gender self to gratify her infantile covetous fantasies. She had had previous treatment in another city and was well prepared for rapid entry into an analysis.

She grew up in an intact family with a brother one-and-a-half years older. She described her mother as a non-empathic, dress-conscious, cold homemaker who "picked on" the patient's father and preferred her brother. She felt her mother would have made her father an invalid if she could have. The patient was fond of her father, a passive man. She disliked her brother who was "better off." Her mother and father were always encouraging and applauding her non-ambitious brother but not the patient.

The history revealed evidence of early childhood problems. She recalled that she had always felt that somehow she had less. At 3, she wanted a hat that her brother had. At 4, she had a severe fear of touching her mother when she handed her food. This fear was so great that her mother had to hand fruit to her on a napkin. She remembered interest in whether worms would regrow after she cut them apart. At 7, her favorite photo was of herself and her brother in similar swim trunks. She felt you could not tell their genders. That same year she began to pull hairs out of her eyebrows and eat them. She joked that, "I'd eat anything that did not eat me first." One memory that proved to be important was that of running out of a theater when the movie showed a man having his head chopped off. Later in the analysis, she felt the same upon watching a cannibalistic scene in a movie.

At 9 years of age, she felt that she and her brother were alike somehow after they did actually exchange swim trunks. She soon entered puberty, and became very conscious of the state of her body. She was dissatisfied, although she was pleased to develop breasts. Excessive eating began just before adolescence. From that time on, there have been cycles of bingeing and anorexia. One summer, late in high school, she lost so much weight that she had trouble working due to lack of energy.

Mrs. Z. felt her body was asymmetrical. She had multiple minor surgeries to remove this or fix that and was looking forward to the next surgery, liposuction. After each procedure there was only a brief satisfaction that her body was now fine.

She was extremely reliable in her homemaking job and in the community. Her capacity for empathy for her young children was marked, and she was thoughtful about their emotional development. Her capacity for empathy for her husband was markedly diminished and their relationship was dominated by her narcissistic needs. When these needs were unmet, she had bouts of anger.

Although she said she had good friends, she rarely expected or asked for help from them and often felt slighted. As it turned out, she had projected her poor sense of self to them and did not expect they would want to help her.

When she presented for analysis, she had an air of superiority. During analysis, this was understood to be the result of her ego's defense against shame and later against the feared covetous fantasies.

The early sessions were filled with a litany of the things that were wrong with her and filled with her anger at others for slights. With recognition of her use of aggression as a defense against drop in self-esteem and shame, she came to realize her pattern of developing anger after she felt humiliated by people who had more or by those perceived as superior. Gradually she was in a better position to be curious about her sense of being less.

At various times, Mrs. Z. avoided even differing (a mild form of aggression) with the analyst through various defense activities. It became obvious that when aggression, in the form of denigration, was not used as a defense against drop in self-esteem, it was almost always conflictual for her and required a defensive maneuver. There were even times when denigration (to defend against a drop in self-esteem) of people important to her became *more* conflictual due to her fears of aggression which were based on fears of abandonment. This is found in the first vignette below. In working with her fears of her aggression, the analysis was focused on the awareness of defense activity to avoid a feared aggressive thought or feeling. Freedom to have aggressive thoughts and feelings would be necessary if covetous fantasies were to become conscious.

The close process attention and defense analysis of the self-esteem shifts and their required defenses as well as the defenses against aggressive thoughts and feelings advanced her observing ego. She was in a better position to be curious about her sense of inferiority and her fears of aggression.

Her sense of being less took many forms. There were extensive worries about her intelligence in spite of good grades and multiple degrees. Her self-concept was one in which she was defective in intellectual and many other spheres due to her gender. Only after months of analysis of derivatives of unconscious fantasies of herself as damaged did a fantasy of having a defective body gradually begin to unfold. Feeling freer to have conscious aggressive thoughts and feelings facilitated the recovery of her primitive covetous fantasies. These emerged secondary to drops in self-esteem which resonated with thoughts of herself as defective. These covetous fantasies turned out to be very early fantasies of repair of the defective body which she unconsciously believed she had.

The development of the body image begins very early. The sense of self, including body self, gender messages, and other senses of the self, are being assimilated even before age 2. By the time of the phallic-narcissistic or infantile-genital phase of development, the issues of male and female parts of the body are prominent. In patients like this one, in whom covetous fantasies involving the body are so frequent, one might consider the possibility of a primary process condensation of many of the gender messages with the ideal body image resulting in these covetous mutative body fantasies.

With continued and increasing freedom for conscious awareness of aggressive thoughts and fantasies, the material in the sessions vacillated between two major themes: (1) the unconscious conviction of being defective and the recovery of extensive details about defectiveness and (2) the recovery of the covetous fantasy, which was an unconscious repair fantasy in response to the unconscious belief in her body being deficient. Naturally, when material is unconscious, it remains with the original childhood interpretations. As this material became conscious, adult thinking could now be applied to the early ideas and more adult interpretations and solutions developed.

In the slow recovery of the covetous fantasies, which were usually of a very primitive aggressive and cannibalistic nature, analysis concerning defenses against aggression and unconscious fears of aggression continued throughout. This facilitated the fuller elaboration of the covetous fantasy. The following are a few clinical vignettes from the case.

The patient's fear of her aggression came into the transference in the early sessions. Mrs. Z. had a fantasy that she had seen my son on the way into her session and that things were perfect for me and in my house. She did not have a son and thought I did. She therefore felt I had more or was better than she was. She developed anxiety, with tachycardia and nausea. Then through a displacement of disparaging thoughts to her mother, her successful defense activity was seen. It took the form of a recollection of being enraged with her mother for letting her daughter get pneumonia a few years earlier. The aggressive devaluation of me, developed as a defense against her diminished self-esteem and her shame when she felt less than me, was too worrisome for her. She developed symptoms. By displacing the defensive devaluation of the object from me to her mother, she avoided her fear of aggression toward me and improved her self-esteem in this displaced way. The anxiety symptoms disappeared.

Interventions about her defenses due to her fears of aggression were repeated over many months. The responses to these interventions raised new and different fears and thus allowed for repeated interpretation of her fears of aggression. As the analysis progressed, she gained increasing freedom to consciously experience aggressive thoughts and feelings as she uncovered the early unconscious fears of abandonment attached to aggression.

She was eventually able to better differentiate between struggling over a critical thought due to fear of abandonment, and using anger to buoy up her fallen self-esteem. She became increasingly interested in the contents of her poor sense of self and in her susceptibility to slights.

With the expanding conscious awareness of the fantasy that her mind and her body were defective, and the greater freedom to experience an aggressive fantasy, she recovered primitive covetous fantasies. These fantasies resulted from the ego's defense activity prompted by a drop in self-esteem with its painful affect of shame. The covetous body repair fantasies unfolded. These covetous fantasies included severing and incorporating parts of other people's bodies. Then she understood why body mutilation scenes had terrified her.

In the transference she had fantasies of cutting and biting off parts of me for herself. She gradually recovered fantasies of breaking off her husband's penis during sexual activity. Visual imagery such as labia and superimposed penis and testicles would occur intermittently as she more clearly outlined these primitive repair fantasies. They involved gaining parts she did not have or imagined she lacked and needed, to make her like her early body image ideal which had been unconsciously retained. Thus, she had continued to have conflictual wishes to be both sexes from early childhood.

From midway in the analysis comes the following material depicting self-esteem issues and covetous repair fantasies in the transference.

> Mrs. Z. reported: As I drove in here, I thought this is the most beautiful land in the city. Yesterday I saw Mr. X., who opened an abortion clinic years ago and now has so much more than we do. But he and his money are really shady. [This was said angrily in an unconscious attempt

to denigrate me since she had a comparison thought in which I had more. The aggressive denigration was defended through displacement to Mr. X.]

    The intervention was as follows: In your thinking, you were referring to my having more than you, but only by dropping me and adding Mr. X. could you go on to add a critical thought and feeling—as if to have an angry critical thought directly toward me was difficult for some reason.

    She responded with: I am having a visual image of a dog biting you. I think that is what I want to do to you. I am remembering some pictures of a boa constrictor who squeezed a rat and then went for its head. It was the kiss of death. Then it swallowed the rat and you could see the lump.

A second intervention referred again to the defensive shift to the snake and pointed out that she could only add the aggressive detail of biting and engulfing something that way, as if to think of it directly was worrisome.

    Mrs. Z. responded with: I have had a fantasy recently that my body is too lumpy. When I put my clothes on, it is untrue. I guess it's in my head and somehow I need to think I have more to me.

    The third intervention was the elaboration of the covetous fantasy which was a defense against the drop in self-esteem and subsequent shame brought on by the idea of body defectiveness. "Thus the fantasy of having more to your body could occur by biting off and taking in by mouth from someone with more. This fantasy was tripped off by the humiliating worry that I had more than you." Actually, she unconsciously felt she was missing parts from both women and men, which has been previously reported in the literature (Fast 1984, Kubie 1974).

At times when the patient felt she was better than others or had more, she would become anxious and therefore altered the thought. Through analysis, it became evident that the anxiety was due to the projection of her own covetous fantasies onto those with less than what she had or thought she was. Thus, when she had more, she would unconsciously fear that someone with less would take it away, or feel aggressive toward her.

Her difficulties with fears of aggression, her sense of being damaged or defective, her aggressive covetous fantasies, and her fears of projected envy became conscious and were worked through in the analysis. Consequently, Mrs. Z. became comfortable in states of feeling more or less as compared to others, was able to be more empathic, and lost the need for many of the compromise formations created through the defensive activities already described. These included the rages and denigrations, primitive covetous fantasies, and haughtiness. She was able to be closer with others, was free to follow her ambitions, and was much more content with herself.

The remainder of the analysis centered around positive oedipal issues which have been omitted as they are not pertinent to this discussion.

SUMMARY

In this chapter, the ego state of envy was examined as a complex consisting of comparisons, a drop in self-esteem accompanied by shame, and a covetous fantasy developed as a compromise formation through the ego's defensive response to the painful affect of shame. Each of these components was described in detail. Because the envy complex most often presents as a compromise formation secondary to the ego's defense activity called forth by the unconscious conflictual covetous fantasy, various defense-generated possibilities were reviewed. A case was presented.

Since defense activity is so common in problems involving the envy complex, the techniques of defense analysis are extremely useful in the analysis of this complex.

References

Edgecumbe, R., and Burgner, M. (1975). The phallic narcissistic phase—a differentiation between preoedipal and oedipal aspects of phallic development. In *Psychoanalytic Study of the Child* 30:161-180. New Haven: Yale University Press.

Fast, I. (1984). *Gender Identity, A Differentiation Model.* Hillsdale, NJ: Analytic Press.

Frankel, S., and Sherick, E. (1977). Observations of the development of normal envy. *Psychoanalytic Study of the Child* 32:257-281. New Haven: Yale University Press.

Freud, A. (1936). *The Ego and the Mechanisms of Defense.* New York: International Universities Press.

Freud, S. (1914-1916). Those wrecked by success. *Standard Edition* 14:316-331.

—— (1923). The ego and the id. *Standard Edition* 19:19-39.

Gray, P. (1994). *The Ego and Analysis of Defense.* Northvale, NJ: Jason Aronson.

Horney, K. (1936). The problem of the negative therapeutic reaction. *Psychoanalytic Quarterly* 5:29-44.

Hutson, P. (1994). *Envy's contribution to fear of success.* Paper presented at the meeting of the Florida Psychoanalytic Society, Miami, FL, June.

Jacobson, J. (1994). Signal affects and our psychoanalytic confusion of tongues. *Journal of the American Psychoanalytic Association* 42:15-42.

Joffe, W. (1989). A critical review of the status of the envy concept. *International Journal of Psycho-Analysis* 50:533-545.

Klein, M. (1957). *Envy and Gratitude.* New York: Basic Books.

Kohut, H. (1972). Thoughts on narcissism and narcissistic rage. In *Psychoanalytic Study of the Child* 27:360-400. New Haven: Yale University Press.

Kubie, L. S. (1974). The drive to become both sexes. In *Symbol and Neurosis,* pp. 191-263. New York: International Universities Press.

Moore, B., and Fine, B., eds. (1990). *Psychoanalytic Terms and Concepts.* New Haven: Yale University Press.

Morrison, A. (1989). *Shame: The Underside of Narcissism.* Hillsdale, NJ: Analytic Press.

Olinick, S. (1964). The negative therapeutic reaction. *International Journal of Psycho-Analysis* 45:540-548.

Rochlin, G. (1973). *Man's Aggression: The Defense of the Self.* Boston: Gambit.

Roiphe, H. (1968). On an early genital phase. *Psychoanalytic Study of the Child* 23:348-365. New York: International Universities Press.

Rosenblatt, A. (1988). Envy, identification, and pride. *Psychoanalytic Quarterly* 57:56-71.

Sandler, J., Holder, A., and Meers, D. (1963). The ego ideal and ideal self. *Psychoanalytic Study of the Child* 18:139-158. New York: International Universities Press.

Spielman, P. (1971). Envy and jealousy: an attempt at clarification. *Psychoanalytic Quarterly* 40:-59-82.

Spillius, E. B. (1993). Varieties of envious experiences. *International Journal of Psycho-Analysis* 74:1199-1212.

Tyson, P. (1980). A developmental line of gender identity, gender roles and choice of love object. *Journal of the American Psychoanalytic Association* 30:61-86.

Tyson, P., and Tyson, R. (1990). *Psychoanalytic Theories of Development.* New Haven: Yale University Press.

9

The Place of Empathy in Analytic Listening

LUCIE S. GREENBLUM, M.D.

INTRODUCTION

In this chapter I will illustrate the type of empathic attunement called for when using close process attention as described by Paul Gray (1994). This technique definitely requires the disciplined use of intuitive processes and the incorporation of nonverbal data at certain critical junctures. It is not a cold, intellectual, mechanical endeavor as has sometimes been suggested.

I will also contrast Gray's use of empathic listening with that of Evelyne Schwaber (1981, 1987), who also emphasizes empathic listening. I will use illustrations from my own clinical work, which is informed by the principles of close process attention technique, and from the published work of Schwaber (1983, 1992).

Inderbitzin and Levy (1990) have already defined Gray's and Schwaber's different *surfaces* and also mentioned "areas of overlap" in their paper on the analytic surface. They said that Gray's surface is one focusing on defenses, with particular emphasis on "those elements in the material that can be observed by both analyst and analysand" (p. 379), whereas Schwaber's surface consists of "moments in the therapeutic dialogue when there occurs a divergence between the analyst's and the patient's experience of the patient's psychic reality" (p. 382).

The moments Schwaber has chosen as a surface consist of shifts in mood, the appearance of ego states or symptom formation in reaction to a disappointment in the analyst's response. Gray's listening mode provides a different view from some of Schwaber's sensitively described dilemmas and from her attempt to "be carefully attuned to the analyst's participation as perceived by the patient" (Inderbitzin and Levy 1990, p. 383).

Gray and Schwaber have different theoretical vantage points. We know that "the way we listen and look ... determines the nature of our data" (Spencer and Balter 1990, p. 394). But Schwaber's and Gray's listening stances and goals are sufficiently similar that comparing their different use of empathic listening in the details that clinical vignettes can provide is a useful way to clarify and delineate their different models of the mind and the related differences in their technical approaches to the challenging moments of deprivation Schwaber has chosen to study.

Schwaber (1983) described her listening stance as follows: "my focus is sharpened on the more experience-near, on the immediate vicissitudes of the patient's state of affect, on shifting defensive patterns, and on her [the patient's] perceptual experience" (p. 523).

Schwaber also stated (1987):

> augmenting the focus on moment-to-moment verbal and affective cues, and on their possible connection to how

the patient perceives our participation—silent or stated—may serve to narrow the leaps of inference we must make, facilitate the patient's capacity for self-observation, while simultaneously bringing to light a further range of experiential and defensive phenomena. [p. 275]

These statements imply a form of very focused attention and perception, moment-to-moment listening, interest in self-observation and defenses, all of which is very similar to what the close process attention analyst does—namely, hearing and processing "moment-to-moment affective cues" (Schwaber 1987, p. 275) and listening for defensive shifts.

I will begin by quoting a passage taken from *Tropism* by the French novelist, Nathalie Sarraute. She captures beautifully what Gray and Schwaber attend to:

> These movements, of which we are hardly cognizant, slip through us on the frontiers of consciousness in the form of undefinable, extremely rapid sensations. They hide behind our gestures, beneath the words we speak, the feelings we manifest, are aware of experiencing, and able to define. They seemed, and still seem to me, to constitute the secret source of our existence, in what might be called its nascent state. These movements seemed to me to be veritable dramatic actions, hiding beneath the most commonplace conversations, the most everyday gestures, and constantly emerging up to the surface of appearances that both conceal and reveal them. [p. vi]

This is a felicitous description of the rapidity and fluidity of cues to the ego's maneuvers. Sarraute also captures the quality of being potentially conscious (the "nascent state," the "frontier of consciousness") and the continually changing compromise formations ("appearances" that simultaneously conceal and reveal) emphasized by Gray.

In his review of empathy, Levy (1985) found that most writers understand empathy to be a "special form of identification characterized by its transient, consciously or preconsciously determined, nonregressive, easily reversible" (p. 355) nature.

Empathy is used in a very focused, continuous manner by the close process attention analyst. Affective cues such as body postures, tone of voice, and rate of speech need to be continuously observed because they provide clues to the data required for close process attention.

It is through empathy that the analyst knows of the appearance or disappearance of drive derivatives into or out of consciousness. It is also through empathy that the patient's receptivity to intervention can be assessed. For close process attention there is a need to continuously monitor the patient's availability for comment because the analyst intervenes relatively more frequently than in other analytic styles. The attempt to minimize suggestion and influence requires the search for opportunities to demonstrate moments when a drive becomes conflicted in front of the analyst so that patients can study their superego projections. Gray (1994) has underlined the importance of adding "experiential insight" to "cognitive insight" in order to provide the ego with "progressive opportunities to gradually take on varieties of drive derivatives" (p. xx).

The additional attempt to keep the focus on "data essentially limited to inside the analytic situation" (Gray 1973, p. 492) places another burden on the patient's ego and a corresponding increase in the need for the analyst's empathic awareness. That will guide him in formulating *when* and *how* to demonstrate a moment to the patient.

In summary, close process attention requires a continual empathic grasp of moment-to-moment states, drive expression, degree of accessibility to consciousness, potential attentiveness, and receptiveness. Gray stated (1973) that:

> the continuously expanding importance of ego analysis as a major component of our technique has imposed in-

creasing tasks upon analytic listening and perceiving. . . . It is certainly true that the most necessary capacity for analytic listening is that complex of functions which allows for the recognition of drive derivatives. Whether this capacity is described as the unconscious . . . as an instrument (Freud 1912b, p. 116) . . . or as listening with the third ear (Reik 1948) . . . or as . . . empathy . . . the reference is to essentially nonpurposeful processes. On the other hand, recognition of the *defense against* drive derivative—that is, ego analysis—usually involves a different kind of perceptual attention and intelligence from that required strictly for awareness of the drive derivatives themselves. [The] observation of the ego's defensive ways . . . involves a greater degree of purposefully directed thinking . . . [and] a different aspect of the analyst's perceptual apparatus. [p. 475]

Here, Gray is emphasizing intellectual processes, whereas what I wish to emphasize is that nonpurposeful processes are also essential for close process attention.

In his attempt in 1973 to begin to delineate techniques that would rely more on a set of observable data than on sensing the unconscious, Gray gave less emphasis to nonpurposeful empathic processes. The emphasis on defining the observable makes it a disciplined form of empathy.

Fliess's definition of the four steps in the empathic process (as summarized by Levy 1985) is most illuminating: "(1) the analyst is the object of an unconscious striving in the patient; (2) the analyst temporarily identifies with the patient; (3) by virtue of this brief identification, the striving becomes the analyst's striving; (4) the analyst projects the striving back onto the patient after he has tasted it" (p. 354). The close process attention analyst adds a fifth step, because he attempts to define what is mutually observable (Paniagua 1985) so that the patient can study and verify (or reject) the analyst's conjecture through conscious verbalizations. This *is* the "purposefully directed thinking" Gray referred to (1973). It involves naming the affects, their sequences, following the flow of defenses, and processing the thematic content of associations.

While following associations is always an aspect of defense analysis, the attempt to focus on what is objectively definable for the patient (what I have called the fifth step) increases the analyst's observing capacity. If one thinks of the experiencing and observing ego functions described by Sterba (1934), close process attention can be described as sharpening the analyst's observing ego functions. This becomes both challenging and useful at certain junctures, in particular at the moments Schwaber has chosen as a surface. Because it involves striving to *look* at and *define* the *patient's* data, it helps the analyst to avoid getting stuck in step 3. Thus, it is useful to avoid countertransference enactments.

Schwaber studies moments that frequently consist of fantasies developed during a perceived silence. The analyst is heard as silent. This can occur during an actual silence (the patient no longer speaks and the analyst has not intervened) or while the patient speaks.

In the perceived silence, narcissistically vulnerable patients can easily develop fantasies of the analyst as disapproving, distant, disagreeing, or withholding because the search for confirmation or some contribution from the analyst is particularly intense. Frequently, the patient continues to act (body movements, sighs, movements of the head) according to his transference fantasy. At those moments, one countertransference potential is for the analyst to feel that he knows what the patient feels and to act on the impulse to verbalize the fantasy for the patient. Another countertransference potential is to empathize because the analyst feels the patient's distress. Close process attention technique, with its emphasis on defining the observable, helps the analyst to master the countertransference. Since the focus is on observing what the patient *does* that causes one to feel, it decreases the over-identification. Gray emphasises the search for techniques that permit the analyst to be tactful at those moments, yet restrained.

Silences also occur when patients who are not necessarily narcissistically vulnerable place the analyst on the receiving end of some active drive derivative such as questions or demands. Fantasies quickly develop in the ensuing silence. The analyst might be perceived as angry, in a battle of wills, frightened, or dumb. It can be challenging to find techniques that will permit the patient to verbalize the transference fantasy. In addition to this, the analyst may temporarily feel impatient, anxious, or dumb, and thus has to analyze as a transference fantasy what has just been a real feeling. Here also Gray emphasises the search for neutral yet tactful techniques that preserve the patient's ability to grasp the fantasy and gradually permit him to become freer to maintain an active stance with the analyst.

CLINICAL MATERIAL

Before moving to Schwaber's clinical vignettes, I will provide vignettes of my own work to illustrate the place of empathic listening in close process attention. The first vignette illustrates the use of vicarious introspection (Kohut 1959) to capture the sequences of expression of drive derivatives.

A patient in her first year of analysis stated: "It's been seven months that I have been coming here" (tone of voice mildly disappointed until the next word); "it's not so long" (she now sounds reasonable). "I'm learning a lot" (she pushes the reaction formation a little further and her tone of voice is flat).

To identify the changing affects—that is, the drives *and* defenses against them—analysts combine empathy as a mode of observation to identify the affects with their knowledge of defense. The "tasting" is the recognition of the drive (here the aggressive drive) through the analyst identifying briefly with the patient by fleetingly recalling moments of similarly flavored disappointments followed by insistence that everything is fine in front of a perceived authority. The next vignette illustrates the use of vicarious introspection to assess the patient's availability for comment. It also demonstrates how Gray's inner focus complicates the task for the patient and the analyst and requires an evaluation, through empathy, of the patient's ability to hear the analyst.

Ms. B. spent many years of analysis stoically struggling against any mention of the occasionally severe back and hip pain she experienced while speaking. She was still very far from knowing that it protected her against wishes for maternal care and passive homosexual wishes, but this day for the first time she was briefly free of her usual restraint and mentioned that she had just noticed that the pain increased as she spoke. She shifted from telling me about her body to telling me generally about her life. While I wished to further her awareness of her defense against telling me about her body, I also "sensed" that she had, a mere half second later, already repressed her observation of herself. An attempt to link her current perceptions to that moment would have felt to her as if I was "coming out of left field." She would have struggled to suppress the aggression that such comments cause. This patient would not have permitted herself what some patients, less conflicted about their aggression, have said to me at such moments—namely, "What on earth are you talking about?" The analyst has to find a way to attract the patient's attention and bring the patient back to the sequence to be explored. "Sensing" that the patient would feel a remark came "out of left field" is due to an automatic scanning the analyst does of an internal image of the patient.

Schafer's concept (1959) of *generative empathy* is useful here even though it refers to a *gradual* building of an internal image, whereas I am referring to an image built over the preceding few seconds. Schafer spoke of the gradual formation of an internal image of the patient, which becomes easily available to the analyst and contains a "hierarchic organization of desires, feelings, thoughts, defenses, controls, superego pressures, capacities, self-representations . . ." (p. 345). He described it as requiring "perceptual attention or vigilance to elusive cues, difficult to conceptualize, in motility, verbalization, affective expression, and tempo" (p. 318).

Schafer's concept can also be used to account for the subliminal knowledge an analyst, who works closely with defenses, has about the characteristic defensive shifts each patient is likely to have. When patients surprise the analyst with a change in the defensive shifts, we frequently come to realize (after the fact) that they have reached a new level of compromise formation.

The following vignette concerns such a change. It is also chosen because it contains a consciously verbalized disappointment in what the analyst provides, and thus parallels one of Schwaber's vignettes reproduced below in which the patient protested the analyst's not answering questions.

Mrs. X. was in the fourth year of analysis. In her early childhood, she had had a depressed, unavailable mother. In general, there had been sessions (particularly during the first couple of years) in which she suddenly became anxiously aware of the analyst's silence. Concerned, she would suddenly say, "Are you there?" When I inquired about the picture that caused the anxiety, a frequent answer was a variant of "You're in analytic Lalaland." Her thoughts would then turn to her mother's withdrawal. My inquiry not only explored her views of me but also let her know that I was, in fact, listening. Thus, I used empathy to dispel the fantasy that I was withdrawn, a transference, while continuing to facilitate the patient's capacity to study it.

Toward the end of an hour in which I had said nothing, she suddenly began to complain about the lack of productivity in the analysis, subtly began to reproach herself for it, and then became silent. While I was still considering whether and how to intervene, expecting her usual anxiety, she again said, "Are you there?" Expecting anxiety, I spoke and called her attention to her rapid turning on herself the moment before. The hour soon ended. After she left, I realized that her tone of voice in the "Are you there?" had not been frightened but sarcastic and that she was beginning to be freer to experience aggression at the deprivation in the analytic situation. This was confirmed in subsequent months when she became able to let me know with contempt just how useless I was to her in certain sessions.

Some automatic anxiety had diminished. Chused (1991) has observed that "enactments are often the first sign of a shift that caught the analyst by surprise and makes him a participant in an emerging transference paradigm he is not yet able to objectify and observe" (p. 636).

The vignette of my own work that follows introduces the second part of this chapter by providing another example of the surface Schwaber works with.

Ms. Z. was in her first year of analysis. She had hesitated to use the couch because "it is in people's faces that I read their cues." She saw herself as very independent and was surprised when the following pattern emerged. She began to speak of certain opinions in a firm tone of voice, then hesitated, possibly reading disagreement in my silence, and slowly adjusted her opinion as if to take into account the disagreement she heard in my silence. Then she arched her head toward me, as if to get some confirmation, and then became silent while her head fell back on the couch. The analyst "felt" she had given up. When this narcissistically vulnerable patient was aware of a silence she immediately developed the transference fantasy that the analyst was disapproving.

Through the process of "empathic sampling" (see Fliess in Levy 1985) I became aware that the patient was, in the absence of confirmation, developing a transference to a disapproving authority. I waited for the end of the sequence and instead of saying, "You seem to feel as though you just gave up," said, "You just fell silent; can you sense what might be happening?"

Similarly, if it had been appropriate to intervene at the prior moment, I could have pointed out to the patient the change of tone as she spoke her opinions and inquired as to her sense of what had happened. In other words, the focus remained on what was observable by both patient and analyst.

At moments in the sequence, I had to restrain the impulse to intervene since I felt as if I was withholding something the patient needed. The automatic focusing on what caused me to feel so strongly helped set aside my momentary identification with the patient's distress and my impulse to be overly empathic. Yet the verbalization of some of my observations (her opinions followed by silence) was sufficient to communicate that I was listening (dispelling the anxiety-producing fantasy of a disapproving authority) and thus permit her to observe the data I was presenting for study. The gradual analysis of many of these moments eventually enabled this patient to state her opinions and even disagree with me without the regression just described. This is very close to Schwaber's intention to "focus on how the patient perceives our participation—silent or stated . . . to narrow the leaps of inference and facilitate the capacity for self-observation" (p. 275).

I will now present two vignettes from Dr. Schwaber's work (1992).

> Two sessions before the summer break, Ms. T. (given to recurrent periods of silence) was quiet much of the time. She began the next hour, again silently. When she spoke,

she said she worried that something might happen to me and I would not return, and she stopped. Then she said, "You're always more quiet before you go away. I want you to talk to me and you don't and I get angry. Before you go away, I want to establish a stronger connection, and I feel you want to establish more distance." [p. 1048]

The patient got quiet again. The analyst then said, "It seems you're wanting me to reach more actively to you." [p. 1050]

The patient agreed. The analyst noted that she sounded more relaxed. The intervention corresponds to Schwaber's goal of "active search for the [patient's] perspective" (1992, p. 1051) and "effort at systematic elaboration of . . . the patient's perceptual experience" (1983, p. 522). She uses empathy as a way to grasp another's reality and, in the process of reflecting this reality to the patient, she also empathizes with her. The patient felt, and was, understood. She was gratified in her wish for the analyst to speak. As in the vignette of Mrs. X. quoted above, the patient may indeed need to hear the analyst's voice because, as Schwaber says, "a moment of my quiet, continuing after she had finally ventured her frightened concern, might understandably be felt as distant" (1992, p. 1049). The patient may become so anxious that she can no longer observe. Using the data gained through silent empathic recognition, one can dispel the patient's fantasy, as in the vignette of Mrs. X., and speak using a more neutral statement of inquiry.

Schwaber's stated goal is similar to that of Gray: to learn about the patient's reality. But the method she employs does not focus on the obstacle that prevents the patient from telling about her experience. For example, an intervention such as "You got quiet after mentioning a disappointment in me" provides the needed gratification more neutrally. The patient would temporarily register that the analyst is listening attentively, if she was aware of the silence. Schwaber includes her thinking process. It provides a further clarification of her different approach, and the different data she attends to. There are also similarities with Gray. Schwaber says:

> "I want [to establish] more distance?" I thought to myself. But she has become quiet; she seems to be distancing herself. I did not feel particularly quiet or distant, but responding just as I always do, to her. My sense of myself was jarred. I was certain I was not the one retreating. Perhaps she is placing her feelings onto me so she will not have to bear them. . . . It would be easy now to find an explanation; after all, I was going away. That could be reason enough, I thought, for her to experience what I saw as my attentive response in this "distorted" fashion—a projection of her own withholding feelings. . . . Then I recognized that I was feeling a sense of certainty about what was only my supposition, as though I had already understood the meaning of her experiences and maybe I had not. Observing this temptation for closure, I shifted my position to try to listen more attentively to what she was telling me. . . . [1992, pp. 1048–1049]

Schwaber is sensitive to her preformed opinions concerning an upcoming interruption of the analysis. She is also sensitive to the closure imposed by her turning to her scrutiny of her own experience of the patient.

The next vignette, from the same article, shows a similar intervention. The patient ended up crying after feeling understood by Schwaber, though it seems to me that he had begun to be annoyed with her.

> A patient, fairly new to analysis, asks me if I have seen a certain play in town—not an unusual kind of question for him. I do not answer; he waits, becoming upset that I do not respond. "What can be the harm in it?" he asks, as he makes a compelling case for my simply telling him.

> ... If I were just to tell him I saw it, he suggests, it would save him the time of recounting it; ... What can possibly be "served," he goes on, by my not saying? "It feels so impersonal." [p. 1041]

In her comment, Schwaber says, "You mean it feels like it doesn't serve anything for you; it's not for you, personally—like uncaring—that I don't tell you about my life outside here?" "Yes," he says, "that's right." Schwaber comments that the patient's tone was calmer, that he became reflective and said, "But I see now, where would it stop? I'd want to know where you're going when you go away and all sorts of other things about you. ... " At some point, the patient wipes his eyes and says, "I know I've cried here when I've felt understood by you" (p. 1041).

Schwaber's intervention, by "empathic recognition" of the patient's reality, shifts him away from the beginning frustration at the analytic abstinence. One could have intervened in the silence immediately following the question, if prior experience with this patient (as is implied in Schwaber's comment that asking questions is not unusual for him) had informed the analyst that when the patient asked questions, he was likely to develop anxiety-provoking fantasies of the analyst. For example, an intervention such as "Would this be a moment when the picture of me is ... " would dispel the transference while preserving the very notion that it is a transference. Another option is to wait, and intervene only if the patient becomes too anxious because of the frustration. A likely next association for this patient would be turning on the self, since at the end of this vignette he could be heard as reproaching himself for his voracious curiosity about the analyst. Could he be heard as complying with another silent transference in which someone has conveyed the idea that he ought not to be curious about the analyst?

DISCUSSION

I have used contrasting vignettes to illustrate that close process attention requires a degree of attunement that places it close to Schwaber's mode of listening. Both perspectives utilize a combination of attention to moment-to-moment cues and vicarious introspection.

Schwaber has chosen the preconscious, the experience-near, as a surface of choice, and so has Gray (Pray, 1992 personal communication). Gray attends to the preconscious because he is interested in the "live" drive (preconscious) and its conflicted fate in the presence of the analyst. Schwaber does so because she attends to the disappointment in the analyst the patient has just experienced.

Both listening perspectives emphasize an awareness of the subtle shifts related to the patient's experience of the analyst. Gray attends to superego projections; Schwaber attends to the shifts caused by narcissistic injuries and deprivations. Both want to move away from a hierarchical, authoritarian mode of intervention that labels the patient's experience a misperception. Both have understood, in the line of Kohut's contribution, the subtle regressions that an analyst's interventions or abstinence may provoke. Thus, their ways of listening are in many ways closer to one another than either is to those of analysts who listen to the unconscious such as Brenner and Silverman.

The following excerpt is taken from process material published by Martin Silverman (1987), who listens to the unconscious. Brenner wrote a critique (1987) of Silverman's clinical paper. Pray (1994) has pointed out that though Brenner does not publish detailed clinical material, it is reasonable to extrapolate that Brenner works in a manner similar to that of Silverman. The excerpt illustrates what both Gray and Schwaber object to. Silverman interprets the young woman's unconscious fantasy that she is inferior to men, while he himself assumes a stance of superior knowledge with her.

> *Patient:* I get intimidated with men. I always feel that they know they have the knowledge. They have the brains and I'm dumb . . . and I always feel like I don't know anything and I can't understand and I get intimidated. It's the same thing here. I keep feeling like asking you, what does it mean? I always feel like you know. I feel like asking you now. I know you've told me you don't know anything until I've told it to you, but I don't feel that way. I feel you're always a step ahead of me. You *know*, because you're smarter than I am and all the training and experience you have.
> *Analyst:* I don't think that's what it is. I think you feel I know because I'm a man, that as a woman you don't have the brains. [p. 152]

The concept of empathy could also be used to describe the process used by Silverman to arrive at his hypothesis. Perhaps he scans the "hierarchic organization of desires, feelings, thoughts, defenses, controls, superego pressures, capacities, self representations . . . " that Schafer describes in his concept of generative empathy (1959). Silverman, however, selects different data because he does not "listen to moments of impulse and defense" but listens for a "bigger picture . . . [within which he] . . . targets . . . unconscious, deep, long-standing infantile conflicts" (Pray 1994, p. 102). He is not *attending* to the experience-near; thus, he *cannot perceive* the moment-to-moment cues that would inform him of his enactment with the patient. This is a dramatic illustration of how our theory of technique influences what we perceive.[1]

---

[1] A current principle of neuropsychological research is that perception consists of selective, sequential attention to data which allows the observer

Gray and Schwaber are similar in avoiding what Spencer and Balter (1990) describe as the risk of a mode of observation that ignores the experience-near: "a . . . [potentially] premature, incorrect, useless intervention because too experience-distant" (p. 416). However, within the moments she has chosen as a surface, Schwaber verbalizes the empathic understanding (instead of restraining it) for observation by herself and the patient, and her gathering of data involves a primary reliance on vicarious introspection. In addition, and most important, defensive shifts are not defenses against awareness of drive derivatives. The moments she studies are challenging: the analyst is *heard* as silent in addition to being silent. The patient has just expressed the wish that the analyst speak (to answer a question or to acknowledge a concern). Some appetite has been awakened and the analyst is silent. Schwaber quotes Freud: "It is just as disastrous if the patient's craving for love is gratified as if it is suppressed" (p. 116). Ferenczi (1928) also spoke of the dilemma of "when one should keep silent and await further associations and at what point the further maintenance of silence would result only in causing the patient useless suffering" (p. 89).

The close process attention analyst will choose to speak but in a more neutral way. The analyst's voice needs to be heard. It is a moment when empathy as gratification of wishes furthers neutrality as defined by Inderbitzin and Levy (1992): "A listening and interpretative stance that encourages the emergence of as many of the multiple determinants of conflicts as are discoverable by the analytic method" (p. 996). Thus, empathy is essential when using close process attention. Empathy provides a mode of observing data that the analyst can use to preserve the observing capacity; it is also

---

to choose one of a series of models which are already internally encoded. The models of course are subject to slow modification and improvement over time (Hutchinson, 1992 personal communication).

an intervention that can involve a planned temporary gratification of wishes. Schwaber also wishes to enhance the patient's observing capacity, but as I see it, she tilts more toward empathizing with the patient.

Inderbitzin and Levy (1990) stated, "Schwaber's work, as distinct from Kohut's and that of the analysts of the self-psychology school, poses no reformulations of psychopathology . . . or theory of therapeutic action of psychoanalysis" (p. 382). Yet, it seems to me that the implication of Schwaber's technical stance is in fact a shift to a self-psychological viewpoint. It also seems to me that she forecloses with empathy the exploration of what is beyond the preconscious.

In her attempt to be sensitive to the analyst's participation, Schwaber permits, perhaps unwittingly, a view of the analyst as personally caring for the patient. This is illustrated by the man who became tearful when feeling understood by Schwaber in the vignette cited earlier. Just before her empathetic comment, he had sounded irritable—perhaps on the verge of aggression—when he said, "What can possibly be served by [your] not saying? It feels so impersonal."

As we know, some patients do require that the analyst not challenge their transference to an idealized, caring maternal figure. But Schwaber does not, to my knowledge, state clearly that she has made a diagnostic distinction between patients who can ultimately tolerate a neutral stance and those who need her to remain a benign understanding figure.

An important reason for making such a distinction is that patients who can tolerate the analyst's neutral stance may not become aware of active aggressive wishes and may remain unchallenged in their view that they are victims of their objects. Gray, on the other hand, has integrated some of Kohut's contributions into an ego-psychological approach, which views narcissistic regressions as defensive. Thus, he has utilized Kohut's contributions to develop a method that aims at preserving the patient's capacity to observe his mental scene.

It is interesting that Gray's method achieves what Schwaber strives for. For example, when the focus of analytic intervention is on the obstacles to the patients' telling of their reality, it will *de facto* exclude what Schwaber correctly picks up as an unwelcome intrusion of her own opinions or values on the patient's reality.

A number of analysts, Hartmann in particular, were concerned that if empathy was to be used as a tool "there would be a replacement of the rule of abstinence," and that this could "lead to acting out of the analyst's countertransference with his patient," that "feeling into" would lead to "feeling with" (Basch 1983, p. 110).

One of Gray's significant contributions is to use "feeling into," instead of "feeling with," so that a patient can experience the analyst's neutrality more clearly. As a patient triumphantly said to me recently, "I speak to you more freely these days; now the real analysis can start."

McLaughlin (1991) has written extensively on the need to be attuned to the patient's vantage point. While citing Gray's contribution, he expresses

> essential agreement with Schwaber's observation about many of the crises and complications in our analytic work. . . . She [Schwaber] sees these events as often expressing our prior failures to seek and acknowledge the patient's viewpoint of our behaviors that he or she has found distressing. She notes the cumulative impact of the analyst's further failure to respond and help to articulate the patient's distress. Her data are impressive in pointing to the analyst's lapses as reflecting countertransference issues of conflicts and avoidance, along with defensive needs to adhere to theoretical technical preference. [p. 612]

Gray's contribution is his development of a technique in which the analyst tries to correct the "empathic failures," the unnecessarily burdensome ways of addressing the patient, while continuing to emphasize a focus that permits *those patients who can* to tell us just how distressing we are to them. Gray, like McLaughlin, addresses analysts' defensive needs and would agree that the analyst may well use technique in the service of countertransference. He would, however, differ in his view of what analysts tend to avoid. Gray (1994) defines counterresistance as "an unconsciously motivated form . . . [of resistance within the analyst] . . . directed against the full emergence of analyst-cathected affects and impulses" (p. 58). Gray sees analysts as unconsciously reluctant to fully free their patients to observe them clearly and speak in detail of what they see and how they feel about it.

He emphasizes our need to be protected from the patient's ultimate capacity to subject us to "drive derivatives of a more detailed and intense variety" (Gray 1994, p. 58-59).

As McLaughlin points out (above), the trend to be sensitive to the patient's experience of the analyst is useful for awareness and control of counter-resistance. However, this trend can itself be used for counter-resistance, if not subordinated to a focus on defenses. While close process attention guides the analyst to intervene empathically, and to keep in mind the patient's vantage point, this gentleness is designed to further patients' capacity to observe us and tell us of their distress at our failures, be they real or fantasied. The focus is not only on minimizing patients' distress but on permitting them to understand what keeps them from being able to articulate in our presence their disappointment in us.

References

Basch, M. F. (1983). Empathic understanding: a review of the concept and some theoretical consideration. *Journal of the American Psychoanalytic Association* 31:101-127.

Brenner, C. (1987). A structural theory perspective. *Psychoanalytic Inquiry* 7:167-171.

Chused, F. J. (1991). The evocative power of enactments. *Journal of the American Psychoanalytic Association* 39:615-639.
Ferenczi, S. (1955). The elasticity of psychoanalytic technique in final contributions to the theory and technique of psychoanalysis. In *Selected Papers of Sandor Ferenczi,* vol. III, pp. 87-101. New York: Basic Books.
Freud, S. (1912b). Recommendations on analytic technique. *Standard Edition* 12:111-120.
—— (1915). Observations on transference-love. *Standard Edition* 12:159-171.
Gray, P. (1973). Psychoanalytic technique and the ego's capacity for viewing intrapsychic activity. *Journal of the American Psychoanalytic Association* 21:474-493.
—— (1994). *The Ego and Analysis of Defense.* Northvale, NJ: Jason Aronson.
Hutchinson, J. (1994). Personal communication.
Inderbitzin, L., and Levy, S. (1990). The analytic surface and the theory of technique. *Journal of the American Psychoanalytic Association* 38:371-393.
—— (1992). Neutrality, interpretation, and therapeutic intent. *Journal of the American Psychoanalytic Association* 40:989-1013.
Kohut, H. (1959). Introspection, empathy and psychoanalysis. *Journal of the American Psychoanalytic Association* 7:459-483.
Levy, S. (1985). Empathy and psychoanalytic technique. *Journal of the American Psychoanalytic Association* 33:353-379.
McLaughlin, J. (1991). Clinical and theoretical aspects of enactment. *Journal of the American Psychoanalytic Association* 39:595-614.
Paniagua, C. (1985). A methodological approach to surface material. *International Review of Psycho-Analysis* 12:311-325.
Pray, M. (1992). Personal communication.
—— (1994). Analyzing defense: two different methods. *Journal of Clinical Psychoanalysis* 3:87-126.
Reik, T. (1948). *Listening with the Third Ear.* New York: Farrar, Straus.
Sarraute, N. (1957). *Tropism.* Trans. M. Jolas. New York: Braziller.

Schafer, R. (1959). Generative empathy in the treatment situation. *Psychoanalytic Quarterly* 28:342–373.

Schwaber, E. A. (1981). Empathy: a mode of analytic listening. *Psychoanalytic Inquiry* 1:357–392.

—— (1983). A particular perspective on analytic listening. *Psychoanalytic Study of the Child* 38:519–546. New Haven, CT: Yale University Press.

—— (1987). Models of the mind and data-gathering in clinical work. *Psychoanalytic Inquiry* 7:261–275.

—— (1992). Psychoanalytic theory and its relation to clinical work. *Journal of the American Psychoanalytic Association* 40:1039–1057.

Silverman, M. (1987). Clinical material. *Psychoanalytic Inquiry* 7/2:147–165.

Spencer, J. H., and Balter, L. (1990). Psychoanalytic observation. *Journal of the American Psychoanalytic Association* 38:393–423.

Sterba, R. (1934). The fate of the ego in analytic therapy. *International Journal of Psycho-Analysis* 15:117–126.

10

Consciousness as a Beacon Light[1]

BARRY J. LANDAU, M.D.

The concept of consciousness (and of the unconscious) underwent a number of changes during the evolution of Freud's models of the mind and his views of the therapeutic action of psychoanalytic treatment. Freud's formulation of the structural theory and his revision of the theory of anxiety were crucial developments which removed consciousness from its central role in defining the divisions of the mind and in determining the distinction between health and neurotic psychopathology. These developments also paved the way for major advances in psychoanalytic technique, especially by reorienting the focus from interpretation of drives to analysis of defenses (resistance). Paul Gray has made crucial contributions to the development of defense analysis and to modify-

---

[1] I would like to thank Fred Busch, Leon Hoffman, Marianne Goldberger, and Monroe Pray for their thoughtful and encouraging contributions to the development of this chapter.

ing certain aspects of technique that had interfered with the analysis of superego functioning. Paradoxically, with these developments in defense analysis, the concept of consciousness has returned to center stage. This paper examines that paradox, reviews the evolution of the concept of consciousness, and considers the complexities involved in using consciousness as a "beacon light" in a structural theory approach to psychoanalytic technique.

HISTORICAL PERSPECTIVE

Freud's earliest ideas on the role of consciousness and of "the unconscious"

Freud's work on the neuroses began with an interest in consciousness. He had learned (1893), from the work of Charcot and Breuer, of the use of hypnosis to gain access to memories that were otherwise unavailable to consciousness and were connected with neurotic symptoms. Freud discovered that without hypnosis, a "laborious" effort was necessary to gain access to these memories. From this empirical finding, Freud (1893–1895) formulated his concept of resistance and his theory of defense. He described defense as a psychical force that excluded incompatible ideas from "association" with the dominant mass of ideas in the mind. At this time, Freud equated defense with repression.

Freud explored the difference between the typical reaction to stressful experiences and the neurotic reaction, which he viewed as a consequence of repression (1893, 1900). Ordinarily, when a person is stressed, he reacts verbally or physically to the impact of that experience. He can also think about the insult and put it in perspective. For example, a person may remind himself of his own worth or his enemy's worthlessness. Both of these responses lead to the gradual diminution, or "forgetting," of painful experiences, as time passes (Freud 1893).

By contrast, when the memory is repressed, it appears to have instantly disappeared. In its place, there appears a neurotic symptom—for example, an hysterical symptom, an obsession, or a hallucination. However, when Freud used his (then) new cathartic treatment, he could demonstrate that although apparently gone, the distressing idea was still retrievable, even many years later, along with the same degree of intense emotion as at the time of the insult (Freud 1893, 1900). In order to relieve the patient of his symptom and to re-institute the normal "wearing away" (forgetting) process, the apparent gap in the patient's consciousness had to be resolved. That is, the patient had to be helped to *remember* the insult before he would be able to really forget about it (Freud 1900).

The central, defining role of consciousness in Freud's topographic theory

Freud's original emphasis on childhood traumatic memories gave way to his discovery of infantile sexuality and of the internal nature of psychic conflict. In chapter seven of "The Interpretation of Dreams," Freud (1900) introduced a theoretical picture of how the mind functions. At this time, the quality of being either available or unavailable to consciousness seemed so central, clinically, to what caused ideas to have their pathogenic effect that Freud made this quality the distinguishing characteristic of the topographically arranged mental systems he envisioned. However, as he was formulating this theory, Freud was already uncomfortable with a topographic model of the mind.

For example, as early as 1900, Freud wrote:

> So let us try to correct some conceptions which might be misleading so long as we looked upon the two systems *in the most literal and crudest sense as two localities* in the mental apparatus.... Thus we may speak of an unconscious thought seeking to convey itself into the precon-

scious so as to be able to force its way into consciousness. ... These images [are] derived from a set of ideas relating to a struggle for a piece of ground. ... Let us replace these metaphors by something that seems to correspond better to the real state of affairs ... and *replace a topographical way of representing things by a dynamic one.* [p. 610, emphasis added]

As Arlow and Brenner (1964), Gray (1982), and others have pointed out, Freud's theory during these years (1900–1923) fit well with his technique, which was to make the unconscious conscious. Interpretation was the vehicle for self-knowledge or insight. Freud's interpretations were aimed at establishing "word linkages" to the repressed, unconscious contents. Then they could enter the preconscious, and ultimately gain access to consciousness. Once the preconscious linkage was established, the ideas could be worked over associatively, which, in turn, diminished the intensity of the driving force. In "The Interpretation of Dreams," Freud (1900) put it thus:

... the fading of memories ... which are no longer recent, which we are inclined to regard as self-evident and to explain as a primary effect of time..., are in reality secondary modifications which are only brought about by laborious work. What performs this work is the preconscious, *and psychotherapy can pursue no other course than to bring the Ucs. under the domination of the Pcs.* [p. 578, emphasis added]

The declining importance of consciousness in determining the divisions in the mind associated with intrapsychic conflict

Gray (1982) demonstrated that in the technical papers, written between 1913 and 1917, Freud expressed increasing dissatisfaction with the central role he had assigned to interpretation of unconscious material. Instead, Freud began to emphasize the importance of overcoming the resistances. This change was paralleled by a decrease in the importance he now attributed to consciousness in his theoretical model. In "The Unconscious," Freud (1915b) expressed his dissatisfaction with the use of the characteristic of being conscious or unconscious as the criterion for distinguishing the systems of the mind: "*the attribute of being conscious, which is the only characteristic of psychical processes that is directly presented to us, is in no way suited to serve as a criterion for the differentiation of systems*" (p. 192, emphasis added).

Thus, Freud posed the dilemma vividly: the attribute of being conscious or unconscious was not suited to serve as the basis for distinguishing the systems of the mind, but it was the only basis that he had. Therefore, he continued to elaborate the topographic model of the mind, even as he lamented: "The more we seek to win our way to a metapsychological view of mental life, the more we must learn to emancipate ourselves from the importance of the *symptom* of 'being conscious'" (p. 193, emphasis added).

Introduction of the structural theory: consciousness no longer defines the elements in conflict but has become a "beacon light" that illuminates them

In 1923, Freud indicated his growing awareness of the complexity of assessing the significance of whether a thought is conscious or unconscious, which he had considered to be "the fundamental premise of psychoanalysis; [the only thing that] makes it possible for psychoanalysis to understand the pathologic processes in mental life . . ." (p. 13). He then went on to describe his discovery that the process of resistance, which must emanate from the ego, is unconscious and "*behaves exactly like the repressed*" (p. 17, emphasis added). Because of this discovery, Freud concluded, "We must admit that the characteristic of being unconscious begins to lose it significance for us. It becomes a quality . . . which we are unable to make . . . the basis of far-reaching and inevitable conclusions" (p. 18). Having said this, he immediately added that the characteristic of being conscious or unconscious is nevertheless "in the last resort our one *beacon-light* in the darkness of depth psychology" (p. 18, emphasis added). I wonder whether the ambiguity here is the result of Freud's shifting from a *theoretical* level (when he declared that "we [can no longer] make the quality of being unconscious the basis of far-reaching conclusions") to a *clinical* level (when he reached for the characteristic of whether a thought is conscious or unconscious as "the one beacon-light in the darkness of depth psychology").

The above quote illustrates how difficult it is to avoid using topographic concepts. At the very moment that Freud was introducing the structural theory, he referred to "the darkness of *depth* psychology" (Freud 1923, p. 18, emphasis added), which is, by definition, a topographic concept. Similarly, in his attempt to draw a diagram of the new divisions of the mind, which were now based on functional attributes, he sketched a picture that continued to employ topographical images (Freud 1923, p. 24).[2]

Freud's concept of the ego was defined not by being conscious but by being a coherent organization

In the discussion that introduced the structural theory, Freud (1923) emphasized that the ego is a coherent organization of metal processes. The function of the defenses is "to ex-

---

[2]Chapter II of "The Ego and the Id" is filled with topographic images, for example, "We have said that consciousness is the *surface* of the mental

clude certain trends not merely from consciousness, but also from other forms of effectiveness and activity" (p. 17). He then described the work of analysis as "removing the resistance which the ego displays *against concerning itself with the repressed*" (p. 17, emphasis added). Similarly, in "Inhibitions, Symptoms, and Anxiety," Freud (1926) emphasized that the ego is defined, not by its being conscious, but rather by its being an organization (p. 97). In repression, he continued, "the decisive fact is that the ego is an organization and the id is not" (p. 97). Shortly thereafter, Freud added: "The ego is an organization. It is based on the maintenance of *free intercourse* and the possibility of *reciprocal influence between all its parts*" (p. 98, emphasis added).[3]

ADVANCES IN PSYCHOANALYTIC TECHNIQUE THAT RESULTED FROM THE FORMULATION OF THE STRUCTURAL THEORY

Gill (1963) and Arlow and Brenner (1964) reviewed Freud's transition from the topographic to the structural theory. They documented Freud's revision of the theory of anxiety and

---

apparatus; that is, we have ascribed it as a function to a system which is [conceived of] spatially . . . in the sense of an anatomical dissection. . . ." (Freud 1923, p. 19, original emphasis).

[3]In developing this picture of the ego as a coherent organization, Freud returned to a concept in his discarded neurological model of the mind, the "Project for a Scientific Psychology" (Freud 1950 [1895]). In the "Project," Freud described the ego as an organization of interconnected and freely associated ("constantly cathected") neurons that could transmit and discharge affective intensities gradually via their "contact barriers" (synapses) (Freud [1895] 1950, pp. 322–324). In the psychological model he was formulating in 1923, the ego was an organization defined by its interconnected and freely associated *ideas* (see Strachey 1953, 1966).

the development of his theory of aggression as crucial components of his new conceptualization of mental functioning. Both Gill and Arlow and Brenner concluded that the structural theory has many advantages over and, in fact, supersedes the topographic theory. Numerous authors were cited whose contributions to the development of psychoanalytic technique derived from Freud's articulation of the structural theory, including W. Reich (1928), Sterba (1934), A. Freud (1936), E. Kris (1938), Fenichel (1941), Hartmann (1951), and Loewenstein (1951).

Arlow and Brenner (1964) described how the structural theory enabled them to better appreciate the complexities of the factors in conflict. For example, according to the topographic theory, defense is equivalent to repression, whereas according to the structural theory, repression is one among a number of defensive responses to signal anxiety. Arlow and Brenner pointed out that when defenses other than repression are used—defenses such as isolation, projection and denial—elements can appear in consciousness even while they are being vigorously defended against by the ego. They cited case material to illustrate that a structural theory approach to technique leads the analyst to recognize these additional defenses and, thus, to also recognize the need to focus his interpretation on these defenses and on the conflicts of which they are a part (pp. 106–113).

Anna Freud's method of observing the ego's defensive activities and Gray's contributions to psychoanalytic technique

Anna Freud took a crucial step in the application of Freud's structural theory to clinical practice in *The Ego and the Mechanisms of Defense* (1936). She developed a method of observing and analyzing the clinical manifestations of the defensive activities of the ego. In particular, she described how the ego's defenses could be recognized as they begin to oppose drive derivatives which were coming into consciousness.

However, it was not until Gray's papers, beginning in 1973 and continuing to the present, that Anna Freud's method of observation was applied to develop a systematic clinical methodology to analyze defense (see Pray 1994). Gray (1973, 1986, 1990) used a "microscopic" approach to the clinical material, in which the analyst *demonstrates* to the patient the evidence for the inference that the patient's (unconscious) ego has initiated action to protect itself. This defensive action becomes manifest at the moment that the drive derivatives, having been verbalized, become threatening. Others, including Busch (1992, 1993), Davison and colleagues (1986, 1990), Goldberger (1989), Holmes (in press), Levy and Inderbitzin (1990, 1994), Paniagua (1985, 1991) and Pray (1994) have made contributions that have further clarified or expanded upon Gray's technical recommendations.

In addition, Gray (1987) demonstrated the clinical utility of Anna Freud's (1936) concept of *transference of defense*, in developing a method for analyzing superego functioning. In his 1987 paper, Gray described his analysis of the transference of authority—that is, his analysis of the re-externalization within the analytic setting of images of past authorities. These restraining images had been internalized during early childhood (especially during the oedipal phase) for the purpose of self-control and safety. Because these internalized images of past authorities are transferred onto the analyst, the analyst is perceived to be in the position of the patient's superego.

Gray (1987) described how this transferred superego authority became the source of power for the suggestive influence used by Freud and his followers to overcome resistance to free association. Gray pointed out that this use of suggestion continued even after Freud came to appreciate the central role of resistance analysis. Transferred superego authority has been used as the active agent in a whole series of technical approaches that have relied on the patient's *identifying* with the analyst's "more benign" superego, such as in Strachey's (1934) technique which was based on "mutative interpretations" (see Hoffman 1994a, pp. 165–166).

Gray implied, in his "Developmental Lag" paper (1982), and Pray (1994) has begun to illustrate (using published clinical material), that defenses continue to be bypassed and that transferred superego authority continues to be utilized by the analyst (albeit inadvertently) to overcome resistances, even in contemporary structural theory approaches to analysis (see also Busch 1992, 1993). For example, Gray (1982) argued that:

> The analyst who makes interpretive remarks referring to unconscious matters of which the patient cannot become aware has left the patient to take the interpretation "on faith".... This is an authoritative approach that relies heavily on suggestion to influence rather than on *analysis* of the resistance. [p. 631, emphasis added] The idea here is that current standard analytic methods rely on the analyst's use of his own unconscious as a crucial component of the analyzing instrument (and, thus, use data which are not available for the patient to observe). Therefore, interpretations based on such methods bypass defenses and are accepted by the patient because of the suggestive influence of transferred superego authority.[4]

By contrast, Gray's method of helping the patient to observe and analyze moment-to-moment defensive operations by the ego offered a fundamentally new approach,

---

[4]Hoffman (1994b) pointed out that Gray's thesis is supported by clinical observation—that when the analyst interprets unconscious drive derivatives there is an intensification of superego manifestations; whereas when the analyst addresses unconscious defenses, there is less tendency for superego manifestations to occur.

whose aim was to minimize the role of suggestion, because of "its greater dependence on confirmable observation" (1990, p. 1095). This method was designed to provide an opportunity for developing a greater degree of voluntary, active participation by the patient than had previously been possible. This more active role for the patient, in observing and analyzing, stands in contrast to a more submissive role that Gray concluded is inevitable when the patient is the recipient of interpretations of material that has not already entered consciousness and, therefore, is not directly observable by the patient. The goal of Gray's method is to help the patient to regain the "use of his objective self-observing functions" (1990, p. 1098), and thereby to achieve the autonomous use of his own analyzing capacity and the autonomous regulation of his drives. These functions were formerly pre-empted by the patient's superego, and were therefore readily surrendered in favor of identifying with the (transferentially authoritative) analyst's interpretive opinions.[5]

REFLECTIONS, QUESTIONS, AND DIRECTIONS FOR FURTHER STUDY: COMPLEXITIES INVOLVED IN CENTERING A STRUCTURAL THEORY APPROACH TO PSYCHOANALYTIC TECHNIQUE ON CONSCIOUSNESS

Gray (1982, 1987, 1991) stated clearly that he regards his technical methods to be clinical applications of the structural theory. In his 1982 paper, Gray offered several reasons to

---

[5]This capacity for self-observation is characterized by its freedom from self-critical, inhibiting fantasies [and, with Gray's 1991 paper, freedom also from dependence on approving, permissive fantasies] that are associated with superego functioning (1990). Such functioning becomes autonomous because it no longer depends on *internalizing* a fantasy of an inhibiting,

explain the "developmental lag" that prevented psychoanalysts from making more consistent use of the potential inherent in the structural theory for the development of psychoanalytic technique.

Among the reasons Gray (1982) mentioned for this lag, one (merely hinted at in his paper) is the inherent difficulty the ego encounters in observing and thinking about its own functioning. I cite this issue as a possible clue to what otherwise emerges as a paradox in Gray's methodology: Gray's method is based on the structural theory, the essence of which is to divide the mind on the basis of whether or not mental elements are associated with one another—that is, whether the elements are integrated within the (organized) ego. This distinction stands in contrast to the one that defines the topographic theory, which is based on whether or not mental elements are accessible to consciousness. However, as has just been demonstrated, the central feature of Gray's technique is to focus analytic attention on mental events that take place in consciousness, where the ego's contents are illuminated and thus can be observed by both patient and analyst. This emphasis on consciousness seems characteristic of the topographic theory, the abandonment of which was a crucial step in the chain of events upon which Gray's technical innovations are based.

Thus, in formulating his technical advances that were based on the structural theory, Gray included elements that are more consistent with the topographic theory. This transition parallels similar ones associated with earlier attempts

---

critical authority or of an approving, permissive authority. Therefore, it does not depend on the presence of another person who represents transferred authority. Instead, it is self-perpetuated. And, as the patient uses these autonomous capacities, he learns that he has them—that is, he "acquires insight . . . (experientially) into the reality that his adult ego" has these capacities (Gray 1990, p. 1094).

to formulate a structural theory approach to psychoanalysis. For example, Freud returned to topographic concepts at the very time he was introducing the structural theory in "The Ego and the Id" (see above). Similarly, Anna Freud (1936) used the structural theory to define a new concept of technical neutrality, in which the analyst tries to remain equidistant from id, ego, and superego. Immediately after having done so, she then described the goal of analysis as making each psychic agency *conscious*. Pray's (1994) observation that Anna Freud included aspects of both the topographic and the structural theory is relevant here.

Arlow and Brenner (1964) also distinguished the analytic goal according to the structural theory as no longer making the unconscious conscious (abrogating repression), as it was according to the topographic theory. Arlow and Brenner stated that, with the advent of the structural theory, the analytic goal became *analyzing* rather than circumventing the defenses, "permitting the *integration* of previously warded-off instinctual drives and memories associated with them into the normal parts of the ego" (p. 54, emphasis added). Arlow and Brenner stated emphatically that the new goal of analysis was no longer to make the unconscious conscious but rather, quoting Freud: "Where id was, there shall ego be" (p. 54). However, having made that distinction so clearly, Arlow and Brenner shifted into language that seems more consistent with the topographic model: "According to the structural theory, it is important to make the patient *conscious* not only of the instinctual aspects of his conflicts but of their defensive and superego aspects as well...." (p. 55, emphasis added). Like Freud and Anna Freud, once they had defined the new mental agencies of id, ego, and superego, they felt a need to include a reference to consciousness, even though it was no longer the crucial characteristic that distinguished ego from id.

Use of the concept of ego-syntonicity: An attempt to resolve the theoretical conundrum posed by consciousness

The 1989 paper by Apfelbaum and Gill, "Ego Analysis and the Relativity of Defense: Technical Implications of the Structural Theory," provides a point of departure that may be useful in this regard. The paper explores Gray's contributions to psychoanalytic technique, in the context of specifying the differences between the structural theory and the topographic theory.

Apfelbaum and Gill stated that, from the structural point of view, any mental content can serve as defense—that is, that there is nothing *intrinsic* to a content which determines whether it will function as defense or as that which is defended against. They then went on to demonstrate that the concepts of defense and wish are relative by illustrating how a dependent wish can be threatening at one moment (and thus be defended against), while the same dependent wish can itself be a defense against an aggressive impulse at another moment (when the aggressive impulse is experienced as threatening).

The crucial point in Apfelbaum and Gill's article for the present study is the application of the structural theory to psychoanalytic technique, including some of Gray's major contributions, without emphasizing the issue of consciousness.[6] Instead, they concluded that the structural theory is

---

[6] The technique Apfelbaum and Gill described has the following elements in common with the technical measures Gray recommends: a "microscopic" moment-to-moment focus of interpretation; a consistent defense-before-drive approach to material *throughout* the analysis; and use of the above technical features with the aim of analyzing resistance rather than overcoming it. The need to use superego pressure was thereby eliminated and an *analysis* of superego functioning became possible.

characterized by the concept that anything can be used as a defense at certain moments and by the ego-syntonicity or ego-dystonicity of the elements in the mind.

Apfelbaum and Gill (1989) specifically stated that the concept of ego-syntonicity can be used as a criterion for distinguishing defense from that which is defended against—that is, for distinguishing ego from id. Or, perhaps more precisely, for distinguishing ego aspects of mental elements from id aspects (see Apfelbaum 1966, Waelder 1936). They added that ego-syntonicity can also be used as a criterion for determining on which of their patient's ideas they should focus their interpretations (p. 1080).

Apfelbaum and Gill did not define what they meant by ego-syntonicity. From the context in which they used it, I infer that ego-syntonicity designates characteristics of a mental element which the ego can integrate relatively easily whereas ego-dystonicity refers to characteristics which the ego can integrate only with great difficulty or not at all. Use of the concept of ego-syntonicity in this way has great theoretical appeal. It is consistent with the structural theory, in contrast to using the quality of consciousness for this purpose, which is more consistent with the topographic theory. For example, it is consistent with the aphorism, "Where id was, there shall ego be," which characterized the revised goal of analysis after the introduction of the structural theory. Restating the aphorism as: "Where ego-dystonic elements were, there shall ego-syntonic elements be," would not only be consistent with the structural theory but would also highlight the idea of the ego as an organization, which integrates syntonic elements but which, in its defensive mode, dissociates elements that are dystonic. Through analysis of the defenses, and specifically analysis of the (imagined) dangers that cause anxiety and trigger defensive reactions, mental elements are rendered less ego-dystonic, more ego-syntonic, and thus more capable of being re-integrated within the ego.

Furthermore, a technique of analyzing conflict over derivatives that are relatively ego-syntonic would be consistent with Gray's emphasis on technical measures that do not bypass defenses. Ego-dystonic derivatives are the ones against which strong defenses are maintained. Ego-syntonic derivatives, being relatively conflict-free, have relatively minimal defenses maintained against them. Thus, the concept of ego-syntonicity could be used to express (with imagery more consistent with the structural theory) the essence of what Gray and others are conveying when they refer to analyzing material "at the surface" of the mind (the latter imagery being more characteristic of the topographic theory).[7]

Clinical complexities of a technical focus on consciousness and the concept of ego-syntonicity

Focusing psychoanalytic technique on moments of conflict over drive derivatives which have entered consciousness—that is, which have been verbalized—seems integral to Gray's contributions. It is the fact that the drive derivatives have been verbalized (and have then been acted upon by the unconscious ego defenses) that makes it possible for the analyst to observe evidence of this mental activity and demonstrate it to the patient. It is the fact that this *evidence* of unconscious mental activity can be demonstrated to the patient that makes it possible to engage the patient as an active participant in the analysis of the transference of superego authority. Gray

---

[7] I am using the term *ego-syntonicity* as a theoretical concept, referring to characteristics of a mental element that lend themselves to being integrated by the ego. The observable manifestations of ego-syntonicity would then need to be specified in order to use this concept in a clinical setting. Such specification could lead to a greater degree of objectivity in characterizing clinical phenomena that are currently perceived via intuition or empathy (see below for some of the complexities involved in applying this concept clinically).

has pointed out that, without this evidence of (unconscious) defenses acting upon drive derivatives that have already been verbalized, transferential superego authority has to be used rather than analyzed because the patient has no alternative but to accept interpretations on faith. In other words, until a drive derivative has entered into consciousness, the patient is in the dark about it.

Gray stated that even when the analyst correctly infers an unconscious wish, and conveys it to the patient, the patient still feels in the dark and has to rely on the analyst's authority as the one with superior vision. However, once the idea or feeling has entered consciousness—that is, once the patient has verbalized it—*it is as though a light has been shined on it*. Then, if the analyst points it out, the patient can be in a position to acknowledge it. More important, if the patient verbalizes a drive derivative, and then initiates a defensive measure, the defense will be manifested clinically by opposition to further expression or by efforts to mitigate the effect of the verbalized derivative. Then the analyst is in a position to demonstrate this evidence of unconscious ego-defensive activity and the patient is in a position to see it for himself. It has thus seemed self-evident that accessibility to consciousness, based on verbalization of the derivatives, is the *sine qua non* for active cooperative participation by the patient and, thus, for optimal analysis of the transferential use of the analyst as external superego figure. The concept of ego-syntonicity would be more difficult to use to accomplish these goals because it is more abstract and less precisely definable.

In addition, because Gray's method relies on data that are readily observable, it is more likely to be reproducible by other analysts. The method's reliance on observable data also creates the potential for research studies evaluating psychoanalytic process and its results. Again, it has seemed self-evident that accessibility to consciousness is the *sine qua non* for these advantages as well. Again, applying the concept of ego-syntonicity for this purpose seems a much more complex and difficult undertaking.

However, a major concern with regard to basing psychoanalytic technique on elements that have entered into consciousness is that the significance of accessibility to consciousness is likely to be overrated. The whole history of psychoanalysis has been a testament to man's over-estimation of the significance of that which is in his consciousness. Freud's early work was needed to document that all that is psychical is not necessarily conscious (Freud 1900, 1915a). The treatment method he originally developed had as its primary goal to expand the domain of consciousness. The development in Freud's thinking that led him to formulate the structural theory was a further step in his recognition that the attribute of being or not being in consciousness was not so crucial a distinguishing characteristic in the study of mental conflict as he had considered it to be when he formulated the topographic theory. This development led, in turn, to a more sophisticated understanding of the functioning of the ego. Psychoanalytic treatment now had new tools and a new goal: the primary goal became expanding the domain of the *ego*, while expanding the domain of consciousness became a secondary goal, a *consequence* of expanding the realm of the ego.

As he was formulating the structural theory, Freud recognized that the *quality* of consciousness continues to have a very special importance. Freud related its importance to its usefulness as a "beacon light [to help find one's way] in the darkness of depth psychology" (1923, p. 18). Gray's technique, in turn, has been to exploit the "beacon light" function of consciousness (along with the more sophisticated understanding of the ego and its defense mechanisms) in a somewhat different, albeit related way: to illuminate, for analyst and patient, evidence of unconscious ego-defensive activity which otherwise would be obscure and, therefore, difficult to demonstrate.

Nevertheless, the light that allows one to see must be distinguished from the subject matter that is illuminated by the light. While verbalization of a drive derivative is, in itself, evidence that there has been some ego integration, it does not provide evidence of the *degree* of integration. That full ego integration has not been achieved is confirmed by the very fact that the derivative is quickly defended against by the ego. A beacon light has been shined on a moment of drive–defense interaction. For a brief period of time, the drive has established contact with the ego (it has gained access to consciousness) and then the ego reacts to banish the drive from its organization once again. Thus, the fact that the derivative has been verbalized does not establish the degree to which ego integration of that drive has occurred.

This issue is reflected in Anna Freud's comment in published conversations with Joseph Sandler (1985):

> *Anna Freud:* "The defenses work in the dark ... and once they are brought into consciousness ... they cease to work with the same efficiency.... At least, that is what the hope was at the time I wrote [*The Ego and the Mechanisms of Defense*]."
>
> *Sandler:* "You sound as if you are not quite so optimistic about it now."
>
> *Anna Freud:* "Well, it doesn't always work. Some people go on employing the same mechanisms." [pp. 55–56][8]

---

[8]Sandler continued: "One has the hope, of course, that the process of working through enables people to become their own policemen in regard to the defenses they employ" (p. 56). The implication in Sandler's remark is that something else must occur—something in addition to having the thought come into consciousness, something that Sandler refers to with the imprecise clinical term "working through" (see Brenner 1987)—before a derivative is fully integrated by the ego.

I believe that Gray's (1991) use of the term *full consciousness* when describing the goal of his analysis of the ego's superego activities (p. 11) is also related to this issue of the variable degree of integration by the ego of derivatives that have been in consciousness.

The difficulty in determining the degree of ego integration of a drive derivative that has been verbalized leads to a particular consequence for technique—namely, it is also difficult to determine the degree to which the ego is "ready" to "recognize" the verbalized derivative or the defenses against that derivative. This distinction is illustrated in the contrast between, on the one hand, the relative ease with which our Tuesday evening study group[9] can reach agreement in identifying ego-defensive shifts in the written transcriptions we examine with, on the other hand, the difficulty the group acknowledges it would have in trying to determine which of those defensive shifts would be useful for the analyst to comment upon. Here the concept of ego-syntonicity could be useful to characterize the nature of the data that would help to determine which defensive shifts to address.[10]

---

[9]Reference here is to an on-going study group on technique, which includes Paul Gray and a number of other contributors to this volume, and which is currently focusing on a research approach to demonstrating unconscious ego-defensive activity and the effect of defense analysis on that activity.

[10]As noted above, I am using the theoretical concept of ego-syntonicity to designate those mental elements, and the defenses against them, that the ego is "ready" to "recognize." The concept itself is a general one and is manifested clinically by phenomena usually perceived via intuition and empathy. The clinical characteristics that correspond to an element being ego-syntonic would need to be specified in order to approach them more objectively. Whether or not an element has been verbalized is one important clinical indicator. The advantage of using a general term, such as ego-syntonicity, is that it leaves room to specify other indicators once we conclude that having been verbalized is not sufficient, by itself.

Thus, the fact of having been temporarily in consciousness is a quality of certain drive derivatives, which makes them particularly useful for psychoanalytic observation. Nevertheless, the distinction between an element being observable *by the analyst* because it has entered consciousness and being recognizable and usable *by the patient* needs to be kept in mind. This distinction highlights the fact that a derivative having been in consciousness is a necessary, but not a *sufficient*, basis upon which to construct a psychoanalytic technical methodology. The concept of ego-syntonicity could be useful in furthering the articulation of such a methodology.[11]

Some additional clinical examples follow to illustrate this point. It is common clinical experience that the patient does not always react with ready and comfortable acknowledgement and interest when the analyst attempts to reconstruct what the patient has just said. The patient may react to the analyst's repetition of the very same words the patient himself has just said with surprise bordering on shock, accompanied by intense affect (denial or disbelief), as though having just experienced a premature interpretation. What defines the comment as premature is that the ego is pesented material of a greater degree of dystonicity than it is ready to deal with.

Some patients react to a demonstration of defensive activity, including tactful comments focusing on derivatives expressed and then resisted, with narcissistic injury, feeling criticized, and a tendency to project their own emerging impulses onto the analyst. Externalization of an authoritarian image has occurred on the spot. An example of this type of reaction is displayed by the patient who says: "You're never satisfied with what I say. No matter how much anger I express [or some other affect], you always want more!" Or:

---

[11] The same considerations elaborated above (Footnote 10) apply here as well.

"You're never interested in what I say! You only pay attention to what I leave out!" A large variety of such reactions is encountered among different patients and within the same patient at different points in the analysis. The difference among these reactions appears to depend on the constellation of defenses utilized, in particular the degree to which repression, rather than isolative or projective mechanisms, is relied upon as a major defense. The degree of dystonicity of the element commented upon (which in turn is affected by such issues as the nature of the transference) is a significant variable, as well.

The clinical consequence of a patient verbalizing material also varies widely. For some, it will seem to have a profound effect, occurring almost immediately. For others, despite a great deal of facility with verbalization, little therapeutic impact is noted for long periods of time. Patients who rely heavily on isolation and projection can readily verbalize ideas, and thus apparently have these ideas in consciousness, before important resistances have been analyzed, in contrast to patients who rely more heavily on repression. Again, the amount of conflict the ego experiences in integrating the material, which can be expressed in terms of the degree of ego-dystonicity, is a crucial variable.

Thus, the issue of whether or not a mental element has been verbalized has varying significance for the patient, depending on the kinds of defenses the patient has been using and on how dystonic the element is. These observations are consistent with the structural theory; in particular, with those aspects of the structural theory that indicate that the ego is not synonymous with consciousness.

The significance of verbalization of a mental element is relative. By focusing attention on the moment when ego-defensive activity begins, Gray can demonstrate the evidence for his inference that the immediately preceding verbalizations became "dangerous" to the patient. Thus, the technique involves observing momentary changes in the ego's tolerance for those verbalized derivatives. But it is clear that in addition to verbalization one needs to include other qualities to conceptualize the ego's conflict over integrating dystonic drive derivatives.

Because verbalization represents a wide spectrum of conscious awareness, the patient can be fully aware of some statements that he has verbalized and almost totally unaware of others, even though he has said them out loud. Paradoxically, there could be derivatives that have not been verbalized that are less dystonic and less strongly defended against than some that have been verbalized.

A method with an exclusive focus on conflicts that have been verbalized has the strength that the data are observable to both patient and analyst. However, the method might leave out other data that may be available to the patient, such as feelings, memories, and impulses which have not yet been verbalized.[12]

Furthermore, if we think of consciousness as an ego function that can become embroiled in conflict, then we can think of the ego using that function according to its multiple purposes, including those that serve mastery and integration, as well as those that serve defense. That is, there would be reason to question an assumption that derivatives come into consciousness only because they are sufficiently free of conflict to be able now to reach the surface of the mind. Such an assumption would be a literal application of the topo-

---

[12] Up to this point, I have used the concept of a thought having been verbalized interchangeably with the concept of a thought having been in consciousness, although it is not always accurate to do so. A thought may be conscious but not verbalized. Also, as illustrated above, a thought may have been verbalized, yet not be in full consciousness. Therefore, I think there is an advantage in consistently using the *descriptive* phrase, "having been verbalized," because it is more accurate in designating what is being referred to.

graphic theory (see Freud 1900, p. 610). By contrast, a structural theory point of view would require that the question of why certain derivatives come into consciousness, and why others do not, become the subject of analytic exploration.

SUMMARY AND CONCLUSIONS: CONSCIOUSNESS AS A BEACON LIGHT AND ITS RELATIONSHIP TO EGO-SYNTONICITY AND EGO INTEGRATION

Gray has developed a psychoanalytic theory and technique which maximally exploits the "beacon light" function of consciousness. This technique is an application of Anna Freud's (1936) method for observing psychoanalytic data that was developed in the context of Freud's (1923) structural theory. I have tried to demonstrate that, from a structural theory perspective, ego integration is the goal of analysis. From this perspective, analysis of the imagined dangers that cause drive derivatives to be ego-dystonic (and therefore defended against by the ego) allows these derivatives to be gradually perceived as less dangerous. In turn, the ego regards them as relatively less dystonic and the ego defends itself less vigorously against them. Ultimately, the ego integrates them within its organization.

By highlighting the advantages of clinical methods focusing on what has been verbalized, Gray's technical recommendations illuminate the need to address the complex role of accessibility to consciousness within the structural theory. In particular, we need to better understand how the clinically observable phenomenon of verbalization is related to ego-syntonicity and ego integration. The ego has, in consciousness, a beacon light which it can shine on some of its contents. The patient makes that illumination available to the analyst as well, when he attempts free association in the presence of his analyst. Gray provides a method whereby patient and analyst use consciousness and verbalization as evidence of the conflict the patient is encountering.

My clinical examples demonstrate that the intensity of the beacon light's beam can not be used, by itself, as a measure of ego integration. This distinction also follows from the very reason that Freud needed to go beyond the topographic theory and develop the structural theory. Without the beacon light afforded by consciousness (verbalization), ego-syntonicity and ego integration are obscure theoretical concepts that can leave us in the dark as we try to develop our psychoanalytic technique. We need to find a way to understand the complex relationship between the beacon light of consciousness and the nature of the ego's conflict over integrating dystonic drive derivatives—that is, between the clinical indicator of having been in consciousness (verbalization) and the concepts of ego-syntonicity and ego integration. Work in this direction offers the best chance of most fully exploiting the advantages of Gray's contributions to psychoanalytic technique.

References

Apfelbaum, B. (1966). On ego psychology: a critique of the structural approach to psychoanalytic theory. *International Journal of Psychoanalysis* 47:451–472.

Apfelbaum, B., and Gill, M. M. (1989). Ego analysis, and the relativity of defense: technical implications of the structural theory. *Journal of the American Psychoanalytic Association* 37:1069–1095.

Arlow, J. A. (1961). Silence and the theory of technique. *Journal of the American Psychoanalytic Association* 9:44–55.

Arlow, J. A., and Brenner, C. (1964). *Psychoanalytic Concepts and the Structural Theory.* New York: International Universities Press.

Brenner, C. (1976). *Psychoanalytic Technique and Psychic Conflict.* New York: International Universities Press.

——— (1982). *The Mind in Conflict.* New York: International Universities Press.

―― (1987). Working through: 1914-1984. *Psychoanalytic Quarterly* 56:88-108.

Busch, F. (1992). Recurring thoughts on the unconscious ego resistances. *Journal of the American Psychoanalytic Association* 40:1089-1115.

―― (1993). In the neighborhood: aspects of a good interpretation and a "developmental lag" in ego psychology. *Journal of the American Psychoanalytic Association* 41:151-177.

―― (1994). Free association and technique. *Journal of the American Psychoanalytic Association* 42:363-384.

Davison, W. T., Pray, M., and Bristol, C. (1986). Turning aggression on the self: a study of psychoanalytic process. *Psychoanalytic Quarterly* 55:273-295.

―― (1990). Mutative interpretation and close process monitoring in a study of psychoanalytic process. *Psychoanalytic Quarterly* 59:599-628.

Fenichel, O. (1941). *Problems of Psychoanalytic Technique.* New York: Psychoanalytic Quarterly.

Freud, A. (1936). *The Ego and the Mechanisms of Defense.* In *Writings* 2. New York: International Universities Press, 1966.

Freud, S. (1893-1895). Studies on Hysteria, *Standard Edition* 2.

―― (1893). On the psychical mechanism of hysterical phenomena: a lecture. *Standard Edition* 3:25-39.

―― (1894). The neuro-psychoses of defense. *Standard Edition* 3:41-68.

―― [1895](1950). Project for a scientific psychology. *Standard Edition* 1:281-397.

―― (1900). The interpretation of dreams. *Standard Edition* 5: 509-621.

―― (1915a). Repression. *Standard Edition* 14:141-158.

―― (1915b). The unconscious. *Standard Edition* 14:159-215.

―― (1923). The ego and the id. *Standard Edition* 19:1-66.

―― (1926). Inhibitions, symptoms, and anxiety. *Standard Edition* 20:75-175.

Gill, M. M. (1963). Topography and systems in psychoanalytic theory. *Psychological Issues* 10. New York: International Universities Press.

Goldberger, M. (1989). On the analysis of defenses in dreams. *Psychoanalytic Quarterly* 58:396–418.
Gray, P. (1973). Psychoanalytic technique and the ego's capacity for viewing intra-psychic activity. *Journal of the American Psychoanalytic Association* 1:474–494.
—— (1982). "Developmental lag" in the evolution of technique for psychoanalysis of neurotic conflict. *Journal of the American Psychoanalytic Association* 30:621–655.
—— (1986). On helping analysands observe intrapsychic activity. In *Psychoanalysis: The Science of Mental Conflict. Essays in Honor of Charles Brenner,* ed. A. D. Richards and M. S. Willick, pp. 245–268. Hillsdale, NJ: Analytic Press.
—— (1987). On the technique of analysis of the superego—an introduction. *Psychoanalytic Quarterly* 56:130–154.
—— (1990). The nature of therapeutic action in psychoanalysis. *Journal of the American Psychoanalytic Association* 38:1083–1097.
—— (1991). On transferred permissive or approving superego functions: the analysis of the ego's superego activities, part II. *Psychoanalytic Quarterly* 60:1–21.
Hartmann, H. (1951). Technical implications of ego psychology. In *Essays on Ego Psychology,* pp. 142–154. New York: International Universities Press, 1964.
Hoffman, L. (1994a). Superego analysis: report of the Kris study group. *Journal of Clinical Psychoanalysis* 3:157–240.
—— (1994b). Personal communication.
Holmes, D. (in press). Emerging indicators of ego growth and associated resistances. *Journal of the American Psychoanalytic Association.*
Inderbitzin, L. B., and Levy, S. T. (1994). On grist for the mill: external reality as defense. *Journal of the American Psychoanalytic Association* 42:763–788.
Kris, E. (1938). Review of *The Ego and the Mechanisms of Defense,* by Anna Freud. *International Journal of Psycho-Analysis* 19:136–146.
Levy, S. T., and Inderbitzin, L. B. (1990). The analytic surface and the theory of technique. *Journal of the American Psychoanalytic Association* 38:371–392.

Loewenstein, R. M. (1951). The problem of interpretation. *Psychoanalytic Quarterly* 21:295-322.

Paniagua, C. (1985). A methodologic approach to surface material. *International Review of Psycho-Analysis* 12:311-325.

—— (1991). Patient's surface, clinical surface, workable surface. *Journal of the American Psychoanalytic Association* 39:669-686.

Pray, M. (1994). Analyzing defense: two different methods. *Journal of Clinical Psychoanalysis* 3:87-126.

Reich, W. (1928). On character analysis. In *The Psychoanalytic Reader*, vol. 1, ed. R. Fliess, pp. 129-147. New York: International Universities Press, 1948.

Sandler, J., with Freud, A. (1985). *The Analysis of Defense: The Ego and the Mechanisms of Defense Revisited.* New York: International Universities Press.

Sterba, R. (1934). The fate of the ego in analytic theory. *International Journal of Psycho-Analysis* 15:117-126.

Strachey, J. (1953). Editor's introduction to the interpretation of dreams. *Standard Edition* 4:xvii-xviii.

—— (1966). Editor's introduction to project for a scientific psychology. *Standard Edition* 1:290-293.

Waelder, R. (1936). The principle of multiple function: observation on over-determination. *Psychoanalytic Quarterly* 5:45-61.

11

Common Ground, Uncommon Methods

CECILIO PANIAGUA, M.D.

> There are often uncertainties as to the governing principles which should be common to all analysts despite differences in personality—if the various methods are still to be called analytic.
>
> O. Fenichel

Quite a few years ago, before I was an analyst, I wrote a doctoral thesis on the types of psychological adjustments found in couples of different nationalities; more specifically, couples in which the husband was an American G. I. and the wife came from a different country. I compared these to couples in which the spouses shared nationality. I found that the heteronational couples could be quite well-adjusted provided they had enough basis for cultural understanding and meaningful communication. One of my more general conclusions was that for the success of the marriage it was crucial that they shared some fundamental values and had sufficient behavioral traits in common to make living together possible, *but* not so many that pervasive concordance led to insufficient stimulation. It seemed to me that the good liaisons were those that managed a reasonable balance between excessive consonance and too much dissonance.

I had something like this in mind as a model when reflecting on the comparisons derived from my years of experience with American psychoanalysis and with the types of analysis practiced in continental Europe. I will quote here the following assessment from Wallerstein (1988):

> Psychoanalysis ... actually succeeded for so many more years in the United States than anywhere else in the world in maintaining an integrated and overall uniform perspective on psychoanalysis, called (and cherished) as the mainstream ... psychoanalysis worldwide today and all within the organizational framework of the I. P. A. consists of multiple (and divergent) theories of mental functioning, of development, of pathogenesis, of treatment, and of cure. [p. 11]

Has analysis remained too consonant in the United States, while it became too dissonant in the rest of the world? Are the choices "petrification or chaos," as Wallerstein (1993) put it recently?

I am one of the few members of the American Psychoanalytic Association in Europe (there are ten of us in the roster, including Israel). In order to establish my credentials as a knowledgeable participant in the intercontinental psychoanalytic scene, I will state that through exposure to scientific meetings and conferences with many European and South American speakers, through participation as a discussant in panels on different theoretical approaches to the same clinical material, through classes and supervisions in my own Association, through participation in all the joint meetings of the American Psychoanalytic Association and the European Psychoanalytical Federation, through my experience as analysand in Spain and in the United States, as a member of the editorial boards of a European psychoanalytic journal and an American one, and as coauthor of papers written with colleagues of different theoretical stances, I have become quite familiar with clinical theories and technical approaches used in various societies around the world (South American and British Kleinian, Bionian, German, Winnicottian, French including Lacanian, etc.). My impressions are additionally based on direct frequent experience in informal discussions, re-analyses, advisorships, and concomitant supervisions. I feel as though in my move from the United States to Europe I went from a very consonant marriage (mainstream contemporary ego psychology) to a very dissonant one.

I am acquainted with the recent overtures of American psychoanalysis to different theoretical schools, and its increasing tolerance of institutional divergences (see Weinshel 1992, p. 329, for instance). This movement and the ensuing dialectics may prove quite beneficial for the growth and consolidation of our discipline; however, it is important that we understand what this heterogeneity might entail. I would like to express here some of my thoughts concerning excessive pluralism and the related hazards of having common ground with uncommon methods.

Much has been written lately about the shared aspects of clinical theory and practice among analysts from different schools. At the 1991 Rome Congress of the International Psychoanalytic Association considerable efforts were made to achieve a sense of "common ground" among its members. A recent issue of the *International Journal of Psycho-Analysis*, "Fifteen Clinical Accounts" (Tuckett 1991), was dedicated to this same endeavor.

I do not believe that the "common ground" topic is an enlightening theme for discussion among analysts from significantly different theoretical schools. We know all along the discussion can be "settled" by restating that we have common ground since we all deal, one way or another, with the clinical phenomena of transference and resistance (see Freud 1914, p. 16). Moreover, don't we all talk about concepts such as psychic agencies, object relationships, unconscious fantasies, repression, symptom formation, and so forth? And don't we all make use of the couch, foster free associations, interpret dreams, etc? However, these and other "common ground" assertions also tend to obfuscate our fundamental differences. We could also think of astronomers and astrologers as having "common ground." Don't they all talk about stars, planets and constellations? I think the question, "Do practitioners from different theoretical persuasions share common ground?" is futile, and cannot lead to meaningful answers. Melanie Klein believed that her theories were a natural extension of Freud's; he simply had not gone far enough. Of course, the same could be said of the early ego psychologists due to their efforts to complete Freud's "general psychology." And this could be stated even more forcefully about Lacan's famous "return to Freud."

It seems to me that the *International*'s emphasis on the common ground theme is based on a wish to promote ecumenism and to foster conciliation rather than on a will to objectively examine our differences. Le Guen in Lussier (1991) have expressed their preference for an International Congress on our *differences.* Probably it would be more enlightening—though more disquieting—to pose ourselves the question, "If we have *common* ground, how come we do such different things—that is, why do we employ such *widely different* methods?" In international circles many believe that we analysts are all "astronomers" and there are no "astrologers" among us; but who can truthfully say that we have won and we should all get prizes, as Lewis Carroll's Dodo diplomatically stated?

In reality, we know that the clinical methodology used

by analysts from different schools can be very dissimilar. We are reminded of this at every International Congress, and Tuckett's *Clinical Accounts* certainly attest to it. To Wallerstein's (1988) question, "Do we have one psychoanalysis or many?" we should answer without hesitation: "Many!" We should seriously examine our motives for entertaining the belief that there is significant commonality in the clinical work of different schools or component groups in the *International*. Although I agree with Wallerstein (1988) that our goal should be to attain "a unitary clinical theory that is empirically testable" (p. 17), I do not agree with a few of the points in his comprehensive and inspiring presidential addresses at the Montreal and Rome International Congresses. I have difficulties accepting his assertion that "adherents of whatever theoretical position within psychoanalysis all seem to do reasonably comparable clinical work and bring about reasonably comparable clinical change" (p. 13).

There are other (overlapping) means besides introspection through which clinical change can be achieved in *different forms* of psychoanalysis. There is the corrective emotional experience; the influence of a holding environment or an atmosphere of safety or containment; the active supportive elements (see Wallerstein 1986, p. 730); symbolic realizations; covert deconditioning; manipulation (in the sense Bibring 1954, gave to this term); and, above all, the powerful, ever-present, and multifarious use of suggestion (see Gray 1988, p. 44). Analyses utilize different principles to varying degrees, depending on the practitioners' orientations, and the different mixtures of therapeutic techniques result in different consequences. Therefore, it is difficult to think that the clinical work can be reasonably considered comparable, as Wallerstein stated.

The argument that treatments heavily based on therapeutic principles other than insight cannot be considered psychoanalysis proper seems to ignore the fact that a good number of them are conducted this way in regular practice and training analyses. Therefore, I must disagree also with Wallerstein's (1990) opinion that "our clinical interventions (apart from differences of style and of theory-drenched languages) reflect a shared clinical method" (p. 11). This seems to go against the evidence. Analysts from different schools do not necessarily share the same clinical methodology. It has been my first-hand experience that, in practice, our interventions do not "rest on a shared *clinical* theory of defense and anxiety, of conflict and compromise, of transference and countertransference," as Wallerstein (1990, my italics) wrote, and I doubt very much that they "evoke comparable data of observation, despite our avowed wide theoretical differences" (p. 11).

We all seem ready to grant (how could we deny it?) that our meta-theories are rather different. Why is it so difficult to admit that our clinical theories are also quite different and their application produces disparate results? Recently, Stein (1991) wrote eloquently about the obvious effects of theoretical preferences on the analyst's clinical activity. Wallerstein (1990) also expressed his disagreement with Arlow and Brenner's (1988) position that, "Perhaps all analysts do not use the same technique, even though all call the technique they use by the same name. This raises a serious problem, since it is obvious that *differences in the method* employed in studying any set of phenomena will produce very different sorts of data" (p. 10, my italics). However, this reasoning is perfectly cogent, and it certainly coincides with my "field observations." Disparate clinical methods influence differentially not only therapeutic outcome but also the quality of the material elicited in patients. Some techniques are more abstinent or "contaminate" the material less than others, which is to say that methods also affect our efficiency as scientific researchers.

Differences in method should not be understood simply as our diverse preferences for general theoretical concepts. Few American-trained analysts would find any significant difficulty in understanding—or even using—concepts such as "bizarre objects," "container," the Jungian "imago," or the Lacanian "signifier," or "phallus" (as the intra- and inter-subjective symbolic representation for "penis"). It is easy to learn, for instance, that when a Kleinian analyst talks about "psychotic mind" he or she is referring essentially to primary process thinking, or when a French analyst talks about *fantasmes* he or she means unconscious fantasies, or that the French term *clivage* (splitting) refers to a more encompassing concept than does its English translation. All these types of concepts have correspondence with clinical realities, and are more or less translatable from one psychoanalytic taxonomy to another. There is nothing wrong with developing a melting pot of terms from various sources, a "metapsychological polyglottism," as De Urtubey (1985), a Uruguayan-French analyst called it; although, of course, we all may have our preferences and dislikes. We may discuss the relative heuristic value of any of the above-mentioned concepts, just as we may discuss ego-psychological concepts such as "neutralization" or "conflict-free sphere." All this is what Wallerstein (1988) called our "chosen array of metaphor" (p. 16).

In very heterogeneous psychoanalytic societies, such as mine, with members trained in different European and South American institutes and using disparate metapsychological frames of reference, candidates benefit significantly from being exposed to these different concepts and terminologies. Kernberg (1986, 1993) has articulated a similar opinion. Pine (1990) wrote on the dangers of tunnel vision based on rigid theoretical commitments, and the helpfulness of having a multiplicity of models. Pulver (1993) has written convincingly on the positive aspects of eclecticism, and on the advantages of adopting precepts from different schools of thought as guiding principles for clinical understanding. However, I disagree with Pulver's argument that "psychoanalytic schools are not as different from one another as they are commonly supposed to be, particularly in matters of technique" (p. 339). As I stated above, in my experience they can be very different indeed in matters of technique.

Differences in method refer to alternative *clinical uses* of our disparate theories of technique. These theoretical convictions may be acquired through patient trial and error, sober inductive reasoning, and years of apprenticeship and experience, but they could be acquired and maintained also on faith and scant evidence. The rules of correspondence used in connecting experiential or intraphenomenological concepts to functional or extra-phenomenological concepts (see G. Klein 1976, p. 50) are the crux of the matter here. The techniques that ensue are deductively derived from these convictions. For instance, an analyst may believe that children have inborn fantasies about parental coitus and, as a consequence, feel justified making sexual interpretations about supposedly allusive material in the child's play. Or, using a very different example, when an analyst believes that a rational alliance is an essential ingredient in any well-conducted analysis, he or she will try to induce in his or her patients an ego dissociation conducive to (quasi) objective self-scrutiny.

The disparate nature of our methods has to do with the differences in what we consider clinical evidence, how we make deductions from our observations, what we judge to be valid inferences, what steps we follow in formulating our interventions, what factors in our interpretations we deem mutative, what we consider analytic progress, and whether we consider that our main job is revealing to our patients the contents of their unconscious or the facilitation of their own discovery of their psychic truths. Is the analysand supposed to "just associate" while the analyst "just interprets," or are the analysand's and the analyst's observing egos supposed to be sharing the analytic enterprise? (see Busch 1992). The practical consequences of applying different methods can be quite divergent. The following words written by Strachey (1934) sixty years ago seem still valid:

> We are told that if we interpret too soon or too rashly, we run the risk of losing a patient; that interpretation may give rise to intolerable and unmanageable outbreaks of anxiety by "liberating" it; that interpretation is the only way of enabling a patient to cope with an unmanageable outbreak of anxiety by "resolving" it; that interpretations must always refer to material on the very point of emerging into consciousness; that the most useful interpretations are really deep ones; "Be cautious with your interpretations!" says one voice; "When in doubt, interpret!" says another. [p. 282]

Have we, analysts from different theoretical persuasions, progressed much in regard to these conflicting general technical recommendations we give our students?

Due to their practical importance we spend long years learning about the intricacies of technique through courses and supervision. How can we then dismiss the technical disagreements between different schools of clinical theory as "only diversity in frames of reference," or "just a matter of styles," as some do, meaning that there exists underlying correspondence in our disparate methods after all? Sometimes the argument is heard that we do indeed practice different forms of psychoanalysis, but *vive la différence*! This attitude cannot be considered responsible since different methods of inquiry elicit different clinical material, and dissimilar technical procedures could produce different therapeutic results. Certainly, we don't cheer the "epistemic richness" of having disparate schools of thought in surgery. We want to know whose anatomical concepts are more accurate and whose techniques are more reliable.

In order to assess these matters appropriately it is probably essential to see them from a historical perspective. We are a young discipline, a "protoscience," as Kennedy (1959) called it. A hundred years is not much for a field of study as complex as ours. Perhaps in another hundred years, as evidence accumulates and our profession becomes better able to fix its concepts and operationalize its procedures, it will become apparent who of us were closer to being "astronomers" and who came closer to being "astrologers." The one thing we can be sure about is that our future colleagues will not consider us all "astronomers" (or "protoastronomers"). Our theoretical and practical differences are such that we cannot all be right. For instance, it does not seem defensible to assume that a clinical theory that favors interpreting mostly according to preconceived psychogenetic formulas can have the same validity as a clinical theory that proposes using close-process resistance analysis (see Gray, 1986).

In order to illustrate these ideas, I will use excerpts from six discussions of a clinical paper of mine with the title "Reconstructions in a 'Castrated' and Castrating Woman," which I presented orally and in written form to a series of well-established colleagues belonging to different theoretical schools. I will not supply my own clinical material here, for I do not consider it necessary for my main purpose of illustrating the differences in these comments. I would like to draw attention to the degree of abstractness in the technical recommendations, and to the difference in the correspondence between the material and preconceived theory. I do not consider it relevant to comment here on which critiques I found helpful or fair.

I do not mean to imply that I believe all adherents to one or another school practice homogeneous techniques;

however, I think these excerpts are fairly representative of my experience with these different groups.*

A colleague influenced by Bion and certain French authors wrote:

> I try to direct my listening toward the unconscious fantasy. For the noun "fantasy" I would use simply the adjective "unconscious," and not "deep," which for Paniagua has a pejorative meaning as synonymous of "premature, incomplete or incorrect."
>
> The fundamental fantasy I have heard in this patient is illustrative of the universal preoccupation of women with their bodies, increased in each phase of psychosexual development, which has been repeatedly observed in the psychoanalytic literature.
>
> There is a normal feminine hypochondriasis of a defensive nature produced by an underlying confusional state. In this patient, this hypochondriasis has become pathological, remaining fixated: "I have this feeling of abnormality inside," "I have the conviction that I have something abnormal in there."
>
> In my opinion, the patient illustrates very well the cloacal fantasy described by Freud in 1908, denoting the undifferentiated state of the anal and vaginal orifices, and their corresponding bodily cavities. [In my paper I said that the analysand remembered exploring her perineal orifices at age six.]

A Spanish-trained analyst, stated:

> The manifestations of this patient's demandingness and anger toward others would be linked indeed to the conflict produced by defective parents who, once transformed into defective internal objects, fostered object relations and

---

*The following comments are from colleagues who, with the exception of Dr. Evelyne A. Schwaber, prefer to remain anonymous.

transferences characterized by unhappiness due to the regression inherent in the repetition compulsion.

This would all then require interpretation of the rejection of her femininity so related to the inhibition of the epistemophilic impulse; as well as interpretations aimed at the recognition of her rejecting-rejected [castrating-castrated] attitude that so interfered with her own integration.

In Paniagua's clinical presentation the theme of femininity could have been approached with different interpretations touching deeper into that emptiness, that feminine hole which is, nevertheless, filled with that creativity indispensable for life.

An Israeli Kleinian-influenced analyst, said:

> The patient's mother reassured her that there were other holes in the body, besides the nose and mouth, that one could breathe through, and she thought right away her mom was referring to the vaginal hole. [As a child, the patient had a nightmare of asphyxiation, and this was then her actual belief.] This reflects her mother's envy: she did not want her to know the facts of life, thwarting her womanly strivings and motherly potential [no evidence for this in the material]. She introjected all this, and she is wondering if you are going also to mislead her like her mother did [no evidence in the verbatim material for this either]. She mistrusts you now, and is afraid of you.
>
> When the patient sighed at the beginning of a session, you said, "What's that sigh taking the place of?" but a sigh is not in place of anything. The message you gave her then was like "a sigh is not good enough." You were responding countertransferentially to something you were not aware of at the moment. What in her evoked that intervention in you?
>
> Also, when you said "I want you to observe" ["how you don't finish the sentence, how you hesitate to say the

precise words when you are talking about sexual matters"] it is as though you were giving her permission. I would have said "I feel like. . . ." You sound removed when you say "observe."

Now we could contrast the above critiques with these from American colleagues, mainly as to closeness of clinical theory to the material.

A colleague from Atlanta, observed:

> My impression is that the analyst is involved in a sadomasochistic (power) struggle with the analysand and that this is not being addressed in the transference as the leading resistance. Obviously, you are in touch with the theme, "This is the topic we are familiar with. Who has the power to do what to whom, and under what circumstances." This transference theme is present throughout and from the very beginning: After telling you, "Your command to talk about everything is impossible to be carried out," she pauses, and you ask, "You have met an obstacle. Are you aware of what's the nature of it?" It seems to me that she has already told you that she experiences you as a commander and that your commands seem impossible for her to follow.

Evelyne A. Schwaber, who wanted to be cited by name, wrote:

> You tell her, "What happened to you an hour ago could be too fresh, too immediate to talk of," but she is telling you something even more immediate—namely, right now she is having difficulty talking. . . .
>
> She tells of the possibility of (her tiredness) being related to her genitals, but says "maybe" and also says "a little related." In other words, she is suggesting that it may be something else, though I would say the suggestion in this material is that she thinks you think it has to do with her genitals. It is hard to tell how much of the sexual

material has to do with her view of that being in your agenda....

You say, "She was patronizing and exacting with him." Did she feel this? You speak of her "castrating behavior." Was this her assessment, or yours? You say, "After one year of analysis she became more considerate"—her view or yours? ... When you say, "She often tended to ignore my interventions; through this obvious defensive maneuver she also tried to devalue and castrate me," you now attribute experiential meaning to her behavior. How it seems to you is not the same as how it is experienced by her.

An analyst from Washington, D. C., stated:

Dr. Paniagua relates to us an intervention, in response to his patient's candida infection, which she believes she can withstand better than her husband, whom she says she infects periodically. Here Dr. Paniagua comments that it is reassuring to the patient that her genital is stronger than her husband's. He has indeed commented empathically, for he has put into words his patient's view of her more powerful genital, and the fact that this view reassures her. Then this allows the analysand to associate further to her feelings about intercourse, and the "third hole" she uses for it. This continues the next day when she indicates that there is a childhood fantasy that her "third hole" is not possessed by others. She then elaborates on that fantasy.

Probably, international forums should discuss more persistently what kind of clinical evidence warrants what kind of interpretations. As I expressed elsewhere (1985), as the analyst "enters the *terra incognita* of the analysand's unconscious, he is in a better position to explore its singular contents equipped with a method and a healthy capacity for surprises than with the wrong maps" (p. 314).

At times, some characteristics of the International Psycho-Analytical Association have made it resemble the Royal Society of Newton's time. Then they had philosophers, astrologers, and physicists discussing the same observable phenomena. Like us, they had "common ground" and "theoretical pluralism." But also like us, they did not have common methods. The most important scientific function of the Royal Society in its beginning was experimental demonstrations before the members. Alas, we psychoanalysts have had a hard time emulating the deeds of better-established scientists. We are all familiar with the special difficulties (intrinsic or not) we have found adhering to time-honored yardsticks of science, such as clear correlation between theoretical concepts and observables, reliable predictions, criteria for confirmation of our hypotheses (i.e., interpretations), use of independent observers, or statistical studies. We have not even been able to reach agreement on what kind of clinical material constitutes optimal *workable surface* for analytic interventions (see Paniagua 1991). These difficulties have resulted so far in a level of intraprofessional communication that might well be described as "Babelian."

Traditionally, learned men have felt that the study of mental life should include consideration of only conscious processes. Freud's theories were, of course, a reaction to the philosophy of the conscious represented by the so-called "academic psychology." Apparently Freud's momentous reaction was interpreted by a good number of followers as an invitation to disregard in their theorizing the laws of valid inference of traditional philosophy, thus throwing the baby out with the bath water. Some of us have had a hard time formulating, or communicating, our ideas in a language fully compatible with formal logic. Perhaps this has been due to the fact that some psychoanalytic findings seem odd from a rationalistic viewpoint. By this I mean findings such as the functioning of primary process, the need to defend against instinctual drives coupled with their ability to serve defensive purposes, the existence of intrasystemic contradictions, and the fact that the superego is a compromise formation, although it is simultaneously conceptualized as a structure or, in Brenner's (1982) words, the fact that "the superego is both a consequence of psychic conflict and a component of it" (p. 120). By now we are quite aware that all these and other seeming contradictions have rational explanations, and that the study of deep psychology in general is not incompatible with the systematic use of logical propositions. Fenichel (1941) had it right when he reminded us that the purpose of analysis was to investigate unconscious mental processes "for the cause of reason." He said, "The subject matter, not the method, of psychoanalysis is irrational" (p. 13). Esman (1979), in a more modern rendition, wrote, "[If] the unconscious is structured as a language, we should take care that our literary language not be as unstructured as the unconscious" (p. 630).

Perhaps, between readings of our analytic classics, we should take an occasional look at works like John Stuart Mill's *A System of Logic* (1843). We might find Book V, *On Fallacies*, particularly interesting. Mill stated that these are of five classes: fallacies of simple inspection or prejudice, of observation, of generalization, of ratiocination, and of confusion. It is a humbling lesson to realize to what extent the examples provided in this book apply to the inductive (and even the deductive) reasoning used in many of the clinical papers published in psychoanalytic journals. I agree with Yorke's (1985) observation, "Any issue of almost any psychoanalytic journal will express a number of viewpoints that flatly contradict each other. To some extent, this may be inevitable in a discipline as inexact as psychoanalysis, but the contradictions are not mere disagreements of a kind healthy to growth and development. Rather, they hinder progress as often as they promote it" (pp. 236–237).

Few would dispute that in scientific meetings and clinical presentations we still often resort to so-called theory-driven explanations, and other indulgences in *petitio principii*. Generalizations grossly overruling the material are still too widespread in clinical theorizing, and we have to wonder why. At times our logic seems so vitiated that the reasoning sounds bizarre, even delusional as we can end up talking, as G. Klein (1976) used to say, about "witches and unicorns" (p. 51), in some sort of *folie à plusieurs*. There is a spectrum in the apperception of clinical facts ranging from emotional resonance to dispassionate observation. The above tendency seems stronger in psychoanalytic groups where the emphasis in the understanding of unconscious dynamics is tilted toward the intuition pole rather than toward the objectivity pole.

The following statement from the philosopher Mill on the difficulties in observing nature remains quite applicable to us psychoanalytic observers:

> The observer is not he who merely sees the thing which is before his eyes, but he who sees what parts that thing is composed of. To do this well is a rare talent. One person, from inattention, or attending only in the wrong place, overlooks half of what he sees; another sets down much more than he sees, confounding it with what he imagines, or with what he infers; another takes note of the kind of all the circumstances, but being inexpert in estimating their degree, leaves the quantity of each vague and uncertain; another sees indeed the whole, but makes such an awkward division of it into parts, throwing things into one mass which require to be separated, and separating others which might more conveniently be considered as one, that the result is much the same, sometimes even worse, than if no analysis has been attempted at all [p. 380].

Indeed, one may arrive at the conclusion that the lack of commonality of our psychoanalytic methods is mostly based on the diversity in our repertoires of logical fallacies used in clinical theories, and in our theories of technique. These fallacies vary in quality and quantity; *chacun à son goût*. Certainly, not all inferences are equally valid, and not all theories of technique can have the same veracity or hold equivalent heuristic value. Freud (1912) wrote, "Let me express a hope that the increasing experience of psychoanalysts will soon lead to agreement on questions of technique and on the most effective method of treating neurotic patients" (p. 120). I think Freud's hope does not stand a chance of fulfillment unless we discipline ourselves to communicate according to *ars artium* (Bacon's epithet for logic: "the science of science itself").

In the development of our theories, concepts have proliferated at all levels of abstraction, with little regard for construct validity. There have been highly influential "excursion(s) . . . into the shadowy past, while much that could be more satisfactorily proved and that is indispensable for analysis has been left unregarded," as Waelder said in an indirect reference to Kleinian theory. There have been pseudo-explanations and, at times, dialectic convolutions seemingly created for the purpose of disguising the deficiencies in our knowledge. It needs to be pointed out, as Schafer (1994) did recently, that Melanie Klein has not been the only one in our history "trying to explain too much too fast, confusing preconceptions and postulates with evidence. . . . The same can be said of the way Freud worked in his early years as a psychoanalyst, as did Karl Abraham, Ferenczi, and others" (p. 363).

As scientists, one of our main tasks is to examine and "break apart" complex psychic realities into their component elements: this is what "analysis" means literally (see Rangell 1983, p. 162). However, at times one gets the impression that the opposite process is taking place: some theoreticians seem to make efforts to render esoteric that which is simple. This is not as strange as it may sound. It is a common experience in psychoanalytic groups where cult of personality ranks as high as dedication to science. Then, one of the foremost values sought for is the elicitation of awe in junior colleagues.

Related also to omniscient claims and other unresolved narcissistic issues in analysts are: the interpretive use of psychogenetic equations and formulas, and other grand clinical theorizing; the tendency to assume, instead of demonstrate, conclusions; the belief in the infallibility of countertransferential intuitions; and the propensity to "enlighten" analysands through interpretations instead of jointly discovering dynamics. This, in turn, is often related to cultural factors. The point could well be made that these attitudes have a lot to do with some historical inertias and sociological, extraanalytic phenomena such as short democratic traditions, expectations of authoritarianism, and other social forces promoting filial dependency into adulthood, but a detailed study of these would go beyond the scope of this discussion.

We have tended to rely on authority (mostly Freud's) as a substitute for proof of theoretical tenets (the *magister dixit* argument). Not rarely, psychoanalysts have confused figurative and literal meanings (see Paniagua 1982). Not infrequently we have been taught to use a declarative style in our interventions instead of the tentative style of hypotheses in search of confirmation. "An analyst does not ask questions; he interprets," goes the dictum. Usually, this approach is a result of the belief (avowed or not) that the clinical theory of choice is sufficiently established as to need no corroboration from emerging material. Observations and inferences then get stretched into the procrustean bed of the analyst's *a prioris* of choice. The practitioner favoring this approach ends up "never finding anything but what he already knows," as Freud (1912, p. 112) put it. It is not unusual to read reports and meet colleagues who never question the correctness of interpretations. If these do not produce the desired mutative effects, it is argued, it is only because they were "too deep" (i.e., not inaccurate for some logical or technical reason). This attitude has important clinical repercussions, for it tends to indoctrinate analysands, either reinforcing their natural resistance, or promoting their submissive compliance. The result is that their unique dynamics do not get appropriately explored. Kaiser (1934) already pointed out that this type of approach actually prevented patients from experiencing the repressed impulse itself.

There are other common erroneous ideas which have untoward consequences in our clinical methodology: the confusion of the concept of transference with the patient's justified reactions to unwarranted interventions by the analyst; "the gathering of data from what the analyst *feels*, rather than from what he *observes*," in Gray's words (Goldberger 1991, p. 10); and the tendency to fuse the analysand's associations with those of the analyst, generally conveyed through so-called "content interpretations," i.e., interpretations of presumed content, or through the "interpretation of absent content," as Searl (1936, p. 476) called it. Equally adverse for our procedures are the inadequate notion and application of analyzability criteria, together with the use of a standard technique for most cases, regardless of their degree of pathology or cognitive abilities; the tendency to interpret all intra-clinical events as transference allusions, and the related faulty exploration of genetic and extratransferential dynamics; and, finally, the technical emphasis on the concrete implantation of parts of the analysand's self into the analyst's during the sessions, bypassing the latter's awareness, with the consequent blurring of the concept of countertransference. Of course, these ideas and techniques are much more frequently applied in Kleinian analyses. It is interesting to note Schafer's (1985) categorization of Klein's clinical methodology as originally practiced by her and her early followers as "a systematized form of wildness" (p. 289).

An essential cornerstone in the Kleinian theory of technique seems to be the explicit or implicit belief that the analysand's thoughts and feelings get reliably transmitted to the mind of the well-analyzed analyst, and are experienced as such by him or her via projective identification. The analyst's main task then would not be analyzing the resistances opposed to the progression of unconscious contents toward consciousness and verbalization. Rather, the analyst's attention would be primarily directed toward the reading of the impressions produced by what is considered the analysand's truthful unconscious communication upon the wax slab of one's own mystic writing-pad, to use Freud's (1925) famous metaphor. According to many Kleinian analysts this provides the most reliable basis for the subsequent formulation of accurate interpretations.

In an address in 1952, Knight pointed out that "calling each other orthodox or deviant is not an attractive [spectacle]" (1953, p. 219), and I think one must agree with the good sense of this disposition. However, a saying I learned in my years in America was: "One should have an open mind, but not so open that the brain falls out." Curtis (1992) also addressed this general issue:

> [The] greater tolerance for new hypotheses is certainly a salutary development and represents a maturational step in our field. However, this tolerance has often led to a kind of critical laziness on the part of some analysts who seem to accept all models as created equal. . . . [This] approach may have the ecumenical virtue of tolerance, reasonable dialogue, and avoidance of rivalry, but lacks the scientific virtue of judging the relative empirical value. [p. 648]

Forty years after Knight's words, another president of the American Psychoanalytic Association had to remind us of the risks of "flabby relativism," that is, the indiscriminate acceptance of theories, and an uncritical eclecticism.

Before we are able to obtain harder data through comparative longitudinal studies concerning the effectiveness of various methods, we can and should resort to disciplined inference-making, "improving the presently poor quality of reasoning about the relation between hypothesis and evidence" (Edelson 1984, p. 55). This is the way to base our clinical theories on firmer epistemological grounds. The methods that best facilitate—or least interfere with—valid inference-making should prevail. I think it might be pertinent to make mention here of a rather common philosophical stance that, in my opinion, seriously hampers the aspirations of psychoanalysis to scientific status. A significant number of analysts think that *realistic* assessments of the object world and the self are inherently impossible, and not just confounded by neurotic conflict. As a result, they do not believe that mental health is definitely related to accuracy in the assessment of reality, or that psychoanalysis permits an asymptotic approximation to objectivity.

Perhaps in the future the International Psycho-Analytical Association will consider it worthwhile to dedicate more of its efforts to seriously examining the clinical consequences of the methodological differences of its members. For this purpose, the model the editor of the *International Journal of Psycho-Analysis* intends to use for the seventy-fifth anniversary celebration on *The Conceptualization and Communication of Clinical Facts* may be a good one. Other models that seem likely to yield positive results are those aimed at exploring different theoretical perspectives on the same clinical material (such as Panel 1992, Pulver 1987, or the previously cited commentaries on my case by colleagues), and Fine and Fine's (1990) comparative study on alternative schools of interpretive interventions. Even more promising for the examination of outcomes brought about by competing clinical paradigms might prove to be Wallerstein's current research at Langley Porter on the assessment of psychic change through the application of "theory-free" scales. Studies of this type may not promote global professional cohesion, at least in the short run, but they will advance " [the] prospect of scientific gain," considered by Freud (1926) "the proudest and happiest feature of analytic work" (p. 256).

References

Arlow, J. A., and Brenner, C. (1988). The future of psychoanalysis. *Psychoanalytic Quarterly* 57:1-14.
Bibring, E. (1954). Psychoanalysis and the dynamic psychotherapies. *Journal of the American Psychoanalytic Association* 2:745-770.
Brenner, C. (1982). *The Mind in Conflict.* New York: International Universities Press.
Busch, F. (1992). Recurring thoughts on the unconscious ego resistances. *Journal of the American Psychoanalytic Association* 40:1089-1115.
Curtis, H. C. (1992). Psychoanalytic ecumenism and varieties of psychoanalytic experience. *Journal of the American Psychoanalytic Association* 40:643-663.
De Urtubey, L. (1985). Fondamentale métapsychologie, inévitable polyglottisme. *Revue Française Psychanalyse* 49:1497-1521.
Edelson, M. (1984). *Hypothesis and Evidence in Psychoanalysis.* Chicago: University of Chicago Press.
Esman, A. H. (1979). On evidence and inference, or the Babel of tongues. *Psychoanalytic Quarterly* 48:628-630.
Fenichel, O. (1941). *Problems of Psychoanalytic Technique.* New York: *Psychoanalytic Quarterly.*
Fine, S., and Fine, E. (1990). Four psychoanalytic perspectives: a study of differences in interpretive interventions. *Journal of the American Psychoanalytic Association* 38:1017-1047.
Freud, S. (1912). Recommendations to physicians practising psychoanalysis. *Standard Edition* 12.
—— (1914). On the history of the psycho-analytic movement. *Standard Edition* 14.
—— (1925). A note upon the "mystic writing-pad." *Standard Edition* 19.

—— (1926). The question of lay analysis. *Standard Edition* 20.

Goldberger, M. (1991). A conversation with Paul Gray. *American Psychoanalyst* 24(4):10–20.

Gray, P. (1986). On helping analysands observe intrapsychic activity. In *Psychoanalysis: The Science of Mental Conflict. Essays in Honor of Charles Brenner*, ed. A. D. Richards and M. S. Willick. Hillsdale, NJ: Analytic Press.

—— (1988). On the significance of influence and insight in the spectrum of psychoanalytic psychotherapies. In *How Does Treatment Help?*, ed. A. Rothstein. Madison, CT: International Universities Press.

Kaiser, H. (1934). Problems of technique. In *The Evolution of Psychoanalytic Technique*, ed. M. S. Bergmann and F. R. Hartman. New York: Basic Books, 1976.

Kennedy, G. (1959). Psychoanalysis: protoscience and metapsychology. In *Psychoanalysis, Scientific Method and Philosophy*, ed. S. Hook. New York: New York University Press.

Kernberg, O. F. (1986). Institutional problems of psychoanalytic education. *Journal of the American Psychoanalytic Association* 34:799–834.

—— (1993). The current status of psychoanalysis. *Journal of the American Psychoanalytic Association* 41:45–62.

Klein, G. S. (1976). *Psychoanalytic Theory*. New York: International Universities Press.

Knight, R. P. (1953). The present status of organized psychoanalysis in the United States. *Journal of the American Psychoanalytic Association* 1:197–221.

Lussier, A. (1991). The search for common ground: a critique. *International Journal of Psycho-Analysis* 72:57–62.

Mill, J. S. (1843). *A System of Logic, Ratiocinative and Inductive*. London: Routledge & Kegan Paul.

Panel (1992). Freudian and Kleinian theory: a dialogue of comparative perspectives. H. B. Levine, reporter. *Journal of the American Psychoanalytic Association* 40:801–826.

Paniagua, C. (1982). Metaphors and isomorphisms: analogical reasoning in "Beyond the pleasure principle." *Journal of the American Psychoanalytic Association* 30:509–523.

—— (1985). A methodological approach to surface material. *International Review of Psycho-Analysis* 12:311–325.

—— (1991). Patient's surface, clinical surface, and workable surface. *Journal of the American Psychoanalytic Association* 39:669–685.

Pine, F. (1990). *Drive, Ego, Object, and Self: A Synthesis for Clinical Work.* New York: Basic Books.

Pulver, S. E. (1987). How theory shapes technique: perspectives on a clinical study. *Psychoanalytic Inquiry* 7(2).

—— (1993). The eclectic analyst, or the many roads to insight and change. *Journal of the American Psychoanalytic Association* 41:339–357.

Rangell, L. (1983). Defense and resistance in psychoanalysis and life. *Journal of the American Psychoanalytic Association* (*Supplement*), 31:147–174.

Schafer, R. (1985). Wild analysis. *Journal of the American Psychoanalytic Association* 33:275–299.

—— (1994). One perspective on the Freud-Klein controversies 1941–1945. *International Journal of Psycho-Analysis* 75:359–365.

Searl, M. N. (1936). Some queries on principles of technique. *International Journal of Psycho-Analysis* 17:471–493.

Stein, S. (1991). The influence of theory on the psychoanalyst's countertransference. *International Journal of Psycho-Analysis* 72:325–334.

Strachey, J. (1934). The nature of the therapeutic action of psychoanalysis. *International Journal of Psycho-Analysis* 50:275–292, 1969.

Tuckett, D. (1991). Editorial. Fifteen clinical accounts of psychoanalysis: a further invitation. *International Journal of Psycho-Analysis* 72:377–382.

Waelder, R. (1937). The problem of the genesis of psychic conflict in earliest infancy. *International Journal of Psycho-Analysis* 18:406–473.

Wallerstein, R. S. (1986). *Forty-Two Lives in Treatment.* New York: Guilford.

—— (1988). One psychoanalysis or many? *International Journal of Psycho-Analysis* 69:5–21.

—— (1990). Psychoanalysis: the common ground. *International Journal of Psycho-Analysis* 71:3–20.

—— (1993). Between chaos and petrification: a summary of the Fifth I. P. A. Conference of Training Analysts. *International Journal of Psycho-Analysis* 74:165–178.

Weinshel, E. M. (1992). Therapeutic technique in psychoanalysis and psychoanalytic psychotherapy. *Journal of the American Psychoanalytic Association* 40:327–347.

Yorke, C. (1985). Finding the Freuds: some personal reflections. In *Analysts at Work*, ed. J. Reppen. Hillsdale, NJ: Analytic Press.

12
What's at Stake in the Truth Controversy?

LAWRENCE FRIEDMAN, M.D.

When a new idea is introduced, analysts argue about whether it is a more correct way to think about mind and treatment. And so it should be: ideas in general are considered for their intellectual adequacy in relation to their subject matter. But that is not the only way to judge psychoanalytic ideas. Treatment is an event, and one can always ask what effect it would have on that event for an analyst to believe a new idea. Such an estimate, however, is not easily made. Treatment itself is often described in theoretical terms and as a consequence, the debate about practical effects is likely to simply repeat the intellectual debate about the validity of the new ideas.

These days we see several critiques converging on a new skepticism about structure in the mind and reality in treatment. I suggest that, in addition to the systematic, philosophical, psychological, and empirical issues that are raised by this skepticism, we can also ask what treatment issues are at stake.

The purpose of this paper is to speculate about what practical implications this skeptical trend might have on future treatment if it should take hold in the profession. In order to picture the effect of the ideas without judging their validity, I will select some gross, experiential features of treatment on which to imagine the new ideas operating. I make no claim for methodological purity in this endeavor. It is just a rough way of guessing futures in order to make choices clearer.

THE RISE AND FALL OF REALITY

In its earliest form, psychoanalysis gave patients a clear task. To some extent it was a task of their own making; to some extent the task was dictated by early psychoanalytic theory, which in turn had roots in the practical successes and theoretical conveniences of hypnotism.

Analytic technique developed in mutual interaction with psychoanalytic theory, and the patient's assigned task was transformed in tandem with such ideas as ego, resistance, and system unconscious. It wasn't long before the patient's assigned goal ceased to be the recovery of traumatic memories. Now the goal was to remember childhood wish configurations, and, more generally, to integrate wishes in a way that would prevent them from compelling a person heedlessly and peremptorily.

That is the aim of the patient's task. But, though they may trade places from time to time, a task's nature and its aim are two different things, especially in psychoanalysis, which is famous for its indirectness. Having stated its aim in a very general way, we must ask what is the *nature* of the analysand's task? We can easily give it a formula, but its essence is hard to capture. The fundamental rule was clearly stated at the birth of psychoanalysis and has remained firmly in place throughout its history. (But see Busch, this volume.)

One could say that the essence of the fundamental rule is to assume an attitude of disciplined passivity before oneself. After the primacy of transference was recognized, a larger significance was recognized in the rule: a combination of closeness to—and distance from—an analyst-audience, and a willingness to risk the emotional investment in an analyst with whom one is passionately involved, in order to appreciate a distant—that is, an objective—truth.

The paradoxical nature of this task was always evident: the patient is supposed to keep in mind the aim of the task and, at the same time, to act aimlessly. Those two aspects of the task are brought together in the image of a patient conscientiously watching the reality of his mind in natural free motion. The patient's passivity, therefore, is that of an empirical scientist in love with the truth, but (according to Freud) it is the affective closeness that enforces the required distance: love of truth follows love of the analyst.

Freud retained this sense of what inspires the patient to carry out his task, undisturbed by his increasingly sophisticated theory of motivation. Gray (1994) has pointed out that Freud continued to rely on the same forces he had counted on for hypnosis. Indeed, I think that even in his rapidly developing theory, advances beyond the model of suggestion were overtaken and almost vanquished by his galloping skepticism about human rationality, finally leading him to doubt the very existence of an ego (a sad consequence, since its ego was the only thing that endeared humanity to him).

However, in the 1930s and '40s, the same complexities that challenged a treatment based on rationality inspired other analysts to enrich the hypnotic model rather than to reject treatment; they happily looked over the various *types* of influence the analyst had at his disposal (see the papers from the Marienbad Conference published in the *International Journal of Psycho-Analysis* in 1937). Freud was always comfortable with the analyst's influence, but that was only because—and just so long as—it was an influence exerted in a single, austere direction. He saw authority as a force for clearing the ego, and despaired when he found so many egos to be permanently altered. Man's freedom from automatic mental functioning was the only goal of treatment he cared about, and that required a discrimination of objective truth. The younger theorists were comfortable imagining themselves influencing patients in a variety of ways, and they were not as discouraged by blemishes on the ego. Less austere in their treatment goals, they saw an opportunity to work those other influences into the theory of cure. As a goal of treatment, facing reality was now becoming subtly shaded—and therefore compromised.

These younger analysts were developing a model in which the analyst actively shapes the patient's objective outlook rather than persuading him to face a simple, objective truth. They were thinking in terms of realistic *attitudes* and realistic *perspectives*; of a composite *orientation* arranged by a well-integrated psychic apparatus (Waelder 1936). Even as they were exploiting the new structural theory, these new theorists were, I suggest, readying the ego for Brenner's recent dismissal, since disappearance is what awaits an organ as it becomes identified with the mere act of integration.

What happened to the patient's task during this evolution? For Freud, the task had been closeness in distance, with the distance (disinterested objectivity) being a clear aim enforced by the closeness. The later analysts, looking at their many-channeled effects on the patient, found it hard to imagine their influence to be so narrowly focused; whatever it was that they were pushing the patient toward, it couldn't be so simply defined. And I presume that this did nothing to reassure them about reality as a target of treatment.

In other words, both psychoanalytic theory and the intuitive sense of practice combined to cloud over the idea of reality. (I refer always to both the reality of the world and the reality of one's mind.)

I suggest that in the 1960s this led to a crisis in the theory of treatment, a crisis directly involving the patient's assigned task. The road was leading toward a treatment in which the reality the patient was asked to face was no longer a simple one; his task was murky and confused, and treatment was conceived of as basically manipulative. A fundamental feature of treatment was thus in danger of falling by the wayside, and it is not surprising that mainstream analysts decided to call a halt to the journey. They did so by an enhanced dogmatism about "interpretation," which now had the mission of preserving the patient's task of distance in closeness. No matter what uncertainties the concept of reality might fall prey to, an interpretation could be relied on as the distant (objective) view of what the patient was closely (passionately) involved with, and the patient's task would be to allow this view to be visible first to the analyst and then to himself. The uniqueness of an analytic interpretation as a type of communication would be a counterpart to the uniqueness of free association as a thought process. And its clear reception would correspond to the definition of the ego (as apotheosized in Eissler's paper of 1953). Thus, the authoritativeness of interpretation was invoked to *minimize* the role of manipulation: that is one of the great paradoxes of psychoanalysis.

The central problem in this model is, of course, resistance. The distant (objective) view, which contrasts with the patient's passionate, wishful thinking, is supposed to be the view that is truthfully represented in an analytic interpretation. But the ego was, by definition, that which appreciates just such a view. Interpretation and truth and ego are almost synonymous. The two central problems of psychoanalysis arise directly from this: Why does theory talk about an impaired (defended, altered, unconsciously collusive) ego instead of a relatively absent ego? And how could an absent ego be expected to respond to treatment? Freud almost gave up on the first challenge. As for the technical challenge, "analyzing resistance" can mean almost anything, but one thing it had to imply, for those who wished to stay within the tradition, was insistence on the correctness, at least, of the analyst's interpretation of the reception accorded his interpretations. Unlike Freud, most of his contemporaries and the succeeding generation of analysts did not want to think of themselves as using personal influence to persuade the patient that his view of reality was distorted by personal interest. They hoped that the simple correctness of their interpretive pattern, taken all together, would somehow do the trick. They would somehow avoid manipulating the patient by employing impersonal (objectively true) yet personal (from the analyst) communications.

But "somehow" isn't good enough. And today one can see a reaction to a weak treatment rationale that relied on the analyst's authority uncoupled from his authoritative influence. Later analysts, squinting at the doctrine, saw the claim to authority clearly enough, but failed to find the alleged absence of influence. And so it looked to them like authoritarianism.

I don't mean to say that there is only one reason for the present revisionist climate in psychoanalysis. There is also the spirit of the times. We see a general egalitarianism in the family and schools, and a relativism in philosophy and literary criticism. But I think we can also find a separate thread of concern about the nature of inner vision and how it comes about. Nowadays there are many contributions from a wide variety of theoretical perspectives that picture the analytic scene more as a dialogue or a discussion than as the delivery of interpretations, and the therapeutic impact is often envisioned simply as an analyst disturbing the patient's psychic equilibrium.

Manipulation is acknowledged and models are constructed to show how an inevitable manipulation is defused—and finally dissolved—by frank and flexible discussion between analyst and analysand (Leavy 1980).

THE DEMAND STRUCTURE OF TREATMENT

What happens to the patient's task in the course of this theoretical shift?

Some current schools of thought assign no task whatever. Brenner, and probably Arlow as well, are, in theory, opposed to the idea of a patient's task. (Patients will do whatever it is that patients do and analysts will do what analysts do, and the conjunction will change the patient.) Other models are less explicit but just as opposed to the idea of a patient's task. In some quarters, the whole idea of an analytic *procedure* is in disfavor.

Although theory is an important ingredient in treatment, doctrine alone does not decide whether the patient will have a task or what that task will be. A far more important determinant is what is *implied* by the goings-on. People have a sense of the direction of any activity in which they are involved, and if their partner is important to them they will be especially alert to what he is after. They will always ask, "What does he want from me?" I believe that in psychoanalysis the vagueness of the answer to this question, and the ambiguity—indeed, on the manifest level, the actual non-existence—of an answer to this question, is important to the treatment process. But a therapist of whatever stripe will inevitably betray the direction of his work. And therefore one vital feature of every talking treatment is what might be called its *demand structure*, by which I mean the implicit requirement or expectation that is laid on the patient.

From the beginning of Freud's work to the end, the demand structure of psychoanalysis implied the existence of an objective external and internal reality. In its most general form, Freud's demand on the patient was the recognition of objective reality. The patient would see all the analyst's efforts converge on that. All of the analyst's actions and arrangements point that way: free association, the splitting of passionate action from distant contemplation, the addressing of the ego, the use of authority—patients would feel all of these to converge on the recognition of an objective reality of his or her mind and the world around it. The patient could not fail to sense that he was expected to recognize that there was such an objective reality and that he hadn't succeeded in his work until he recognized its truth. The particulars varied as Freud's theory developed: at various times "reality" might refer to a traumatic incident, or the feeling attached to that incident, or a fantasy of many uses, or a nuclear complex, or a childhood neurosis, or the actual passage of biographical time, or the difference between a child's vulnerability and an adult's, or how one ignores a perception in order to indulge a wish. But one way or another, there was always an objective reality to be faced up to. Kohut was certainly right that Freud's treatment was built around a truth morality.

When analysts began to see themselves as exerting various sorts of influence, this structure of treatment necessarily came into question. The integrative goals of psychoanalysis now appeared to be the only plausible ones, while detached recognition of reality became problematic. The patient's task was becoming more and more obscure. The fundamental demand structure of psychoanalysis was threatened, and although one generation sought to save it by a return to a strict reliance on interpretation, the rescue was only temporary, and the demand structure of psychoanalysis is on the block again today.

DESCRIBING AND POINTING

Looking back at this (admittedly very speculative) history, one is tempted to see as the critical juncture the moment when analysts attempted to reinforce the status of interpretation by idealizing both its communicative and its purely propositional nature. In doing that, they were postulating a human interaction that was unique in being free from suggestion or manipulation. They were, in effect, trying to shore up the demand structure of analysis (which requires the patient to take a detached look at objective reality) by supposing that the truth value of the analyst's verbalization would allow it to be picked up and accepted in a detached fashion. But the analyst does not make propositions; he makes statements. And his statements, like all human statements, have manipulative, attitudinal, perspectival, and relativistic aspects. In J. L. Austin's (1962) terms, they have illocutionary force. In other words, the demand structure of psychoanalysis was still in jeopardy.

Well then, is there no escape from the jeopardy which has threatened the traditional truth-seeking mission of psychoanalysis? Indeed, there is another approach: one can think of the analyst's communications as pointers. By pointer I mean an act that primarily *directs* attention, in contrast to a description, which primarily *characterizes* a matter in an effort to influence the way it is perceived. The critical stage in analytic theory was reached when analysts realized that they were influencing and not just pointing. Their initial reaction was to pretend that in addition to those influences, psychoanalysis possesses a descriptive influence that acts *just like a pointing*, namely a psychoanalytic interpretation (see Fenichel 1941). That was indeed the original model of psychoanalytic treatment, and it is a valid model when the search is for discrete, traumatic memories. But descriptions will no longer be pointers if there is no discrete object to be found.

In this larger field of psychoanalytic surveillance, it seems to me that the act of pointing is just the sort of communication that will reinforce the old demand structure of psychoanalysis, since it conveys the idea of an objective structure of the mind together with an expectation that the patient will apprehend it. And here, I think, is the terrain that has been mapped by Paul Gray.

Of course, I realize that the distinction between pointing and describing is not a distinction in logic: it reflects the balance of a speaker's motives and the psychological thrust of his action. Logically speaking, every particular description points to something or other. And every pointing—even a non-verbal gesture—declares something, since it must specify what it wants noticed, and can do that only by characterizing it in some way, at least implicitly. But psychologically there is an important difference in the degree of influence and suggestion between, "Look at that picture over there!" and, "Look at the way Matisse uses pure color to make forms."

Gray's method is designed to minimize the analyst's influence and prepare for the patient's independent use of his mind. It is a matter of degree. As Gray (1994) indicated, the analyst's influence can never be totally eliminated (pp. 224–225). Even the selecting of an important moment in the patient's speech is descriptive and therefore an influencing force, as Lacan understood when he decided to "punctuate" the hour by ending it according to what the patient had just said. When the analyst calls attention to a shift in tone, or suggests that something is happening instead of something else, these are descriptive influences, but minimally so when compared with elaborate descriptions of wish, fantasy, and defensive structures. I suppose we could classify technique according to the degree to which the analyst's interventions are designed to characterize or to point.

Since our objective is to speculate on practical implications we should now turn our attention to what is at stake in these differences.

The most pertinent issue is the one elaborated by Gray: the issue of manipulation. Pointing and characterizing involve different degrees of manipulation on several different levels. On the face of it, as already mentioned, when someone characterizes a subject, he attempts to mold its perception, whereas when someone mainly points, his characterizing has an *ad hoc* pragmatic air—it is anything that will orient attention, the ultimate characterizing being left to the perceiver. Compared to the pointer, the characterizer is more a manipulator of perception and thought.

But in psychoanalytic treatment such obvious manipulation is the least important effect of characterizing. Indeed, we probably overestimate the power of that sort of manipulation since, instead of characterizing the patient as intended, the analyst's comment may be more significant to the patient for the way it points to the analyst's attitude, or perhaps it is felt to point to what the patient is mainly concerned about in himself (see Michels 1983) rather than characterizing what the analyst intended. In other words, the *analyst's* description may be used by the *patient* mainly to point, within himself and to the analyst.

But if the content of the description is not always as powerful a manipulator as we might have thought, the same cannot be said about the *act* of describing. More influential than the direct propaganda of a description, the *relationship* with his partner that is set up by a describer is in marked contrast to the relationship induced by a pointer. That is what Gray has called our attention to. By asking someone to accept a description of himself, especially of a sort that he would ordinarily reject, the analyst implicitly asks to be invested with power and trust, and, as Gray has emphasized, he thereby invites all the other uses that a patient can make of such a figure.

We should note that at this authoritarian end of the interactive spectrum, manipulation is at a maximum, but it is unclear who is manipulating whom, and, of course, we must finally conclude that it is a mutual manipulation. The fear that they were losing out on both sides of this mutual manipulation may have been partly what disturbed analysts in the

1940s. On the one hand, they had become increasingly aware of their entanglement with the patient's patterns and needs (for example, Stone, Gitelson, Loewald). On the other hand, their authority seemed unwarranted if the reality they rule on is not a remembered event, but a synthesis of interests represented by various institutions of mind.

Nor is it just a matter of authority. The descriptive style of interpreting (if I may call it that) necessarily emphasizes a dramatic presentation of the image of the patient. When it comes to human behavior, description is almost equivalent to dramatization. But dramatization will always express a personal, slightly moralizing attitude by the analyst and thus, ultimately, a departure from analytic neutrality. Schafer (1983) has attempted to confront this problem head-on by acknowledging the dramatization (and thus implicitly the moralizing) while attempting to restore neutrality by a philosophical skepticism about all attributions.

These features of authority and dramatic moralizing bear on a third difference between the descriptive style and the pointing style. It is an aspect which might be called the *audience effect*. I have already commented on the basic psychoanalytic principle of detachment within intense involvement. Putting the task into terms of dialogue, one might say that the patient has to move between addressing a particular, personal audience and a more generalized, virtual audience. (The more generalized audience is internal and abstract; it corresponds, for example, to Kohut's developed selfobject, and to Piaget's equilibrated perspective.) What is crucial in treatment is the degree to which this behavior is fostered by the analyst as an actual audience. Gray has taught us that the inclination or disinclination of an analyst to deliberately speak from within a transference role influences the patient's chance of moving from a personal to a more generalized audience. Such a movement will be proportionately retarded by the analyst's readiness to adopt a dramatic, and therefore moralizing stance. There are probably several reasons for that retarding effect. The most obvious reason, of course, is that such a stance colludes with the patient's demand for a personal relationship—indeed, it may invite such a relationship. But, in addition, a dramatic moralizing attitude on the part of the analyst may retard the patient's treatment because it fails to *model* the more abstract audience that the analyst wants the patient to develop and to address.

CHOICES AND VISIONS OF THE FUTURE

Now let us return to our speculation about the outcome of current trends. Perhaps the most common feature of new analytic theories is disbelief in the mind considered as an object, with a consequent softening of the rules of treatment that were designed for that now-vanished object. All concepts are affected by this movement, but perhaps none more than ego and resistance. Structure in general is in disfavor.

What this trend will do to treatment depends on two unknown factors: (1) What we see is a shift in *theory*. We do not know what effect, if any, that shift will have on the demand structure of the *treatment*. (2) If the theoretical preferences have an effect on the demand structure of treatment we do not know what effect that will have on the patient. What would treatment look like with a different structure of demand?

Theoretical innovations obviously affect theory more than they do treatment. And that's not just because theory is conceptual before being practical; it is also because psychoanalytic treatment is more directly shaped by its own tradition than by its rationale. We are not surprised to find Schafer recommending a classical analytic procedure despite his startling dissolution of all theory of the mind, and we do not expect Brenner's interpretive style to change when he no longer thinks about an ego. If a patient sees an analyst who seems to be after The Truth (a truth of any sort), the demand structure of that treatment is likely to remain much the same, regardless of what the analyst *writes* about Truth.

In the short run, the largest effect of a theoretical change is probably the analyst's *reaction* to his own departure from traditional theory. If, for example, the analyst is convinced that his implicit truth-seeking is a distortion of discourse, incompatible with psychological reality, he may experience his customary treatment as intolerably manipulative, and then his discomfort may affect the treatment. Or if the analyst is persuaded that there is no such thing as objective truth, he may worry that his attentiveness can be read by patients only as an intimate personal attachment, which may force him to imagine novel forms of intimacy that appear more therapeutic than sociable (for example, the so-called holding environment).

Finally, let us turn to the long-term speculation. What might a therapy look like with a different demand structure? I stress here the word "different." If treatment forces do not converge on discovering and facing up to some sort of truth, then they will converge on something else. We are not trying to imagine a treatment with *no* demand structure. A treatment in which a patient can imagine no desired task will not be a psychotherapeutic procedure, though it might be a medical or psychopharmacologic one, since these are not, in principle, cooperative ventures.

My guess is that there are two possibilities: If the therapist is not asking the patient to see something, then he is asking him to be something. Or, to put it differently, if a patient cannot sense that he is supposed to discover some truth, then he will feel that he is supposed to discover a role. And what might that be?

Again, there seem to be two possibilities: One demand is that the patient "be well," whatever that means. The patient comes looking for a better way of living or feeling, and he may sense that the treatment requires him to *find* it, so to speak. He should be less afraid of people, more willing to take chances, more self-accepting, less irritable, more successful, more assertive, and so on. Another version of this might be a demand that the patient see things more "appropriately," but in the sense of *reacting* more appropriately rather than seeing things for whatever they are.

Let us look more closely at this last possibility: The ambiguity of the word "appropriate" is the tip-off that these treatments might simply feign the old demand structure. Appropriate behavior may be advertised as realistic, but if it is unaccompanied by a conception of objective truth, appropriateness refers simply to a recommended role. Treatments such as this include cognitive therapies, and educative efforts for "wider scope" patients. Economic and social pressures will doubtless foster these therapies in the future, maybe exclusively. Would it be unfair to say that this option leads back to the pre-analytic realm of moral therapies? In any case, it is not a mysterious road and we don't need to speculate about what it would look like.

More interesting is the demand that the patient be a certain way in relation to the analyst. It is that sort of demand that will probably be instituted if analytic styles are retained while the demand structure is altered.

The patient thinks: He doesn't seem to want me to discover something, so I guess he feels that this relationship will heal me. I am being asked to feel something for him, to get something out of knowing him, to pick up some personal quality of his, to see him in a certain way.

Of course, analysts have always talked about "transference cures." But what I am referring to here is not the patient's preferred use of the analyst, but the destination to which the analyst seems to be urging the patient. These are two sides of the same coin: those features of analytic treatment that make the transference possible may legitimately be described as *inviting* the transference, implicitly telling the patient that such a relationship is what is demanded. Indeed, a close relationship *is* actually demanded in Freudian analysis, but I am envisioning a future treatment that not only includes this feature but seems to focus all its forces on its development. It is my belief that all psychoanalytic treatments tend to covertly convey to the patient that the analyst is involved with him in an intimate and family-like way. Balancing this illusion, analysts in the past have been able to indicate that it is the patient's acknowledgement of objective truth that will cure him, and this keeps the illusion of intimacy from advertising itself also as the vehicle of cure.

In order to get an idea of how the situation would shape up without that balance, we should examine the self psychology paradigm, as it is implemented, and Schafer's (1983), Gill's (1988), or Hoffman's (1991) paradigm in its implications, as well as the many other object-less "discussion" or "dialogic" models of treatment.

Like most analytic innovators, Kohut long maintained traditional analytic customs. It was hard for him to drop the insight rationale; he held onto the importance of a "lesson" until shortly before his death, when the logic of his position (and probably reflection on his experience) led him to declare that it is the relationship that heals, and not stories about disappointment.

I think self psychologists are now essentially in the position of Thomas French (1958) who, in effect, arranged a field of forces in which the patient's alternating hopes and discouragements will automatically (unconsciously) integrate themselves finally into a more secure pattern of aspiration. Other developments than that may go on during self psychological treatment, but I think that over time, its practice will converge on that rationale. And what will the patient then feel pushed toward? What will he feel is demanded of him? Self psychology's enemies argue that patients will feel obliged to idealize their analysts, even though self psychologists are taught to seize on disappointment and highlight it.

In my opinion, the situation is somewhat more complicated, and lies between the declared mission of the school and the criticism of it. Patients of self psychologists are indeed being asked to trust the analyst, and the concentration on moments of disappointment is designed not to reinforce the disillusionment but to mend distrust, as Kohut explicitly stated. But when all is said and done, the trust that is asked for is not absolutely vague and general. It is trust that one can take a relationship *from* the analyst and carry it away. That is the larger demand that is being made of the patient; that is the long-line expectation that he feels required to fulfill. The patient is asked to behave with the analyst *as though* the analyst had an intimate concern *and* a strength that can be transferred.

What about the conversationalists, intersubjectivists, and constructionists, the conventionalists and the relativists, if they were to carry over their verbalized philosophy into the atmosphere of treatment rather than using it merely to prod the patient into exploring an implicitly objective reality? What will their demand be?

My guess is that on a general level it would be the demand to be creative, and, on a specific level, it would be the demand that the patient be interested in the analyst. In that respect, the demand would resemble one half of the Freudian demand, which is to be interested in the analyst while also giving up that interest by abandoning one's wished-for role. The difference is that in the constructivist paradigm there is no objective-truth demand to distract from the personal interest. In order to balance the invitation to a personal relationship, the treatment would have to find a new distraction—something that would take the place of the hunt for truth. What would it be? Perhaps it would be playfulness.

How would the demand for playfulness compare with the objective truth demand? Without an implicit truth demand, will the analyst feel entitled to take up various, unserious relationships as play progresses? Where will he get his confidence that the patient's response is just play and that the patient will play differently tomorrow?

And what about the patient who is subjected to this new demand? Why would he be playful without a realistic goal in mind? Won't he simply feel teased? Or will he welcome this as an unusually safe freedom?

Let us be clear about the difficulties in this position. If the analyst actually conveyed his skeptical relativism to his patient, he would be labeling his interventions not as perspectives on reality but as personal reactions. He would be advertising his behavior unashamedly as attempts to influence in response to being influenced. The patient would be asked to make use of the analyst's personal behavior toward him. I think this is likely to be read as a demand for a personal "fitting in" with the analyst, though perhaps in paradoxical ways. How that demand would affect a program of playfulness, I am not sure. An elusive therapist might appear to be asking for a "fitting in" which, at the same time, he never allows. A Zen-like treatment of that sort is an intriguing prospect; it might be a pure culture of one of the standard components of psychoanalytic treatment. But it would not look much like the psychoanalysis we know.

In conclusion, I remind the reader that I have been trying to imagine only the shape and vector of therapies with new demands. I have not considered the validity or therapeutic power of the various possibilities. That is a separate subject.

References

Austin, J. L. (1962). *How to Do Things with Words,* 2nd ed. Cambridge, MA: Harvard University Press.

Brenner, C. (1993). *Psychoanalytic Technique and Psychic Conflict.* New York: International Universities Press.

Eissler, K. R. (1953). The effect of the structure of the ego on psychoanalytic technique. *Journal of the American Psychoanalytic Association* 1:104–143.

Fenichel, O. (1941). *Problems of Psychoanalytic Technique*, trans. D. Brunswick. New York: Psychoanalytic Quarterly.

French, T. (1958). *The Integration of Behavior*, vol. 3. Chicago: University of Chicago Press.

Gill, M. M. (1988). Converting psychotherapy into psychoanalysis. *Contemporary Psychoanalysis* 24:262–274.

Gray, P. (1994). *The Ego and Analysis of Defense.* Northvale, NJ: Jason Aronson.

Hoffman, I. Z. (1991). Discussion: toward a social-constructivist view of the psychoanalytic situation. *Psychoanalytic Dialogues* 1:74–105.

Leary, S. A. (1980). *The Psychoanalytic Dialog.* New Haven: Yale University Press.

Michels, R. (1983). Contemporary psychoanalytic views of interpretation. In *Psychiatry Update,* vol. 2, ed. L. Grinspoon, pp. 61–70. Washington, DC: American Psychiatric Press.

Schafer, R. (1983). *The Analytic Attitude.* New York: Basic Books.

Waelder, R. E. (1936). The problem of freedom in psycho-analysis and the problem of reality-testing. *International Journal of Psycho-Analysis* 17:89–108.

13

An Interpretation of Transference

JONATHAN LEAR, Ph.D.

THE SOCRATIC INHERITANCE

"The unexamined life," Socrates famously said, "is not worth living." Now it is almost commonplace to view Socrates as the great ancestor of psychoanalytic method; after all, he fashioned a method of cross-examination designed to elicit conflicts which had hitherto remained unconscious inside the interlocutor. Like the cathartic method, this inquiry was meant to be therapeutic. His was not an abstract inquiry into, say, the nature of piety, but a practical attempt to help the "analysand" live a better life. For Socrates, "How shall I live?" was the fundamental question confronting each person; his peculiar form of examination was intended to help a person to answer it well. Therefore, Socrates had his own fundamental rule: state only what you believe. The "analysand" was not allowed to try out a debating position, but had to bring his own commitments to the inquiry. If the inquiry led to contradiction, it was not the *reductio* of an abstract position with no putative owner, but of the "analysand's" own commitments.[1] That is also why Socrates, like a contemporary psychoanalyst, disavowed knowledge of how the "analysand" should answer the fundamental question: the point of Socratic examination was to help people to ask and answer the question for themselves.

Socrates does, then, have a claim to be recognized as an ancestor. But, before we let this family romance proceed further, it is worth noting that this Socratic dictum was among his last words; they were uttered in his own defense, while on trial, charged with introducing new gods and corrupting youth. His defense was not a success, at least by any standard measure: he was found guilty, sentenced to death, and ultimately executed. It is easy enough to blame the Athenian *demos* for this outrage, but is it not also an indictment of Socrates's therapeutic method?[2] His cross-examination was meant to make people better, but it provoked the *demos* to act out its mur-

---

[1] At first sight, it might appear that nothing could differ more from Socrates's fundamental rule than the fundamental rule of psychoanalysis: try to state whatever comes into your mind without censorship. However, if one believes, as Freud did, that a person's psychic commitments have their own upward thrust—that the contents of the unconscious will tend to get themselves expressed unless prevented from doing so by inhibiting psychological forces—then, in trying to state whatever comes into consciousness, one tends to state one's 'beliefs', at least in the extended sense of psychic commitments. Freud discovered that, if one enlarges the scope of psychological commitments, Socrates's fundamental rule is too narrow to elicit them. Stating only what one believes, in the narrow sense, can be a way of hiding and inhibiting unconscious psychic commitments. But the fundamental rule of psychoanalysis is an emendation and extension of the Socrates's rule, not a reversal; it plays an analogous role in eliciting psychic commitments.

[2] Perhaps blame is too easy; it is certainly controversial, as is almost any serious claim one might wish to make about the ancient world. For a fascinating attempt to recover the historical Socrates as an anti-democrat

derous impulses. Whatever else one might want to say about the death of Socrates, one must admit that it represents, in the short run at least, a psychotherapeutic disaster.

Socrates's mistake, it seems in retrospect, was to ignore transference. He thought one could go up to anyone in the marketplace and begin a cross-examination. The only effort he made to determine the current psychic state of the "analysand" was to elicit his (conscious or preconscious) beliefs. He acted as though the meaning of his activity would be transparent to others, and thus provoked a transference storm. He argued, for instance, that it is better to suffer injustice than to be unjust, but he seemed oblivious to the fact that within the marketplace of fifth-century Athens such an argument would be experienced as an unjust attack. What to Socrates seemed like helping a person to continue the inquiry into how to live, seemed to his accusers to be introducing new gods and corrupting the youth. These are very different perspectives on the same activity, and Socrates seems to have lacked a systematic understanding of how that gap could be possible. Before we go further in claiming Socrates as our ancestor, we ought to recognize that the concept of transference, fundamental to psychoanalytic method, is one that Socrates, to the peril of all concerned, did not possess.

PLATONIC REVISIONS

Plato is well known for his defense of Socrates and his condemnation of Athenian democracy, but there is implicit in his work a recognition of Socrates's therapeutic failure, and

---

see Stone (1988), and, for a plausible rebuttal, see Vlastos (1979, 1983). For a more persuasive and less flawed presentation of the anti-democrat thesis see Hanson (1980). (This will be translated into English and published in the proceedings of the United Nations conference on the origins of democracy, Athens, [1992].)

a revision of the theory of the psyche to accommodate it.[3] Curiously, these revisions bear a family resemblance to developments within psychoanalysis during its first forty years. One suspects that both theories were coming up against and responding to something fundamental in the human psyche. For Socrates, like Freud, began with an essentially cathartic method. He did not have an account of a structured psyche; while a person might have conflicting beliefs, and thus experience conflict *within* the psyche, there was, for Socrates, no room for conflict of the psyche with itself.[4] Overcoming conflict could, for him, only be a matter of eliciting and expelling false belief. For Socrates, the psyche was little more than a container.

Plato can be credited with the invention of psycheanalysis, at least in the sense of being the first to give a systematic account of a structured psyche. He does this against a background assumption that the human psyche has a characteristic activity: to create a meaningful world in which to live. The members of a community constitute themselves in the creation and maintenance of a social–cultural–political world, the *polis*. Humans, Plato says, are polis animals. The polis provides the only environment which is fit for human habitation. That is one reason why Socrates refuses to flee

---

[3] A scholarly defense of this interpretation of Plato is beyond the scope of this paper, but I do attempt such a defense in Lear (1992, 1994). Readers interested in textual support for the interpretation offered here should consult *Republic*, II.377A-B, II.378D-E, 381E, III.395C-E, 401D-E, II.395D, IV.424C-D, IX.590E, IV.435C, VIII.544D-E, II.358B, 366E, IV.435E, VIII.554B-555B, IX.577C-578C, VII.519D-521B, II.376E-377A, 382B-C, II.382B-D. See also Lear (1988) for an interpretation of the Platonic legacy to Aristotle, and Lear (1990) for a discussion of the Socratic–Platonic concern with individuation and its relation to psychoanalytic theory.

[4] This is why, for Socrates, knowledge is sufficient for virtue, bad acts can only be committed out of ignorance and thus *akrasia* (so-called weakness of will) is impossible.

Athens, with all its faults: life outside its boundaries would, for him, be meaningless. Indeed, the polis, for Plato, has a deeper claim on humans: they are dependent on it for the very constitution of their psyches. Humans are born with a capacity to internalize cultural influence: this is why Plato spends so much time discussing the stories which mothers and nurses should be allowed to tell their children, the art that should be allowed in the polis, and the content of children's education. At stake is the shape and content of the human psyche. In maturity, humans raise families, work at their jobs, engage in civic life—all the while externalizing the cultural influences they had previously internalized. The social-cultural world is the joint externalization of the psyches of those who live within it. This cultural habitat is an enlargement and reflection of the structure of the psyches of the historically significant actors. Therefore, Plato thinks, in studying the structure of the polis we can discover the structure of the psyche "writ large." In studying the world it inhabits, the psyche will find itself reflected back to itself in its own characteristic activity.

Plato thus invented the first systematic object relations theory: a dynamic theory of the relations between the psyche and the world it inhabits. Plato thought he was living in a sick society—after all, Athens had just put to death its best citizen—and, given his dynamic theory, he knew this sickness had to be traceable back to the psyche. Following the basic fault lines he saw in the polis, Plato devised a structural theory of the psyche. The psyche, he thought, is divided into three parts: appetite, characterized by its basic desires for food and sex; a narcissistic component, which Plato called "spirit," concerned with pride, honor, and anger; and reason, which desires knowledge. These parts are distinguished not only by their distinctive types of desires, but by the possibility to enter into fundamental forms of intrapsychic conflict with the others. Plato even devised a theory of pathological character types which were the manifestations of typical forms of intrapsychic conflict. So, for example, oligarchical character disorder was the outcome of appetite dominating the other parts and creating a division within itself, whereby certain appetites were encouraged and others were forcibly held down. The oligarchical personality would tend to create an oligarchical society which was itself divided between the rich and the repressed poor. It was a sign, however, of a pathological structure that an oligarch could not entirely succeed in his characteristic activity, and would only produce a conflicted structure that would eventually collapse of its own contradictions.

Pathology of character, Plato knew, had to be reflected in pathology of outlook. The tyrant, for example, thinks he is living the best life, even though he is living the worst. In general, people are trying to answer the question "How shall I live?" as best they can; since they are doing such a poor job, their methods of inquiry must be distorted. Plato devised a theory of fantasy to explain these distorted perspectives. In his famous metaphor of the cave, people are bound at certain levels, exposed only to distorted images which they mistake for reality. The cave is often taken to offer but a bleak prospect for human life, but I think it is the most optimistic metaphor in Western philosophy. Although our experience may be permeated by distorted images, they are ultimately distortions of something real. Moreover, every distorted form of experience has within itself its own conflicts; that is, even from within a distorted perspective, one can get a glimmer that all is not well. If one were to pursue these conflicts, painful though that would be, one would eventually work through them, and end up better off—at a higher level of the cave.

Only the philosopher, whom Plato thinks is also a psyche-analyst, is able to work through the contradictions at each level of experience and so only he can ascend out of the cave and see reality clearly. Having done that, Plato has his

"Socrates" argue that it is the philosopher's obligation to descend back into the cave to help educate and govern his fellow citizens. This will be an unpleasant task for the philosopher: it will take time for his eyes to get used to the dark and to the fantasy world his fellow citizens mistake for reality. But, in requiring the philosopher to go back down into the cave, the "Socrates" of the *Republic* is issuing a prescription which the historical Socrates ignored. In the *Republic,* Plato recommends that the philosopher-ruler tell the citizens a "noble falsehood." This is regularly, and I believe mistakenly, translated as a "noble lie," and it has generated much discussion about the evils of political censorship. But the point Plato is making is, I believe, essentially psychological: if one wishes to communicate with people whose lives are dominated by fantasy, one must speak the language of the fantasy world in which they live. The noble falsehood is Plato's attempt to say something he believes to be true, but in a form he thinks his hearers can grasp. The translation into fantasy converts a truth into a falsehood; but, for Plato, this is as close as this fantasy level of experience can get to the truth.

THE RECOGNITION OF TRANSFERENCE

In the story I wish to tell, Plato's reflection on the therapeutic disaster of Socratic method led to the recognition of the phenomenon of transference and to the development of its theory. For transference, I believe, is just the psyche's characteristic activity of creating a meaningful world in which to live. This characteristic must be understood against a background of a structured psyche, vulnerable to myriad forms of internal conflicts, dependent on prior internalizations for its structure and content, and regularly dominated by fantasy.

In my analytic work, I have often had the experience of entering, or being drawn into, a world—a world endowed with its own peculiar meanings and structures. I expect many analysts have had this experience; and the question I should like to address in this paper is: what content can be given to such an experience?

This is not a question which the early Freud can pursue, because he assumes the world is already endowed with its own meanings. In *Studies on Hysteria* (1893–95), he introduces the idea of transference as a "false connection." A woman in analysis experiences, to her dismay, a desire that Freud give her a kiss. It turns out that she had previously experienced and repressed such a desire, directed towards another man. As Freud explains:

> The content of the wish had appeared first of all in the patient's consciousness without any memories of the surrounding circumstances which would have assigned it to a past time. This wish which was present was then, owing to the compulsion to associate which was dominant in her consciousness, linked to my person, with which the patient was legitimately concerned; and the result of this *mésalliance*—which I describe as a "false connection"—the same affect was provoked which had forced the patient long before to repudiate this forbidden wish. [p. 303]

Transference, on this interpretation, is the unconscious movement of a desire across space and time from one person in her past to another in her present. What makes this a *false* connection, for Freud, is that a desire which would have been appropriately directed toward her former would-be lover, is merely re-enacted with her current doctor. Similarly, in his case study of Dora, Freud speaks of transference phenomena as

> new editions or facsimiles of impulses and phantasies which are aroused and made conscious during the progress of the analysis; but they have this peculiarity,

which is characteristic for their species, that they replace some earlier person by the person of the physician. [Freud 1905, p. 116]

In this conception of transference, emotions, desires, and fantasies are faxed across a given world, and they re-emerge in the analytic situation, unconscious that they are facsimiles. This is Freud's *Archimedean assumption*: if one holds the world constant, one will see psychological contents traveling across it.

Here, then, are the bare bones of the traditional conception of transference, and it is remarkable how little psychoanalytic understanding is needed to formulate it. The idea that wishes and emotions are transferred or carried over from a previous situation to the analytic situation is there in the *Studies on Hysteria* before Freud had any detailed grasp of the workings of unconscious mental processes. All Freud needed to formulate this conception of transference was the idea of the repression of forbidden psychological contents, and the return of the repressed in the analytic situation. In this interpretation, one can see transference in terms of an empiricist model of learning: the analysand is expecting the future to be like the past. The extra fillip which Freud adds to this picture, is that the anticipated future is along the lines of a repressed and rejected past. As Freud came to understand archaic mental functioning, he revised and elaborated this conception of transference. These revisions make room for a more psychoanalytically informed conception of transference.

INTRAPSYCHIC TRANSFERENCE

Freud begins to grapple with the nature of unconscious mental processes in *The Interpretation of Dreams* (1900), and there he introduces the idea of transference as an *intra*psychic phenomenon.[5] Freud wants to explain how dreams use day residues and other preconscious ideas to disguise and express an unconscious wish. As the wish cannot directly enter consciousness, it *transfers* its intensity onto an idea that is already preconscious and thereby gets itself "covered" by it. One might say that, in Freud's view, because the wish cannot transfer *itself* from unconscious to conscious it transfers intensity instead. Freud uses the concept of psychic energy,[6] but the point I wish to emphasize can be made without it. Our conscious thoughts, dreams, and daydreams are linked by webs of associations to unconscious wishes and fantasies. The conscious thought, dream or fantasy becomes a representative of the unconscious wish or fantasy, and its use, even within conscious experience, has to change.[7] There is no reason why this day residue would occur in dreams (daydreams or actings out) other than to do duty for the unconscious wish. "Covering," then, is not mere intensification: it is the covering *over* of one idea by another. The conscious idea has been made

---

[5]This passage, as well as the general topic of intrapsychic transference and its relation to transference as an interpsychic relation, is discussed at length by Loewald (1960), to whom I am indebted. See also Freud (1900), pp. 562–567.

[6]This is in harmony with his conception of the mental molecule as consisting of an idea plus a quantity of energy. (See Freud [1893–95], pp. 86, 166–167.) The idea has to stay where it is, so the energy moves. In practice, Freud recognized that intrapsychic transference was more than a redistribution of energy: it also establishes an *energy line* between the unconscious and conscious idea. In the redistribution of energy, transference necessarily preserves its own history. This shows up as the unconscious idea getting itself *covered*.

[7]Most psychoanalytic work since Freud has been the elaboration of a theory of unconscious fantasy, which allows more fine-tuned analysis among intrapsychic conflicts. As Freud recognized, we regularly find that a conscious or preconscious fantasy serves as a covering for a web of interrelated unconscious fantasies.

into a *covering*—an outer shell, an artifact of the unconscious idea. The conscious idea now has a new meaning due to its links to the unconscious. It has been endowed with unconscious significance: both in the sense that it now expresses unconscious ideas and that this very fact must remain hidden.

These intrapsychic transferences tend to be idiosyncratic. Freud was a master at showing how a chance occurrence of the day—for example, seeing a botanical monograph in a store window—can be endowed with deep unconscious significance. The idea of a monograph will become embedded in a web of associations of which the subject is unaware. Such an embedding will by nature be peculiar. The embedding depends on a chance encounter with the monograph at a time when a certain set of issues were psychologically prominent for this person. It must also somehow "fit in with" the loose associations of archaic mental functioning; that is, it enters a web of associations whose formation depends on a history of chance encounters and loose associations. However common some of the basic problems of human existence may be—helplessness, entrance into the social-sexual world—they acquire their meaning for each person through a web of associations which is idiosyncratic through and through. This embedding is made even more complex and idiosyncratic by condensation. As a result of the fluidity of archaic associations, a single idea or image may do duty for a wealth of conflicts, wishes, and fantasies. The idea will typically be woven into overlapping webs of associations, so the idea of a one-to-one relation between a covering and a covered idea is only a first approximation (see Freud 1900, pp. 279–305, 595–597, 602).

Throughout *The Interpretation of Dreams*, Freud resists the idea that the meaning of a dream can be elicited by a simple decoding of symbols into meanings. Instead, he insists that we do not really understand the meaning of a dream until we understand its location in an entire network of wishes, prohibitions, and associations. This is one manifestation of Freud's *psychological holism*: the full meaning of any particular dream is revealed by its place in the whole web of wishes, desires, and other psychological forces. Therefore, to understand that dream fully, we must understand the (mal)functioning psyche which produced it. In practice, no analysis can be spent explicitly unpacking one dream; conversely, it would not be unusual for an analysis to keep going back to one or two key dreams and endow them with ever more richness and complexity. To understand more about the whole is to understand more about the dreams which are embedded in it.

The lesson of intrapsychic transference is that psychological holism must include the unconscious.[8] Any conscious thought will, typically, be embedded in a wealth of associations which will endow that thought with meanings which are at once both unconscious and idiosyncratic. We do not fully understand the meaning of any conscious thought until we understand the myriad ways in which this thought is functioning as a "covering" for unconscious mental forces—it is these transferences which come to light in an analysis. As we listen to an analysand's associations over the years, we become increasingly aware that though they are adept at speak-

---

[8]Philosophers have been attuned to the holistic nature of the mental: to the fact that the very content of a given belief or desire depends on its relation to other beliefs and desires. But they have tended to concentrate on the holistic nature of the conscious mental, while Freud's crucial point is that holism must include the unconscious mental. (For evidence of Freud's psychological holism see [1900], pp. 97–100, 104–105, 179, 218–219, 280–284, 307–308, 330, 350–353, 652–653.) For a classic exposition of the importance of holism for interpretation see Davidson (1982). However, in "Paradoxes of irrationality," Davidson ingeniously argues that the repressed should be treated as split off, and thus functioning like another mind. I believe that this underestimates Freud's insistence on the holistic relations between conscious and unconscious, even taking repression into account.

ing a shared natural language, in our case English, they are at the same time speaking an idiolect with its own special meanings and resonances. One of the tasks of analysis is to help analysands become consciously aware of the peculiar meanings with which they endow their words.[9]

When Freud introduced the conception of intrapsychic transference, he had not yet formulated the structural theory, but the idea can be readily extended to accommodate it. For, as we find regularly in analysis, a superego voice is serving as a "covering" for an archaic wish or fury. I regularly hear analysands, referring to themselves in the third person, say something like, "—, you ass, just shut up: you're such a jerk." Clearly, this is an attempt to repress or "cover over" an emerging wish or fury, but it is also a "covering" in the sense of being the conscious representative of the repressed. The superego voice, as Freud saw, draws its harsh intensity from the id, and the intensity is reciprocal and dynamic. There would be no need for a harsh superego voice if there were not an intense wish or fury to hold down. One might, thus, say that there is intrapsychic transference between a person's id and superego. Although the superego's task is to repress the id, in that very role it becomes the id's covering: its artifact and representative, "the superego," says Freud, "is always close to the id and *can act as its representative vis-à-vis* the ego" (Freud 1923, pp. 48–49, my emphasis).[10]

---

[9]Geertz (1973) has helped us understand the importance of "thick" concepts in the interpretation of cultures; in those terms one might say that Freud's discovery of intrapsychic transference is the discovery that "thick" concepts tend to be *hyper*thick, though unconsciously so.

[10]Although Freud does not always explicitly extend the concept of intrapsychic transference to include structural theory, it is implicit in his account. See above and also p. 36: "Whereas the ego is essentially the representative of the external world, of reality, *the super-ego stands in contrast to it as the representative of the internal world, of the id*" (1923, my italics).

The significance of intrapsychic transference is that consciousness in general serves as a covering for the unconscious: it has been made over into an artifact and representative of unconscious wishes, fantasies, and furies.

FROM INTRAPSYCHIC TRANSFERENCE TO INTERPSYCHIC TRANSFERENCE

If people endow their words, thoughts, and fantasies with indiosyncratic and unconscious meanings, these must spill over into their daily lives. There is, at the very least, an important relation between *intra*psychic and *inter*psychic transference.[11] As a first approximation, take a classic, if simplified, example: an infantile wish for an incestuous relation may be transferred onto the thought of having an affair with one's analyst. The conscious thought, one might say, has been made over into an artifact, a covering. This is intrapsychic transference, which might be revealed in a dream, but which also might be revealed interpsychically as an experienced erotic desire for one's analyst. Might transference, as it emerges in analysis, be an attempt to turn the analyst into an artifact, a covering? In the throes of a powerful parental transference, it seems to the analysand that the analyst is speaking with a critical voice; a voice which the superego usually speaks intrapsychically. Just as the superego serves as a "covering" for a powerful unconscious fantasy, it seems that the analysand attempts to make the analyst into the statue of the *Commendatore*. In the interpsychic transference, the analysand seems to be attempting to endow the analyst with peculiar, unconscious meaning.

---

[11]Loewald has pointed this out (1960, pp. 247–248), though we should accept that, due to projection, externalization, and related psychological activity, this is not a hard and fast rule.

In Freud's later writings on transference, he seems to move towards such a view. The accent of his writings shifts from transference as a transfer (across a given world) to transference as a repetition. The cost of keeping something out of consciousness, Freud says, is that one acts it out unconsciously: repetition is the return of the repressed, in unconscious form. This re-enactment is inescapable in the transference: "As long as the patient is in treatment, he cannot escape from his compulsion to repeat; and in the end we understand that *this is his way of remembering*" (Freud 1914, p. 150, my italics). The peculiar form of "remembering" is not a form of recollection, but of memorialization; an enactment designed to make the present into an artifact of the past, consciousness into an artifact of the unconscious. In its most general sense, the aim of the enactment is to endow the world with comprehensible meaning. As Freud says, transference is a repetition "*not only onto the doctor, but onto all other aspects of the current situation*" (p. 151, my italics). In the transference, the psyche is engaged in its characteristic activity of trying to create a meaningful world in which to live.

One's view of this activity can be obscured by holding too fast to the idea of transference as a repetition. To see something as a repetition is to see it as "the same thing again"; to understand transference, however, we need to maintain a certain flexibility in the ways we count. Consider, by way of analogy, the soldier, doctor, or shoemaker of Plato's Athens. From one perspective, each was engaged, in his profession, in the same characteristic tasks over and over again. From another perspective, each was living one characteristic type of life, and making his contribution to the maintenance of the social world. In a healthy polis, Plato said, each person will "do his own thing," perform the *one* task for which he is best suited. If, like Plato, one sees the continued existence of the social world as dependent on people performing their distinctive social roles, one will tend to view these roles less as repeated than as *enduring*.[12]

THE CREATION OF A POLIS

Before we can understand what transference within the context of an individual's analysis is, we need to reflect on our joint contributions to the creation and maintenance of the social world. Consider, to begin with, the Athenian polis. On the one hand, it is a psychological creation: who counts as a citizen, and who a slave, who is inside it and who is barbarian, how property is allocated and justice meted out, where and how the boundaries are delineated—all of this reflects the interests, needs, concerns, and outlooks of the participants. On the other hand, it is not just a psychological state or a mere projection: Athens is a creation, an artifact, and it gains a certain independence from the shifting psychological states of its inhabitants. Athens was a real invention, as is the United States, yet the continued existence of these social worlds depends on the enduring willingness of its citizens to defend their boundaries, to go through the rituals which

---

[12]Winnicott makes a related point when, in speaking of a baby's experience, he says: "As observers we note that everything in the play has been done before, has been smelt before, and where there appear specific symbols of the union of baby and mother (transitional objects) these very objects have been adopted, not created. Yet *for the baby* (if the mother can supply the right conditions) every detail of the baby's life is an example of creative living. Every object is a 'found' object. Given the chance, the baby begins to live creatively, and to use actual objects to be creative into and with" (1971, p. 119). Of course, once someone has grasped the creative–enduring aspect of the transference, he can then go back and view it either as a transfer or as a repetition. These formulations are problematic in so far as they obscure our understanding of the creative or the enduring aspects of transference.

lend peculiar meaning to being an Athenian or an American, and to pay for their characteristic activities. Watching the demise of the Soviet Union, we see what happens when there is a collective divestiture or de-cathexis: the polis falls apart and loses meaning.[13] Although the polis is dependent on our enduring commitment, and although it reflects our collective psychic activity, it is not just psychology. Rather, we have created an environment which our psyches can, for better or worse, inhabit.

This is most easily seen in the case of physical artifacts. It is obvious that, say, the houses we build reflect our interests and concerns, our judgment and taste. Yet, though they manifest our psychological states, they achieve a quasi-independent status: a house is at once permeated with our psychology and free-standing. Nor do our meaning–endowing activities require physical construction: a prison may be turned into a museum, a concentration camp sanctified as a church, a set of buildings turned into a university, though little or nothing is done to the physical structures. These transformations usually require certain rituals as well as a shared commitment to use the structures in different ways. In general, social institutions—like law, medicine, the university, the corporation, art—reflect our interests and depend on our enduring commitments, but they cannot be reduced to our psychological states. These institutions are artifacts, and they help to constitute a social world, a polis, in which we locate ourselves.[14]

---

[13] Of course, the literal loss of meaning was preceded by a prolonged and widespread cynicism about the true meaning of the Soviet Union.

[14] Interestingly, Freud uses the polis metaphor to describe the mind and its activity, but as his interest was in capturing the unconscious and infantile mind, he used the image of a *buried* polis. Thus, archaeology became, for Freud, an enduring metaphor for psychoanalytic exploration. (See Freud [1896, p. 192; 1930, pp. 69–71].) However, as psychoanalysis has,

The distinction between subjective and objective can be used to make myriad constrasts, but when psychologists or psychoanalysts speak of someone being able to perceive reality undistorted by fantasy, or of establishing "mature object relations," the reality they are speaking of is social reality. Confusion only arises if one both takes the social world to be objective and, as an archimedean, implicitly assumes that all psychic activity must be subjective. In his discussion of transitional phenomena, for example, Winnicott (1951) used the term "transitional" to designate this form of experience because he conceived of it as *en route* from subjective experience to experience of an objective world.[15] He saw the psyche's activity in the creation of transitional spaces, and he *also* saw that the boundaries between inside and outside, subjective and objective, are blurred. These are two observations, but if one is an archimedean, there will be a tendency

---

in theory and practice, tended to move away from deep interpretations towards working with the transference and detailed texture of the analysand's associations, so perhaps the image of the polis should be replaced by a living polis (standing above the ancient polis). Perhaps too the metaphor of archaeology should be replaced by *topological* archaeology. The topological archaeologist inspects the contours of the land, the flow of the rivers and seas, and has faith in the upward momentum of buried artifacts: as the fields are plowed there will regularly turn up shards of ancient civilizations. By extrapolating from this evidence, the topological archaeologist comes to grasp both what lies buried and its relation to contemporary life. For evidence of Freud's movement in this direction see Freud 1937, p. 259. This movement can also be seen in those influenced by both Melanie Klein and Anna Freud, e.g. Spillius (1983) and Gray (1982, 1986). Furthermore, I do not think there is an inherent conflict in the concepts of analytic surface and analytic space, as does Poland (1992a, b), and I see the conception offered in the next section as harmonious with his thought-provoking description of analytic space.

[15]Loewald has criticized this use because, as he argues, objectivity and subjectivity come to be together with the establishment of a boundary from a previously less differentiated position (1988).

to lump them together and assume that as the boundaries become sharper, the psyche's activity will be located on only one side: inside the psyche. Winnicott asks where cultural experience is located, and he notes that there are certain forms—for example, certain religious experiences—where the boundaries do seem to blur. But I wonder if the question of location is puzzling to him because he recognizes, on the one hand, that culture is permeated with psyche, but assumes, on the other, that the world is not. Once one allows that the psyche informs the social world, it becomes easier to say where cultural experience is located. Some of it may be transitional;[16] but some cultural experience is of a world we create and inhabit. Cultural experience, Winnicott says, is an extension of the idea of play, but he is not able to say in what this extension consists. Roughly speaking, the extension consists in the fact that in play we are playing at creating a world, whereas in cultural activity we are *attempting* in earnest to do so. We are at least *trying* to have our psychological activity move out across the boundary of our psyches and inform the world.[17] For an archimedean, there will be a tendency to

---

[16] The essence of this idea goes back at least to Freud (1930, section I).

[17] When trying to make a difficult point, there is an everpresent danger of being defeated by one's vocabulary. Ultimately, though, the vocabulary used matters less than how it is understood. If we want to say that even the social-cultural world is "transitional," that is fine so long as we do not thereby assume that the boundaries between subjective and objective must be blurred. We should, then, accept that there may be degrees of transitionality which allow for more or less boundary differentiation. Or, if we only want to use "transitional" to describe experience where boundaries are blurred, that is fine too, just so long as we do not thereby assume that "the objective world" is devoid of the psyche's activity. Further, nothing I say in this paper implies that whenever a group agrees it has created something it must be right. There has got to be room for the distinction between social reality on the one hand, and a shared illusion of social reality on the other. Just as analysis is committed to

interpret this activity as projection. Of course, projection is always possible. But when we judge, say, a house to be graceful we need not be projecting grace onto the house (though we can do that too): we may be recognizing grace which has been built into the house.

I am going to suggest that there is something real about the social–cultural world that transference, as it becomes manifest in analysis, lacks. There are many factors which contribute to the reality of the social world but, in broad outline, they can be divided into two categories: firstly, that it is intersubjective; secondly, that it provides a space in which people can live. It is the first hallmark, intersubjectivity, at least in a moderately strong form, which, I shall argue, transference in analysis lacks, so it is worth delineating a few of its features. A social world is open to reflection, to debate, to testing in thought and action, and to the possibility of consensual endorsement. A polis, like Athens or the United States, depends on the willingness of its citizens to defend its boundaries from outside incursions, but the polis can also be tested in thought and debate. The question of whether Athens or the United States should be a slave society is one which was tested inside the boundaries of each polis. Here it is worth noting both the power of a question to shape a world and a classic defense against it. The question, "Is a slave naturally inferior?" and the attempt to answer it, shaped the course of American history. A slave culture can generally not survive the insight that the difference between slave and citizen is purely accidental. Thus, the importance, for the institution of slavery, of stories which

---

denying the omnipotence of wishes in the individual, so it must be in a position to offer a critique of the omnipotence of certain wishes shared in a culture. Though it is beyond the scope of this paper to discuss the distinction between reality and illusion at the social level, I shall simply note in passing that certain inadequate interpretations of Wittgenstein make this distinction impossible by assuming that any shared "form of life" has *ipso facto* its own reality. I discuss problems with this interpretation in Lear (1986).

portray slaves as innately inferior, and the threat of reflective questioning. A classic way to defend against challenge is what I shall call *the barbarian defense*: put the challenge on the outside, treat it as the attack of a barbarian outsider who does not understand. In the United States, the barbarian defense—that Yankees do not understand—was overcome by force. But the most insidious challenge is when the barbarian defense crumbles and there is a realization *inside the culture* that there is no innate difference between slave and citizen. There is no obvious way that slave culture can survive this internal reflective questioning.

Winnicott suggests that it is religious experience in adult life which bears closest resemblance to the transitional experiences of childhood. But there is, nevertheless, an asymmetry. With the myriad transitional phenomena of childhood, the parents instinctively understand that they are not to ask whether the object is found or created, whether the play is a game or real. All such questions are species of the genus "Is this subjective or is it objective?" which Winnicott recognized was the great dissolvent of transitional space. Shared religious experience is, in this way, more like the rest of shared cultural experience than it is like the transitional phenomena of childhood—it is always open to the question of its reality. To take an example Winnicott mentions, the question as to the meaning and reality of transubstantiation shaped Western civilization.

In general, a social-cultural world is always vulnerable to reflective questioning inside the culture. There is a permanent possibility of bringing the meaning of an activity to consciousness and of questioning its validity.

THE CREATION OF AN IDIOPOLIS

The dynamics of intrapsychic transference reveal that even when a person participates in shared cultural activities, they will tend to have an idiosyncratic, unconscious meaning for that person. This, I believe, is one of Freud's greatest discoveries. We have seen that a person's thoughts, words, and activities are embedded in a web of unconscious associations that are both archaic and idiosyncratic. Just as each person, when speaking a natural language, also unconsciously speaks an idiolect, does he not also, as he participates in the culture's activities, unconsciously inhabit an idiosyncratic world? If an artifact gets its shared meaning via its location in a common web of psychological forces, it would seem that each participant, as he plays his role in the shared culture, is also performing an idiosyncratic variation on a theme. For, as we watch how the unconscious uses day residues, condensation, and displacement—all the loose associations of archaic mental functioning—to disguise and express itself, we see that every public ritual, every shared artifact, is permeated with idiosyncratic meanings by each of the participants. One of the deeper consequences of Freud's discovery, I believe, is that each person, as he participates in a shared culture, is also attempting to create and inhabit an idiosyncratic polis—an *idiopolis*–the peculiar lineaments of which are largely unconscious.

There is also room within a culture for people to act out fantasies in private enactments. Imagine a middle-aged man who has never married and lives at home with his aged mother. We can imagine it emerging in analysis that he is acting out a fantasy of remaining with mother in an incestuous relation. All other women are treated as "barbarians"—not to be trusted, dangerous, outside the polis. Has not this person created a micropolis with its own peculiar meanings? Of course, before analysis, the meaning of his activity will have remained unconscious to everyone, himself included, and thus it has been excluded from intersubjective questioning. It therefore fails one of the hallmarks of social reality—though even here one must acknowledge that analysis is itself a form of intersubjective questioning by which the contours of the idiopolis come to light. However, it does possess the other hallmark: the person has carved out an arena in which to live. His environment has a stable system of reference points and associations, people are endowed with idiosyncratic meanings, and the boundaries of this idiopolis are actively defended. One can say in all seriousness that this man has *given his life* to the cause of keeping the barbarians outside the gates.

Transference, as it emerges in analysis, is simply the idiosyncratic, unconscious side of the psyche's fundamental activity: to inform the world with meaning. To paraphrase the novelist L. P. Hartley: transference is a foreign country, they do things differently there. The fundamental demand of all transference is to participate in the idiopolis, and thus lend it reality. To return, for a moment, to Freud's discovery of transference in the "false connection:" what is it about the connection that made it *false*? Is it not Freud's refusal of his patient's invitation to participate in a ritual, to enter a world? Just one kiss, for all we know, might have turned this *mésalliance* into an *alliance amoureuse*. It is not as though the patient was making a simple mistake, she was trying to invest the world with particular meaning—instead of joining in, Freud pointed it out. Freud once said that the transference is a *"battlefield"* (1917, p. 454). What we see here, within the confines of a shared culture, is the battle of two microcultures, at the point where they meet. The patient wants Freud to play the role of lover; Freud insists on playing the doctor.

Freud might have "won" that battle, but it is easier to see what is going on if we imagine him "losing." Imagine, not that he kissed her, but that he misunderstood her wish. Her wish was not to be kissed, but to be rejected. It is she who wished to look on love as a *mésalliance*. She could then defensively justify her isolation as a series of rejections by others. Her problem, as she saw it, was that she was attracted to the wrong sort of person. On this interpretation, Freud unconsciously entered her idiopolis: he actively took on the significance with which she had endowed him. Indeed, the discovery of transference turns out to be the gratification of her wish. The fundamental demand of all transference, underlying all the particular demands, is that the analyst, the other, should participate in a world endowed with peculiar meanings. Missing the transference meaning, as we see in this imagined instance, is tantamount to unconscious compliance with the fundamental demand.

The fundamental demand, then, is at once for intimacy and for a certain intersubjectivity. The myriad transference demands are not *simply* for love: love's required form is that the analyst should travel the hidden byways of a peculiar world. The analyst is to participate in an intimate world, and thereby lend it substance. Nietzsche admonished us to live our lives as though we were creating a work of art; the phenomenon of transference reveals, I think, that each of us is unconsciously trying to do just that. Each of us is trying to create a peculiar polis in which to live and unconsciously demanding that others recognize it and participate in it. This demand, it is worth noting, is not always absurd. The artist, Freud saw, succeeds in having his fantastic expressions appreciated by others. The public recognition of artistic creation lends the creation a reality it would not otherwise possess. There is poignancy in the fact that each of us labors against the background that his or her creation could, just possibly, be recognized by others.

But while all transference demands are implicitly for participation, that is only one part of intersubjectivity, and transference, as it emerges in analysis, typically shuns the other part. Acting out, Freud says, is a *substitute* for conscious remembering (1914, p. 150). It is as though the ritualistic enactment of an idiopolis depends on the absence of conscious understanding. This, I believe, is a hallmark by which a neurotic idiopolis is distinguished: because a neurotic conflict is repressed, it must be acted out over and over again, and this lends the neurotic idiopolis a special rigidity.[18] There is no room for life's passing events to influence the shape of the idiopolis, for they have already been endowed with fixed meanings within it. Ironically, the sense of reality inside a neurotic idiopolis depends on it lacking one of the essential criteria of social reality: intersubjective reflection and testing. Just as the power of dream experience typically depends on there being no room within it for the thought "this is only

---

[18] It remains the project of a future work to capture the unique blend of rigidity and instability of a neurotic idiopolis. Plato argued that a conflicted polis—for example, an oligarchy—was not, strictly speaking a polis at all, but rather, two polis bits: a rich and a poor class. The conflicts prevented there being sufficient integration to count as a polis, properly speaking (*Republic*, IV.422E-423D; VIII.551D; cp.553C-554E). Since, for Plato, there is a basic isomorphism between polis and psyche, it follows that a neurotically conflicted psyche is not, strictly speaking, *a* psyche, but various psychic bits. The isomorphism, Plato thinks, is due to psyche and polis standing in dynamic relations of internalization and externalization (see Lear 1992). This concept has been taken up, elaborated and deepened in psychoanalysis, most prominently by Melanie Klein (1975). By going back to Plato we can gain a clearer understanding of the *political* nature of the inner world: inner strife (civil war) is "politics pursued by other means," and that must affect diplomacy between the inner world and the idiopolis. A neurotic idiopolis is ultimately an unsuccessful attempt to create a meaningful world, and the fundamental conflicts of the polis not only reflect but stand in dynamic relation to intrapsychic conflicts. It is the fault lines in a neurotic polis which contribute to the unhappiness of life within a neurotic world, but which, because of their dynamic relation to the psyche, also provide the possibility for therapeutic action. Nevertheless, despite the conflicts, the rigidity of a neurotic idiopolis lends it a certain durability which, in turn, provides an experience of ersatz unity.

a dream," so the power of an idiopolis depends on there being no room inside for a conscious, communal inquiry into its meaning.[19] Of course, it is no use, as Freud well knew, simply to explain to a person his intrapsychic conflicts. The problem, classically understood, is that the explanation will only register in a person's consciousness; it will be dynamically excluded from making an intrapsychic difference. This is the intrapsychic version of the barbarian defense: the consciously registered explanation cannot communicate with the relevant unconscious representations. But this intrapsychic failure reflects a prior failure of interpsychic communication. The speaker, for his part, is proceeding in ignorance of the listener's idiolect: he has no idea of the intrapsychic transferences which embed these words in a web of unconscious meanings. Thus, the words he speaks drift off aimlessly, unanchored to the idiosyncratic unconscious resonances of his audience. Therefore, just telling a person his or her problem will not make a difference. To the ear of the unconscious, the speaker's words are little more than barbaric noise.

This barbarian defense is the interpsychic version of repression. The question is understanding how it is that saying something could make a difference. Here it is worth returning to three Platonic insights: firstly, a neurotic's idiopolis is not one in which a happy life is possible, because the world itself is essentially conflicted; secondly, it is possible to gain a glimmer of this conflict inside the world; thirdly, it is the task of the psychoanalyst to descend into the cave and speak the truth at the fantastic level at which it can be grasped. The question is how these insights can be applied to the analytic situation.

---

[19] Of course, as Freud recognized, it is possible to dream that "this is only a dream" (Freud 1900, pp. 338, 488–489). See also O'Shaughnessy (1982).

THE RESOLUTION OF THE TRANSFERENCE

The development of the transference in analysis is a single process with two aspects. From the analysand, there is an attempt to metabolize the analyst and the analytic situation. The analysand is performing re-enactments which endow the analyst with important and familiar meanings. Freud says that the transference is "artificially constructed," and the manifest content is that it is being produced, as it were, in laboratory conditions, like a culture of bacteria. But the latent content is that it is an artifice, an artifact: the analyst is being drawn inside an idiopolis.[20] In the "true illness," as in the "artificially constructed" one, the analysand is basically engaged in the same activity. At least in the opening stages, the real difference between the true and the artificial lies not in the analysand's, but in the analyst's activity. Freud speaks of the transference providing "new editions of the old conflicts." By that he does not mean that it is just the *latest* edition, but that it is to be a *revised* edition. As Freud says, "the new struggle around [the analyst] is lifted to its highest psychical level" (1917, p. 454). To understand this upwards revision, we have to understand what the analyst is doing as the transference develops. While the analysand is taking the analyst into his world, the analyst is gaining a clearer understanding of what

---

[20]See Freud (1914, p. 154 and 1917, p. 454), in which he describes the transference neurosis as an "artificial illness." In his remarkable 1972 paper, Bird suggests that in the transference neurosis, the analyst becomes part of the analysand's intrapsychic conflict. It is as though the analyst were being assigned a position inside the analysand's psyche. This insight seems to me both astute and not quite correct. Bird, of course, did not have the concept of an idiopolis which stands in dynamic relation to the psyche. By contrast, Strachey's (1934) classic description of the analyst being brought into the neurotic's vicious circle seems very apt. Indeed, one can read this paper as an attempt to elaborate and explain how a mutative interpretation is possible.

that world is like. By listening to associations and dreams, the analyst gains some understanding of the intrapsychic transferences which endow conscious thoughts with unconscious resonances; that is, he achieves a working knowledge of the analysand's idiolect. Similarly, the analyst is gaining a clearer understanding of the overall structure of the analysand's intrapsychic conflicts. Thus, just as the analysand is getting in a position to listen, the analyst is getting in a position to speak.

Freud speaks of the analytic transference as a "playground" in which repetitions are allowed to proliferate (1914, p. 154). In this playground, unconscious intrapsychic conflicts will be acted out, and thus inadvertently put on display. The idea of the analytic situation as a playground is redolent with meaning: it is on a playground that culture has a dress rehearsal, and the regressive pull of analysis will tend to draw culture back to its infantile roots. But there is another sense in which transference, as it emerges in analysis, stands between child's play and shared culture. On the one hand, the analysand is not just playing at creating a world, but is actually trying to create one; on the other, there is no room in the idiopolis for the kind of reflective questioning which every shared culture must allow. In order to survive, a shared culture must be able to tolerate the relevant version of "is this subjective or is it objective? is this real or only a game? is this found or is it created?" These reflective questions typically dissolve transitional space, and the only way a neurotic idiopolis can cope with them is by employing the barbarian defense—if they are coming from the outside, they can be treated as so much noise.

However, condensed in the image of transference as a playground, there lurks another meaning: the analyst is now inside the game. In a maternal transference, for instance, the analysand has made the analyst into a maternal "covering," while the analyst has been learning the deeper resonances of the "mother tongue," and gaining a view of the dynamic, conflicted structure of psyche and world. The barbarian defense is no longer possible, because the analyst is no longer an outsider making unanchored comments on an observed ritual. It is, for the analysand, as though the ritual itself were speaking. But "mother" has somehow changed her tune. In speaking the "mother tongue" the analyst also tries to reflect back to the psyche an image of itself as a conflicted whole.

No one else in the analysand's world is able to do this; all the other figures have been given limited roles and partial perspectives. The analyst is always cast in a limited role—those are the only roles there are—but he tries to use the language of each role to speak an understanding of the place of that role within the functioning of the whole. One indication of a good transference interpretation is the unique blend of comfort and discomfort it elicits. It is as though the analysand is trying to bring together an experience of recognition—Mama, it's you!—with an experience of irredeemable strangeness—Mama, what has come over you! One might call this a disturbance of memory in the idiopolis. At every stage, in every role, the analyst is trying to import self-conscious understanding into the heart of a world which must, for its survival, remain opaque to itself. However, the basic means of preserving opacity are no longer available. The analyst is no longer outside the world, making comments about it, which is why he is able to give a "new transference meaning" to an analysand's symptoms, rituals and emotions (Freud 1914, p. 154). The analyst enables a characteristic emotional response to speak its own role in the dynamic functioning of the whole.

In recognizing a maternal transference, we see the analysand experiencing the analyst as a not-good-enough mother; but we tend to forget that, in the beginning, mother was the world. For whatever reason, mother was experienced as not-good-enough, disappointing the child too much, too soon, or too often. The child goes on to construct a not-good-enough world, and to experience himself as forced to live within it. It is not surprising, then, that as the fault lines of this world emerge we hear maternal echoes. In my analytic work, I find that I am often treated as a maternal figure around the time that the analysand has dynamic reason for experiencing disappointment. Sometimes there is an external trigger—for instance, I may be about to go on vacation—but often a well-engineered disappointment is constructed to suit intrapsychic needs. Were I to play out the role of a disappointing mother I could help damp down an emerging wish; I could also be the target for the ensuing (often unconscious) fury, and I would thus reinforce and legitimate the background assumption that the world is disappointing.

A well-placed interpretation frustrates all these functions. The drama was meant to act out a disappointment; instead, the analysand is asked to reflect on why he or she needs a disappointment now from me. The interpretation not only gives the enacted experience a name, so that it can be consciously considered *as* disappointment, it also hypotheses the intrapsychic conflicts that give rise to a need for disappointment. It is as though the world not only describes itself, it also describes what is going on across the border—inside the psyche, which requires the world to be the way it is experienced. The interpretation thereby frustrates the attempt to make me into a superego "covering," but it also names the associated wish that the analysand would like covered over, at just the moment when that wish is closest to conscious experience; that is, at just the moment when the wish is most closely linked with its conscious "covering." The interpretation also gives a name to the fury that inevitably follows the frustration of a wish, and describes its myriad uses: to help inhibit the wish, to punish the analysand for having it and to punish the analyst for frustrating it. In short, in my role as "mother," I try to speak, in the mother tongue, my role within this idiosyncratic world. That is why the conflict is "lifted to its highest psychical level." "Mother," one might say, cannot ultimately survive self-understanding of what she is doing here.

Neither, ultimately, can the particular intrapsychic configuration of the analysand. The analysand's psyche stands in a dynamic relation with its world, and if key elements of that world shift, the psyche cannot remain unchanged. Human life must find its way amongst three sets of significant boundaries. The first are those which delineate intrapsychic structure and which collectively separate what is available to consciousness from what is repressed. The second is between what is inside a person's psyche and what lies outside. The third is between what is inside a person's world and what lies beyond the pale. Meaningful contents may travel across a boundary, but each boundary serves as a kind of buffer. Each bounded area is offered limited freedom from the pressures exerted by what lies beyond. So, for example, while it is virtually impossible for someone to hold two consciously recognized contradictory beliefs, it is easier to tolerate living with a conscious belief and an experience in the world which seems to contradict it; or to tolerate a conscious belief and a countervailing unconscious wish. These boundaries provide some respite from the holistic demand that everything fit together. Each boundary permits certain discontinuites to lie on either side.

There are, I believe, both theoretical and clinical advantages in distinguishing between a person's psyche and his idiopolis. Firstly, this distinction helps us to do justice to the psyche's creative, artifact-making abilities. In the transference, the psyche is engaged in the same type of activity as when, in concert with others, it does its part in the maintenance of a social world. Here there is no concert: the psyche is marching to the beat of its own drum. It is, I think, a mistake to treat the idiopolis as a mere projection of the psyche.

Projection is only one of a wide range of psychic tools. So, for example, a person committed to living in a disappointing world may generate disappointment in myriad ways. Genuinely disappointing events may be enhanced, ambiguous events can be given a certain fantastic spin, people may be tricked into unwittingly delivering disappointments, the person may form wishes—such as a crush on a movie star or on the analyst—whose very existence depends on the expectation that they will be disappointed. Projection may also be used: for example, a person may project her sadism on to another both to get rid of it and to experience a cruel disappointment. These are a range of distinctions which tend to get flattened when one speaks of a person's "psychological world."

Secondly, this artifact is experienced by the psyche as though it were a world in which the psyche is located. It is a stable structure which systematically attributes motives, emotions and attitudes to the people in the world. The attributions purport to offer psychological explanations of all the significant actions of all the significant people in this world, the analysand and analyst included. Of course, the psyche is unaware that these purported explanations are dynamically related to intrapsychic needs. In this way, the psyche mistakes its creation for an objective world that is given to it. Although a neurotic world is essentially conflicted, there is, nevertheless, a certain stability, systematicity, and inclusiveness to this creation which distinguishes it from a passing illusion, fantasy or psychological state.

Clinically, it is advantageous to be able to distinguish a person's shifting psychological states from the more or less stable world in which that person lives. A person living in a disappointing world may at various times feel angry, sullen, disappointed, resigned, comfortable, at home, reassured. Theoretically, we see that the boundary between psyche and world lends a certain resilience to the world: it can endure a person's shifting psychological states. That is why merely disappointing an analysand's wish to be disappointed would itself be of no therapeutic value. When an analysand needs a disappointment, for example, virtually anything I do, and countless things I am fantasized as doing, can be woven into a tale of being let down. This stability, in turn, contributes to the experienced reality of the world. Indirectly, the world's stability ensures stability of intrapsychic structure. For while a person may go through a cascade of emotional reactions, they will tend to follow a familiar and intelligible pattern, and they will all be defined in relation to a certain type of unsatisfactory world. The only way to effect a profound shift in the psyche is via a transformation of the world in which it lives. In terms of technique, this account of transference encourages patience on the part of the analyst, and cautions against premature interpretation. If the analysand is engaged in creative activity, the analyst must exert care not to inhibit or disrupt this process. Only after the world has been woven with the analyst inside it can both the analyst and analysand together find their ways around in it.

Psychoanalysis, I believe, distinguishes itself from other forms of "talking cure" by its aim of changing the world. Although analysis may eventually help analysands establish more realistic relations with the common social world, its first task is to help analysands take apart a private world which has held them captive—that is why it is such a long and arduous task. Through repeated interpretations of the need to be disappointed, spoken by the designated disappointer in the appropriate idiolect, the psyche is fed a transference meal which it cannot metabolize in its familiar ways. The analyst is already inside the idiopolis, and he gives his interpretation in a language designed to work its way into the psyche. The interpretation makes explicit the intrapsychic transferences which have hitherto relied for their existence on remaining unconsious. The interpretation is spoken so as to awaken these unconscious resonances and thus to permeate the intrapsychic boundaries. As the intrapsychic transferences are so described, the need for them diminishes. Over time, this helps foster a transubstantiation of intrapsychic structure. As the multiplicity and diversity of the "disappointments" are pointed out and interpreted, the analysand comes to see that he or she is not being acted upon by a not-good-enough world, so much as creating a world in which to be disappointed.

Theorists sometimes write as though once analysands can grasp their conflicted responses, they can choose less conflicted ways to live. There is truth to this, but it tends to portray analysands as smart shoppers: now that they have been given a choice, analysands can choose better psyches than they did the last time around. It is as though the only problem with conflicts is that they are painful; and one is thus better off without them. It is Plato who saw that there are certain types of conflict which, when recognized, are not just bad, but impossible. Not all conflicts are such: the recognition of tragic conflict, for instance, can reinforce a sense of the world's reality: of its painful independence. A neurotic idiopolis is experienced as though it too were painfully independent—subjecting the person, say, to a wave after wave of disappointment—and it cannot survive the pervasive recognition that it is both motivated and created. For it is of the essence of a world to present itself as given. The analysand does not choose a better world over his familiar idiopolis: the old world goes dead.[21]

By the time analysands can recognize their own activity in creating a world, that world is already on the wane. That is why making the unconscious conscious ultimately requires (and is a sign of) the transformation of the analysand's world.

---

[21]There is an interesting analogy in Bernard Williams's discussion of a hypertraditional society in which reflection turns knowledge into belief. (See Williams, 1985, pp. 142–148, 158–159.)

In this process, analysands move from experiencing themselves as passive victims to recognizing their own activity. This is what a person experiences in the deconstruction of an idiopolis. All transference, I have argued, is an attempt to create a world in which to live. But not all attempts are successful, and what analyst and analysand eventually come to recognize jointly as transference are the attempts that do not succeed. The world has gone dead, a sure sign that the transference is all but moribund. Hence, at this stage, it is so easy to think of transference as a merely psychological state. Ironically, by the time analysands can look on transference as their psychological activity, the power of this activity to inform the world has evaporated. In analysis, Loewald says, "the ghosts of the unconscious are laid and led to rest as ancestors" (1960, p. 249). In this chapter, I have tried to describe a process by which a living world is transformed into a remembrance of things past.[22]

SUMMARY

This paper offers an interpretation of the concept of transference. It begins with a re-examination of Socrates's thera-

---

[22]An earlier draft of this chapter was presented at the New York Psychoanalytic Institute on the occasion of receiving their Heinz Hartmann Award—and the presentation helped me to rethink a number of central issues in the chapter. I should like to thank the members of that Institute for their encouragement. I would also like to thank Tyler Burge, David Carlson, Christopher Dustin, Stanley Possick, Al Solnit, Rebecca Solomon and Bernard Williams for their comments on a previous draft. For the six years before he died, Hans Loewald and I met weekly, firstly in a tutorial, later as friends. By the time I finally wrote this chapter, Hans felt too weak to read it, and though I do not wish to claim his support for any particular thesis, I do wish to acknowledge a profound debt to the man and to that extended conversation: a *sine qua non* of this paper.

peutic intent and Plato's revisions of psychological theory in the light of Socrates's failure. In particular, Plato devised an account of a structured psyche, a theory of fantasy, and a complex "object relations" theory, to explain dynamic interactions between psyche and social world. It is argued that these revisions embody a recognition of the phenomenon of transference, i.e. the psyche's characteristic activity of creating a meaningful world in which to live. Freud's early conception of transference—as a transfer of psychological content across space and time—is criticized on the ground that it assumes that the world is already given, independent of any psychic activity. Freud's later conception of transference as a repetition is then explored in the light of the psyche's ability to create artifacts. It is argued that neurotic transference is the unconscious attempt to create an idiosyncratic polis, an idiopolis, in which to live. The resolution of the transference occurs because the analyst is made a citizen of the idiopolis, has learned the idiolect, and can speak in that idiolect of the fundamental conflicts within the idiopolis and their dynamic basis. A neurotic world cannot survive this internal recognition.

References

Adam, J. A. (1929). *The Republic of Plato.* Cambridge: Cambridge University Press.

Bird, B. (1972). Notes on transference: universal phenomenon and hardest part of analysis. *Journal of the American Psycho-Analytic Association* 20:267–301.

Davidson, D. (1982). Paradoxes of irrationality. In *Philosophical Essays on Freud*, ed. R. Wollheim and J. Hopkins, pp. 289–305. Cambridge: Cambridge University Press.

—— (1984). *Inquiries into Truth and Interpretation.* Oxford: Clarendon.

Freud, S. (1896). The aetiology of hysteria. *Standard Edition* 2.

—— (1900). The interpretation of dreams. *Standard Edition* 4–5.

—— (1905). Fragment of an analysis of a case of hysteria. *Standard Edition* 7.
—— (1914). Remembering, repeating and working through. *Standard Edition* 12.
—— (1917). Introductory lectures on psycho-analysis. *Standard Edition* 15–16.
—— (1923). The ego and the id. *Standard Edition* 19.
—— (1930). Civilization and its discontents. *Standard Edition* 21.
—— (1937). Constructions in analysis. *Standard Edition* 23.
Geertz, C. (1973). Thick description: towards an interpretive theory of culture. In *The Interpretation of Culture*. New York: Basic Books.
Gray, P. (1982). "Developmental lag" in the evolution of technique for the psychoanalysis of neurotic conflict. *Journal of the American Psychoanalytic Association* 30:621–655.
—— (1986). On helping analysands observe intrapsychic activity. In *Psychoanalysis: The Science of Mental Conflict. Essays in Honor of Charles Brenner*, ed. A. Richards and M. Willick, pp. 245–262. Hillsdale, NJ: Analytic Press.
Hansen, M. H. (1980). Hvorfor henrettede Athenerne Sokrates? *Museum Tusculanum* 40–3:55–82.
Huizinga, J. (1955). *Homo Ludens: A Study of the Play Element of Culture.* Boston: Beacon.
Klein, M. (1975). *The Writings of Melanie Klein.* London: Hogarth.
Lear, J. (1986). Transcendental anthropology. In *Subject, Thought and Context*, ed. P. Petit and J. McDowell. Oxford: Clarendon.
—— (1988). *Aristotle: the Desire to Understand.* Cambridge and New York: Cambridge University Press.
—— (1990). *Love and Its Place in Nature: A Philosophical Interpretation of Freudian Psychoanalysis.* New York: Farrar, Straus and Giroux; London: Faber and Faber.
—— (1992). Inside and outside *The Republic*. *Phronesis* 37:184–215.
—— (1994). Plato's politics of narcissism. In *Essays in Honor of Gregory Vlastos*. University Park, PA: Pennsylvania State University Press.
Loewald, H. (1960). On the therapeutic action of psychoanalysis.

In *Papers on Psychoanalysis*, pp. 221–256. New Haven and London: Yale University Press.

——— (1988). *Sublimation.* New Haven and London: Yale University Press.

O'Shaughnessy, B. (1982). The id and the thinking process. In *Philosophical Essays on Freud*, ed. R. Wollheim and J. Hopkins, pp. 106–123. Cambridge: Cambridge University Press.

Poland, W. S. (1992a). From analytic surface to analytic space. *Journal of the American Psychoanalytic Association* 40:381–404.

——— (1992b). Transference: "an original creation." *Psychoanalytic Quarterly* 61:185–205.

Spillius, E. B. (1983). Some developments from the work of Melanie Klein. *International Journal of Psycho-Analysis* 64:321–332.

Stone, I. F. (1988). *The Trial of Socrates.* Boston: Beacon.

Strachey, J. (1934). The nature of the therapeutic action of psychoanalysis. *International Journal of Psycho-Analysis* 50:275–292, 1969.

Stone, I. F. (1988). *The Trial of Socrates.* Boston: Beacon.

Vlastos, G. (1979). On "The Socrates Story." *Political Theory* 7:533–536.

——— (1983). The historical Socrates and Athenian democracy. *Political Theory* 11:495–515.

Williams, B. (1985). *Ethics and the Limits of Philosophy.* London: Fontana.

Winnicott, D. W. (1951). Transitional objects and transitional phenomena. In *Through Paediatrics to Psycho-Analysis*, pp. 229–242. London: Hogarth, 1975.

——— (1971). The location of cultural experience. In *Playing and Reality*, pp. 112–121. Hammondsworth and New York: Penguin.

Wollheim, R., and Hopkins, J. eds. (1982). *Philosophical Essays on Freud.* Cambridge: Cambridge University Press.

Credits

The editor gratefully acknowledges permission to reprint material from the following sources:

The International Journal of Psycho-Analysis:
  Chapter 5, "The Importance of Facial Expression in Dreams," by Marianne Goldberger, M.D. (1995), vol. 76, pp. 591–593. Copyright © 1995 Institute of Psycho-Analysis.

  Chapter 11, "Common Ground, Uncommon Methods, by Cecilio Paniagua, M.D. (1995), vol. 76, pp. 357–371. Copyright © 1995 Institute of Psycho-Analysis.

  Chapter 13, "An Interpretation of Transference," by Jonathan Lear (1993), vol. 74, pp. 739–754. Copyright © 1993 Institute of Psycho-Analysis.

Journal of Clinical Psychoanalysis
  Chapter 2, "Two Different Methods of Analyzing Defense," previously titled "Analyzing Defense: Two Different Methods," by Monroe Pray, M.D. (1994), vol. 3(1),

pp. 87–126. Copyright © 1994 by International Universities Press, Inc.

Chapter 6, "The Clinical Use of Daydreams in Analysis," by Marianne Goldberger, M.D. (1995), vol. 4(1), pp. 11–21. Copyright © 1995 International Universities Press, Inc.

Journal of the American Psychoanalytic Association
Chapter 3, "Free Association and Technique," previously titled "Some Ambiguities in the Method of Free Association and Their Implications for Technique," by Fred Busch, Ph.D. (1994), vol. 42(2), pp. 363–384. Copyright © 1994 International Universities Press.

Chapter 7, "External Reality as Defense," previously titled "On Grist for the Mill: External Reality as Defense," by Lawrence Inderbitzin and Steven Levy (1994), vol. 42(3), pp. 763–788. Copyright © International Universities Press.

Excerpts from "Psychoanalytic Theory and Its Relation to Clinical Work," by E. A. Schwaber (1992), vol. 40(4), pp. 1041–1051. Copyright © International Universities Press.

Excerpts from *The Standard Edition of the Complete Psychological Works of Sigmund Freud*, translated and edited by James Strachey, by permission of Sigmund Freud Copyrights, The Institute of Psycho-Analysis and The Hogarth Press, W. W. Norton and Company, Basic Books, and Routledge, UK.

Index

Abraham, K., 308
Absences, timing of intervention, 14
Acting out, timing of intervention, 14–15
Action
   ego analysis, 160–161
   symbolic meaning of, drive states, 157–160
   words as replacement for, drive states, 148–157
Admission of bias, mutative interpretation bias, 31–32
Affect, incongruent, timing of intervention, 9
Aggression
   mutative interpretation bias, 28–29
   turned on self
      mutative interpretation bias, 38
      timing of intervention, 7

Allen, D., 201
Analytic perception, centrality of, xiii–xiv
Analytic relationship, external reality (as defense) and, 205–207
Apfelbaum, B., 115, 198, 276, 277
Arlow, A., xvii
Arlow, J., 73, 74, 92, 97, 125, 126, 202, 213, 266, 269, 270, 275, 296, 323
Assertive-retractive curve, mutative interpretation bias, 35–36
Austin, J. L., 325
Auxiliary treatment modalities, impulse disorders, 169–171
Avoidance, timing of intervention, 12–13

Bacon, F., 308
Balter, L., 242, 257

Basch, M. F., 259
Biases, mutative interpretation, 28–40
Bibring, E., 295
Bion, W. R., 301
Bird, B., 202, 204, 205, 363n20
Blake, W., 75
Blum, H. P., 113
Brenner, C., xvi, xvii, 2, 5, 53, 54, 56, 59, 66, 67, 68, 69, 71, 72, 73, 74, 75, 76, 85, 86, 92, 95, 97, 125, 126, 198, 203, 255, 266, 269, 270, 275, 281n8, 296, 306, 320, 323, 329
Breuer, J., 110, 264
Bristol, C., xvi
Buchsbaum, H. K., 177
Burge, T., 371n22
Burgner, M., 230
Busch, F., xvi, 111, 117, 122, 124, 263, 271, 272, 299, 318

Carlson, D., 371n22
Carroll, L., 294
Charcot, J., 264
Close process attention analysis
impulse disorders and, 131 172. *See also* Impulse disorders
mutative interpretation, 5–6
superego and, xv
Close process monitoring, mutative interpretation bias, 39–40
Common ground theme
international comparison, 294
theoretical schools and, 293–295
Comparisons, narcissistic injury, envy complex, 224–226
Compromise formations
analysis of, defense analysis methods, 85–86
conjectures about, defense analysis methods, 86–88
unconscious conflicts and, defense analysis methods, 82–84
Conflict
consciousness and, 265–266
conscious versus unconscious, defense analysis methods, 58–59
defense analysis methods
Brenner, Charles, 66
Freud, Anna, 59–66
in transference, mutative interpretation bias, 39
Conscious conflict, unconscious versus, defense analysis methods, 58–59
Consciousness, 263–290
ego-syntonicity and ego integration, 286–288
future research, 273–286
historical perspective on, 264–269
overview of, 263–264
psychoanalytic techniques and, 269–273

Covetous fantasy, envy complex, 226–227
Curtis, H. C., 311

Dahl, H., 16, 64, 70
Danger
　mutative interpretation bias, 38–39
　superego and, xv
Davidson, D., 348n8
Davison, W. T., xvi, 2, 27, 31, 37, 271
Daydreams, 179–192. *See also* Dream analysis
　case illustrations, 181–192
　paradigm for, 180–181
　transference daydream, 179
Defense analysis, mutative interpretation and, 1–51. *See also* Mutative interpretation
Defense analysis methods, 53–106
　case illustrations, 76–82
　comparative perspective, 56–57
　comparison table, 103
　compromise formations
　　analysis of, 85–86
　　conjectures about, 86–88
　　unconscious conflicts and, 82–84
　conflict
　　Brenner, Charles, 66
　　conscious versus unconscious, 58–59
　　defenses themselves, 68–70

Freud, Anna, 59–66
　moment-to-moment listening for, 70–74
　perspectives compared, 67–68
　discussion of, 93–102
　overview of, 53–56
　technical scheme, Freud, Anna, 88–93
　technical tasks, 74–75
Defenses. *See* External reality (as defense)
Denial, envy complex, defense activity, 227–228
Denigration, envy complex, defense activity, 228
Destruction, envy complex, defense activity, 229
De Urtubey, L., 297
Dewald, P. A., 215
Dick, M. M., 215
Displacement, mutative interpretation bias, 35
Dream analysis. *See also* Daydreams
　avoidance, timing of intervention, 12–13
　facial expression and, 173–178
Drive states
　action
　　symbolic meaning of, 157–160
　　words as replacement for, 148–157
　generally, impulse disorders, 144–148
Dustin, C., 371n22

Edelson, M., 312
Edgecumbe, R., 230
Ego
  analytic perception and, xiv
  consciousness and, 268–269
Ego analysis, impulse disorders, 160–161
Ego integration, ego-syntonicity and, consciousness, 286–288
Ego splitting, impulse disorders, 161–164
Ego-syntonicity, consciousness and, 276–286
Eissler, K. R., 321
Emde, R. N., 177
Empathy, 241–262
  case illustrations, 247–254
  discussion of, 255–260
  overview of, 241–247
Envy complex, 221–240
  case illustration, 230–238
  components of, 224–227
    covetous fantasy, 226–227
    narcissistic injury, 224–226
  defense activity, 227–229
  discussion of, 238–239
  overview of, 221–223
  treatment, 229–230
Epstein, G., 113
Esman, A. H., 306
Europe. *See* International comparison
External reality (as defense), 193–220
  analytic relationship and, 205–207
  discussion of, 215–218
  extra-analytic contacts, 210–214
  life crises, 214–215
  overview of, 193–195
  technical issues, 207–210
  theory of defense, 198–201
  theory of reality, 195–198
  transference issues, 202–205

Facial expression
  daydreams, 180–181
  dream analysis and, 173–178
Fantasy, covetous fantasy, envy complex, 226–227
Fast, I., 237
Fenichel, O., 53, 54, 55, 56, 65, 94, 119, 135n1, 144, 145, 171, 191, 197, 203, 212, 213, 270, 291, 306, 325
Ferenczi, S., 257, 308
Fine, B. D., 108, 223, 224, 225
Fine, E., 312
Fine, S., 312
Flavell, J. H., 122, 123
Fliess, W., 245, 251
Frankel, S., 222, 223
Free association, 107–130
  discussion of, 123–127
  mutative interpretation bias, 38
  overview of, 107–110
  resistance analysis and, 110–115
  self-reflection and, 115–123
French, T., 332
Freud, A., xvi, 2, 4, 53, 54, 55, 56, 57, 58, 59, 61, 62, 64, 65, 66, 67, 69, 74, 75, 76,

88, 90, 91, 93, 94, 95, 98, 100, 101, 102, 119, 120, 137n2, 144, 145, 198, 203, 225, 270, 271, 275, 281, 286, 353n14

Freud, S., xv, xx, 3, 4, 15, 54, 62, 63, 107, 108, 109, 110, 111, 112, 113, 115, 116, 117, 118, 121, 123, 124, 125, 126, 157, 193, 195, 196, 198, 200, 202, 214, 222, 225, 229, 257, 263, 264, 265, 266, 267, 268, 269, 270, 275, 280, 286, 287, 294, 301, 305, 308, 309, 311, 313, 319, 320, 321, 322, 323, 324, 338n1, 340, 344, 345, 347, 348, 349, 351, 353n14, 355n16, 358, 359, 360, 362, 363, 364, 365, 372

Friedman, L., xix, 5, 13, 118

Galler, F. B., 108, 109
Ganzarain, R., 197, 210, 211
Gardner, M. R., 118
Gaskill, H. S., 119
Geertz, C., 349n9
Genetics, psychoanalysis and, 75
Gill, M. M., 115, 198, 203, 204, 205, 269, 270, 276, 277, 332
Goldberger, M., xvii, 173, 263, 271, 310
Gray, O., 146, 147, 148
Gray, P., xii, xiv, xv, xvii, xviii, xx, 2, 15, 26, 37, 53, 54, 100, 102, 111, 113, 114, 115, 120, 121, 124, 125, 126, 131, 133, 134, 135, 138, 139, 140, 144, 167, 170, 171, 173, 197, 200, 203, 204, 213, 230, 241, 242, 243, 244, 245, 247, 248, 252, 253, 255, 257, 258, 259, 260, 263, 266, 271, 272, 273, 274, 276, 278, 279, 280, 282, 284, 286, 287, 295, 300, 310, 319, 326, 327, 328, 353n14

Greenblum, L., xviii
Greenson, R. R., 111, 119
Grossman, W. I., 63, 101

Hansen, M. H., 338n2
Hartley, L. P., 359
Hartmann, H., 54, 64, 75, 92, 100, 196, 208, 259, 270
Hill, J. C., 62
Hoffman, I., 195n1, 205, 206, 207, 214, 332
Hoffman, L., 263, 272, 272n4
Holmes, D., 271
Horney, K., 226, 229
Hutchinson, J., xvii, 256n1
Hutson, P., xviii, 229

Identification
  envy complex, defense activity, 228–229
  mutative interpretation bias, 33–35
Imagination, avoidance, timing of intervention, 12–13

Impulse disorders, 131–172
  auxiliary treatment modalities, 169–171
  drive states
    generally, 144–148
    symbolic meaning of action, 157–160
    words as replacement for action, 148–157
  ego analysis, 160–161
  ego splitting, 161–164
  overview of, 131–139
  superego analysis, 164–169
  therapeutic applications, 139–143
Incongruent affect, timing of intervention, 9
Inderbitzin, L. B., xviii, 135n1, 214, 241, 242, 257, 258, 271
Inhelder, B., 122
Inhibition, in time recall, timing of intervention, 10–12
International comparison, 291–316
  case illustrations, 300–304
  clinical consequences, 312
  common ground theme, 294–297
  consciousness, 305–306
  consonant/dissonant dichotomy, 292–293
  education, 299–300
  experimentation, 305
  historical perspective, 300
  logic, 306–308
  methodology, 298–299
  overview of, 291–292
  science, 308–310
  theoretical schools and, 293–296
Interpretation, mutative interpretation, 1–51. *See also* Mutative interpretation
Interpsychic transference, transference interpretation, 350–352
Interruption of thinking, timing of intervention, 7–8
Intrapsychic transference, transference interpretation, 345–350

Jacobs, T. J., 205
Jacobson, J., 225
Joffe, W., 222
Jones, E., 94

Kachele, H., 64, 70
Kaiser, H., 310
Kantrowitz, J., 119
Kanzer, M., 108, 113
Kennedy, G., 300
Kernberg, O. F., 297
Klein, G., 298, 307
Klein, M., 222, 223, 294, 308, 310, 353n14, 361n18
Knight, R. P., 311
Kohut, H., 226, 228, 247, 255, 258, 324, 328, 332, 333
Kris, A., 108, 112, 113, 114, 115, 117
Kris, E., 54, 56, 64, 75, 92, 93, 98, 100, 119, 270
Kubie, L. S., 57, 64, 237

Lacan, J., 294, 326
Landau, B., xviii, xix, 126
Langs, R., 149
Language neutrality, mutative interpretation bias, 36–38
Lateness, timing of intervention, 14
Lear, J., xx, 340n3, 355n17
Leary, S. A., 322
Levy, S. T., xviii, 135n1, 241, 242, 243, 245, 251, 257, 258, 271
Lichtenberg, J. D., 108, 109
Life crises, external reality (as defense), 214–215
Loewald, H. W., 121, 328, 346n5, 350n11, 354n15, 371
Loewenstein, R. M., 64, 112, 119, 270
Lussier, A., 294

Mahoney, P., 112, 124
McLaughlin, J., 259, 260
Methodology, international comparison, 298–299
Michels, R., 327
Mill, J. S., 306, 307
Mitchell, S., 205, 207
Moment-to-moment listening, for conflict, defense analysis methods, 70–74
Moore, B. E., 108, 223, 224, 225
Morrison, A., 224, 225, 226
Mutative interpretation, 1–51
biases, 28–40
case illustration, 40–49

close process attention analysis, 5–6
definitions, 2–5
repression, 4
resistance, 3
working through, 4–5
overview of, 1–2
research implications, 15–27
timing of intervention, 6–15
acting out, 14–15
aggression turned on self, 7
avoidance, 12–13
generally, 6–7
incongruent affect, 9
interruption of thinking, 7–8
lateness and absences, 14
nonpayment, 14
posture of patient, 10
repetitive affect, 14
rituals, 13
silence, 8–9
time recall inhibition, 10–12

Narcissistic injury, envy complex, 224–226
Neutrality, language, mutative interpretation bias, 36–38
Nietzsche, F., 360
Nonpayment, timing of intervention, 14
Novick, J., 119
Nunberg, H., 119

Olinick, S., 229
O'Shaughnessy, B., 362

Paniagua, C., xix, 245, 271, 302, 304, 305, 309
Patient perspective, mutative interpretation bias, 32
Perception focus, mutative interpretation bias, 33
Piaget, J., 122, 328
Pine, F., 297
Plato, xx, 339, 340, 341, 342, 343, 351, 361n18, 370, 372
Poland, W. S., 353n14
Polarity emphasis, mutative interpretation bias, 30
Possick, S., 371n22
Posture, of patient, timing of intervention, 10
Pray, M., xvi, 255, 256, 263, 271, 272, 275
Process focus, mutative interpretation bias, 29-30
Process intervention, mutative interpretation bias, 39
Projection
  envy complex, defense activity, 229
  mutative interpretation bias, 33-35
Psychoanalysis, genetics and, 75
Psychoanalytic education, international comparison, 299-300
Pulver, S. E., 297, 298, 312

Rangell, L., 308
Rapaport, D., 54, 62, 92, 100, 196, 197, 208
Raphling, D. L., 216

Reality. *See* External reality (as defense)
  truth controversy, 318-322
Regression, mutative interpretation bias, 33
Reich, W., 270
Repetitive affect, timing of intervention, 14
Repression
  defined, 4
  mutative interpretation bias, 33-35
  unconscious and, 264-265
Resistance
  defined, 3
  mutative interpretation bias, 31
Resistance analysis, free association and, 110-115
Risk, mutative interpretation bias, 38-39
Rituals, timing of intervention, 13
Rochlin, G., 226, 228
Roiphe, H., 225
Rosenblatt, A., 223, 226, 227, 228, 229

Sandler, J., 54, 57, 58, 59, 60, 61, 62, 65, 94, 95, 98, 100, 101, 206, 216, 224, 281
Sarraute, N., 243
Schafer, R., 198, 248, 249, 256, 308, 310, 328, 329, 332
Schwaber, E., xviii, 241, 242, 243, 246, 247, 251, 252, 253, 254, 255, 257, 258, 259, 301n, 303

Searle, M. N., 114, 310
Self-reflection, free association and, 115–123
Shame, narcissistic injury, envy complex, 224–226
Sherick, E., 222, 223
Silence
  empathy and, 247
  timing of intervention, 8–9
Silverman, M., 56, 58, 64, 76, 77, 85, 86, 87, 92, 95, 255, 256
Simon, B., 63, 101
Socrates, xx, 337, 338, 339, 340, 343, 371, 372
Solnit, A., 371n22
Solomon, R., 371n22
Sonnenberg, S. M., 119
Spacal, S., 117
Spencer, J. H., 242, 257
Spielman, P., 223
Spillius, E. B., 227, 353n14
Stein, M., 180
Stein, S., 296
Sterba, R., 117, 118, 120, 246, 270
Stone, I. F., 328, 338n2
Strachey, J., 1, 6, 31, 269n3, 272, 299, 363n20
Strean, H., 210
Success drive, envy complex, defense activity, 228
Superego, analytic perception and, xiv, xv
Superego analysis
  dream analysis, facial expression and, 173–178
  impulse disorders, 164–169

Tarnower, W., 210, 211
Technical tasks, defense analysis methods, 74–75
Thoma, H., 64, 70
Time recall inhibition, timing of intervention, 10–12
Timing (of intervention), 6–15
  acting out, 14–15
  aggression turned on self, 7
  avoidance, 12–13
  generally, 6–7
  incongruent affect, 9
  interruption of thinking, 7–8
  lateness and absences, 14
  mutative interpretation bias, 30
  nonpayment, 14
  posture of patient, 10
  repetitive affect, 14
  rituals, 13
  silence, 8–9
  time recall inhibition, 10–12
Transference
  conflicts in, mutative interpretation bias, 39
  external reality (as defense), 202–205
Transference daydream, defined, 179
Transference interpretation, 337–374
  interpsychic transference, 350–352
  intrapsychic transference, 345–350
  Platonic revisions, 339–343
  resolution, 363–371

Transference interpretation (*continued*)
  social-cultural world, 352–357
  Socratic inheritance, 337–339
  transference recognition, 343–345
  unconscious, 357–362
Transition emphasis, mutative interpretation bias, 30
Truth controversy, 317–335
  describing and pointing, 324–329
  future trends, 329–334
  overview of, 317–318
  reality, 318–322
  treatment structure, 323–324
Tuckett, D., 293, 295
Tyson, P., 225, 230
Tyson, R., 225, 230

Unconscious
  consciousness and, 264
  transference interpretation, 357–362

Unconscious conflict
  compromise formations and, defense analysis methods, 82–84
  conscious versus, defense analysis methods, 58–59

Vlastos, G., 338n2

Waelder, R. E., 277, 308, 320
Wallerstein, R. S., xix, 292, 295, 296, 297, 312
Weinshel, E. M., 3, 119, 120, 293
Weiss, S., 210, 211, 212
Welker, R., xvi
Williams, B., 370n21, 371n22
Winnicott, D. W., 352n12, 354, 355, 357
Working through, defined, 4–5
Wurmser, L., 166

Yorke, C., 306
Young-Bruehl, E., 57, 62, 64